Table of contents

KV-657-694

Preface

This book brings together the work of a team of professionals with different backgrounds on the prevention of HIV infection and care of AIDS patients. The book reflects considerable knowledge gained in a project being carried out in Mwanza Region in the United Republic of Tanzania but also refers to experiences from other countries. It outlines principles and practical advice concerning aspects of prevention and care at district level, including the organization, management, implementation and monitoring of district activities.

Those involved in conceiving, planning, financing and implementing this project are to be complimented. District health systems are the backbone of health care and the implementation units for an integrated assault on health problems. Dissatisfaction with vertically organized health care interventions, which often provide clients with a maze of conflicting and fragmented interventions, is widespread. Such services lead to considerable duplication of effort and are thus not cost-effective. How can these deficiencies be corrected? The Mwanza project is one of the first to begin exploring practical ways of achieving greater cohesion in prevention and control of HIV/AIDS within District Health Development.

While the book provides sound guidance on most issues that are dealt with, it also opens a dialogue and debate on a number of them. For example, it is clear that many poor countries do not have the resources to meet the cost of essential components of HIV/AIDS programmes. While some additional resources are needed from governments, nongovernmental organizations and households, as well as the private sector, donor support will be essential for a prolonged period. Thus, debate and rethinking on the role of donor support to countries are required, ultimately leading to recognition that their extended support is essential and not something to feel ashamed of, as is sometimes the case.

This timely book makes a valuable contribution to the fight against AIDS.

E. Tarimo, M.D.
Director, Division of Analysis, Research and Assessment
World Health Organization, Geneva

Acknowledgements

Field work done by government agencies and NGOs in Tanzania during the past five years or so provides the main basis for this book. Many of the experiences documented come from work in Mwanza Region and Magu District, adjacent to Lake Victoria in northern Tanzania. The main institutional actors have been the government of Tanzania, the TANESA project (Tanzania-Netherlands Project to Support AIDS Control in Mwanza Region), AMREF (African Medical and Research Foundation) and the Royal Tropical Institute in Amsterdam, the Netherlands.

These chapters are the result of collaborative efforts at implementation level, which have involved the Mwanza centre of the Tanzanian National Institute for Medical Research, the Regional Medical Office, the District Medical Offices of Mwanza Region – especially those of Mwanza and Magu Districts, the Regional and District Offices of the Departments of Education and Community Development, and Bugando Medical Centre in Mwanza town.

The book has been made possible by the concerted effort of a large number of people. First and foremost, we want to thank the communities that participated actively in the development of interventions and research activities. We also appreciate the participation and cooperation of district and regional health management teams, particularly in Mwanza Region, and of representatives from other sectors (education, community development and planning). We are also grateful to the numerous local and international reviewers of chapters. Particular thanks go to Maria de Bruyn of the Royal Tropical Institute (KIT), who provided us with many ideas and thorough reviews and a list of further reading and resources.

All of the drawings that illustrate this book are used as discussion starters by our peer educators and professional staff to stimulate discussions among the target audience. They were produced by the late Bernard Gidda Stephen, TANESA artist, who died of AIDS on May 1, 1996.

We would also like to gratefully acknowledge the donors who have made this work possible; in particular, we thank the Netherlands' Minister for Development Cooperation for support to the TANESA project.

Japheth Ng'weshemi
Ties Boerma
John Bennett
Dick Schapink

Introduction

John Bennett, Japheth Ng'weshemi and Ties Boerma

- Why focus on districts?
- How important are sectors other than health in combatting the spread of HIV?
- Where is Mwanza?
- For whom was this book written, and how is it arranged?

There is no doubt that in sub-Saharan Africa AIDS is one of the major epidemics of this century – an epidemic with strong roots in human behaviour and no cure available in the short run. Eleven million people in sub-Saharan Africa were estimated to have been infected with the human immunodeficiency virus (HIV) by 1995. Of these, about 4.5 million people had progressed to acquired immunodeficiency syndrome (AIDS); most then died within a year of becoming seriously ill.

The AIDS epidemic in Africa, largely invisible and insidious as it began, became visible in what first appeared an unlikely place: Rakai, in Uganda. With hindsight, however, it is now obvious how war, poverty, smuggling, movement of people and inadequate treatment services for sexually transmitted diseases (STDs) created the circumstances for a high rate of transmission, leading to an explosion in the number of cases and deaths. The years of quiet dissemination of HIV are now surfacing, as the delayed morbidity and mortality related to AIDS appears all over Africa: it has become clear that the consequences are a disaster, and that there is a great need for care. In fact this need is urgent, visible, increasingly dramatic and costly; aspects related to HIV prevention are not so readily evident to the population. AIDS is more visible in the towns, where HIV testing and hospitalization take place and where the epidemic is fuelled by overcrowding, commercial sex work and movement of people, as well as cultural and economic diversity. Transmission occurs especially along roads, and also with contiguity as people from the towns return to rural areas with HIV infection or to die – rural people attempt to escape rural poverty by migrating to the towns, but retain their original links. There is no area, no matter how rural, that is too secluded or isolated for HIV transmission.

HIV/AIDS has not spread evenly across sub-Saharan Africa. Although data on HIV prevalence are far from satisfactory, it appears that HIV is much more common in large parts of eastern and southern Africa than elsewhere. In West Africa, Cote d'Ivoire seems to be the hardest hit country. The uneven appearance and spread of AIDS in Africa has been a matter of interest and speculation. It has been attributed to many inter-related factors such as an absence of male circumcision, marriage patterns, urbaniza-tion, frequency of untreated sexually transmitted diseases, sexual behaviour, the status of women, economic disparities and poverty, and movement patterns. Areas of high prevalence of HIV and AIDS incidence have been mapped but the picture is changing, both nationally and in districts.

What has the response to the AIDS epidemic been? Generally, countries have been slow to react. Initially, it was hard to convince policy makers and planners of the magnitude of the epidemic, mainly because of the insidious nature of HIV infection. In most countries a national AIDS programme was established in the second half of the eighties and did not become operational until the early nineties.

District focus

Virtually all countries have organized their administration using districts (or *départe-ments*) and regions or provinces. A district generally has a population ranging between 100,000 and 500,000 people; the majority of districts in sub-Saharan Africa can be considered rural. That is, the majority of the population (up to 90%) live in rural areas or small settlements.

HIV is present in all divisions and wards of an average African district, although at varying levels of prevalence. In rural areas the consequences of HIV may not be evident to the average person; preventive measures seem unnecessary. Moreover, HIV testing is too expensive to be readily available. AIDS is a health problem that may be more evi-dent to communities, but the disease presents itself in a way that makes it easy to see it as a disease beyond human control, which can be ascribed to witchcraft. District health managers know they have a ticking time bomb on their hands, but they are in a dilemma – what funds they are given are eaten up by the burden of current AIDS care; they have nothing left to allow them to act in time to prevent the even more massive consequences of AIDS that are almost sure to come later.

In recent decades, governments have attempted to decentralize their administration; districts have become the key administrative unit for health and development program-mes, including efforts to provide HIV prevention and AIDS care. A district health system based on primary health care (PHC) is now the norm in most countries, and in the health sector the district is the main operational unit that supports a PHC strategy. Within a district health system, the district health management team, chaired by the district medical or health officer, is the key actor. The most important PHC strategies are inter-sectoral coordination and community involvement, coupled with bringing together all other relevant parties (including government, private health providers, NGOs and tradi-tional healers) as partners in work related to health. Important partners in district health systems include planning, education, and community development sectors. PHC is also inherently multidisciplinary. Some of the implications of this approach are outlined in the following section.

Multisectoral approach

Research and the resulting literature are increasing rapidly, but the results scarcely filter down to districts. There are few if any mechanisms for disseminating results within the areas where data is collected. Districts need to have this information in a usable form, including its cost implications. Even those decision makers who have access to the literature have difficulty keeping up with the latest ideas, changing concepts and emphasis on particular interventions, as well as their management implications. What is needed is help in selecting priorities for action, for example by providing information on those which have been tried and found to be feasible and cost-effective.

There are numerous constraints to setting up a well-balanced HIV prevention and AIDS care programme, including lack of funds, equipment, trained staff, transport and communication. Poor roads; deteriorating, unmaintained health units; ill-paid, poorly motivated staff; outdated equipment; lack of security for supplies; a non-functional health information system; and an emphasis on curative work over promotion and prevention – longstanding constraints of existing health services – may also hamper the introduction or acceleration of any specific programme.

Sustainability of health activities is visibly and dramatically an area of concern in the districts of Africa. Cessation of donor funds, increasing inflation and changing government funding priorities are the substance of nightmares for health workers and planners. In Africa the supply of condoms for programmes usually comes from donors; training of health workers, teachers and others is often dependent on outside funds; and money, no matter how little, for new cadres such as peer educators are difficult to ensure. Recurrent costs are generally not funded. Yet supplies, processes, skills, transport and allowances have to be sustained.This makes cost containment and cost-effectiveness essential. With or without a research element, a district needs to keep track of expenditures and to record inputs, outputs and outcomes. This implies a functioning accounting system, as well as a health management information system that is capable of monitoring the implementation process. To make the best use of the available resources, district HIV/AIDS programmes are usually in urgent need of improvement in this area.

Despite this catalogue of constraints and problems, however, we must recognize that progress is possible, and is being achieved in many areas. A multisectoral, multi-disciplinary approach is needed: with additional ideas and expertise, all districts could make improvements. First, if the successes and how they are being achieved during practical implementation in the community, as well as the disappointments and their reasons, can be documented, programmes will be able to learn from each other. Second, HIV prevention and AIDS care programmes need inputs from many disciplines, including not only many different fields of health care but also behavioural sciences and education. If research is to be carried out, people with social science, demographic, epidemiological, clinical and computer skills will be needed; these are usually only readily available if there are links with universities, donors or NGOs. If not, the inputs of new ideas have to come via the literature or from visits.

On the other hand, districts typically have no shortage of potential partners for planning and implementation of health services. The potential for HIV/AIDS, STDs and tuberculosis to reinforce each other, leading to a 'synergistic disaster' looming ahead can serve as a rallying point around which district health systems based on PHC can be energized. Networks, coordinating committees, development and planning committees, village government, ward and divisional committees could all accept HIV/AIDS as one of their concerns and put it on their agenda. Other sectors – women's affairs, social welfare, information, community development, education, and local organizations (NGOs as well as other community-based organizations), religious organizations, women's and youth organizations, trade unions, farmers' organizations, village committees, development committees – all include groups that can participate in a social mobilization process. Coordination, obtaining cooperation and establishing networking is difficult, and the structures needed to assist this process are often not operative, but good communication, advocacy, looking for mutual points of interest and good management of the activities that will help to achieve shared goals and objectives can overcome many obstacles.

Purpose of this book

As this introduction should make evident, Africa – with an epidemic that is affecting 5–10% of its rural adult population, and an even higher proportion of its urban population – needs to have a more effective range of activities implemented at district level, which has now become the basis for health interventions. District implementation of HIV prevention and AIDS care programmes is a long, difficult process in which successes and failures are interspersed. To make HIV prevention programmes work, many obstacles will have to be removed; even more will have to be done to improve AIDS care. Districts need ways to work toward developing the skills and planning that will make it possible to implement such activities.

An approach is needed that mobilizes the resources available within communities to meet the multiple challenges HIV/AIDS presents to district health systems. While the AIDS epidemic has been accompanied by an explosion of literature, little has been done with respect to addressing and involving the main actors in the implementation of interventions in the district. Without this, it will be difficult to significantly reduce HIV transmission and enhance coping with the consequences of the AIDS.

The aim of this book is thus to synthesize experiences and tested methods related to the broad range of activities needed to meet the challenges HIV/AIDS poses to district health systems. It is not a manual nor a 'cookbook': the main goal is to serve as a source book, by sharing field experiences, discussing the difficulties encountered, and explaining solutions found. Our hope is to stimulate thinking about AIDS programmes in sub-Saharan Africa and provide ideas for feasible interventions at the district level.

Setting and approach

Much of this book is based on field work done by government agencies and NGOs in Tanzania during the past five years or so. The experiences documented come especially from work in Mwanza Region and Magu District, both situated along the shores of Lake Victoria in northwestern Tanzania. Mwanza Region (see Map 1) covers a land area of 19,500 km^2; in 1995 its population exceeded 2 million inhabitants. The primary sources of income are agriculture (e.g. cotton, rice, maize, cassava), fishing, and a limited amount of industrial production. Mwanza town, the second largest population centre in Tanzania, has about 200,000–250,000 inhabitants and functions as a trading centre. The main roads to Kenya, Rwanda, Burundi and Dar es Salaam cross the region. Within Mwanza Region, one largely rural district, Magu, and one predominantly urban district, Mwanza, were the focus of the development of a comprehensive package of interventions. More specific interventions were developed in places throughout the region.

Although much of the experience described was gained in the districts of Tanzania, a large number of the chapter authors have also worked in other parts of Africa. We have tried to make the book useful for the continent as a whole. Examples are thus drawn from experiences in other countries as well, based either on the authors' personal experiences or the literature. As more parts of the world begin to cope with the HIV/ AIDS epidemic, perhaps these African situations will have even broader relevance.

Also, the authors cover a wide range of organizations, disciplines and backgrounds. They are affiliated with a range of institutions and organizations including AMREF Tanzania; Bugando Medical Centre, Mwanza; the Institute for International Health in Nijmegen, the Netherlands; the London School of Hygiene and Tropical Medicine; the Tanzanian National Institute for Medical Research, in Mwanza; the Regional Medical Office, in Mwanza; the Institute for Social and Economic Research, Rhodes University, Grahamstown, South Africa; TANESA, Tanzania; the Royal Tropical Institute, in Amsterdam; and the World Health Organization. They have had extensive field experience in implementing AIDS and primary health care programmes.

Outline of the chapters

This book is intended for a broad audience, including field staff, such as district health management team members and NGO project staff; regional and national staff; and academics. Some chapters are written primarily with district health personnel in mind, while others are aimed at other sectors. Some are more research-oriented; others deal predominately with interventions.

Chapters are divided into six sections. The introductory chapters relate to Organization, while those following cover Defining and monitoring the epidemic, Behavioural interventions, Health interventions, Consequences of the epidemic, and Financing and sustainability. Each chapter begins with a few questions that are addressed to and may serve as a guide for the reader. Chapters conclude with a list of further reading.

Map 1. Mwanza Region, showing districts

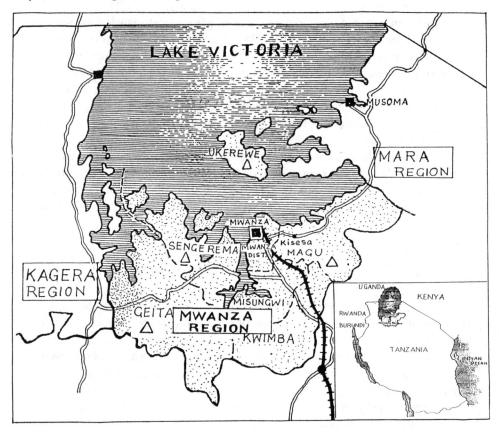

Part I: Introduction

This Introduction gives the context for the development of a comprehensive district HIV prevention and AIDS care programme focused on planning and management aspects, as described in Chapter 1. Chapter 1 outlines the process of developing a district AIDS programme in the context of PHC. This provides a basis for the following chapters and puts them into the perspective of a broad-based district AIDS programme.

Part II: Defining and monitoring the epidemic

Part II presents topics related to the data needed to define and monitor the epidemic. During the planning stage a district situation analysis (Chapter 2) is essential, to assess the magnitude of the HIV/AIDS problem in the district and the resources available for an AIDS programme.

Epidemiological and social science methods can assist in obtaining and analyzing data on HIV, other STDs and sexual behaviour. Chapter 3 suggests ways to use epidemiological methods in a relatively simple way to increase our understanding of the disease, including methods to estimate HIV prevalence and monitor the epidemic.

Since the primary mode of HIV transmission is through sexual activity, understanding the social context and especially sexual behaviour is essential. While this is a difficult task, it is necessary for the development of interventions. Chapter 4 presents some anthropological methods and considerations that can be used to gain insight into these issues within districts.

Gender issues pervade all aspects of the HIV/AIDS epidemic, from HIV prevention to AIDS care. Using examples from across Africa, Chapter 5 demonstrates the importance of taking gender differences into account in planning and implementing interventions. The chapter is made up of questions comprising a gender-based situation analysis, plus related issues to consider at district level, along with a brief discussion of assessing gender sensitivity.

Monitoring and evaluation at district level can range from using a set of priority prevention indicators to simple process monitoring of interventions. Chapter 6 describes the type of indicators that can be used to monitor AIDS programmes and how such data should be collected. Practical experiences with participatory methods are also presented.

Part III: Behavioural interventions
Changing sexual behaviour is considered the key intervention in reducing HIV transmission. Chapters in Part III cover behavioural interventions at community level. This includes work in high-transmission areas such as truck stops, addressing gender issues, working with youth, and condom promotion.

Interventions at community level require a subtle interaction between community and district or project staff. The process developed to mobilize communities to support and participate in community AIDS programmes is presented in Chapter 7. This might include for example health education campaigns, establishment of special committees and training and support for peer educators.

High-transmission areas play a central role in the epidemic. Where resources are limited, focusing predominantly or only on the high-transmission areas within a district may be justified. Chapter 8 describes the experiences in developing a truck stop intervention project in Tanzania, a project that evolved from a target group orientation to a community programme.

In the context of the AIDS epidemic, special efforts are required to strengthen the position of women. Chapter 9 gives examples of how gender issues can be addressed within a district. This entails including gender issues in AIDS awareness campaigns, strengthening the position of women, training drama groups that will focus on gender issues, and developing gender-sensitive health education materials. Experiences in working with women's groups are also described.

Youth need to be the focus of many HIV prevention activities. Programmes in schools, if directed at younger age groups, can reach the majority of youth. However, out-of-school youth are an equally important group who need to be included in district youth programmes. Chapter 10 describes the establishment of a peer educator programme, as well as the implementation of a national curriculum on sex education and AIDS education in district primary schools.

Condom promotion and distribution is another key intervention for reducing HIV transmission. The obstacles and requirements for such programmes are discussed in Chapter 11, including the role of social marketing of condoms.

Part IV: Health interventions

A range of health interventions can be implemented to reduce HIV transmission, including training health workers, reducing medical-care associated transmission, STD control, and HIV testing (Part IV).

Health workers are faced with a new disease, and can play important roles as educators in communities in relation to both prevention and care. In many cases, however, their current knowledge is limited. Special training programmes may be needed; various approaches to training are described in Chapter 12.

Prevention and control of sexually transmitted diseases other than HIV/AIDS are important health interventions in themselves, since STDs are a leading public health problem. Recent data indicate that STD control can bring a dramatic reduction in HIV transmission as well. Chapter 13 describes STD control within the health unit. Chapter 14 focuses on activities a district health management team can undertake to set up an effective STD control programme. These chapters are based on extensive experience with STD control gained in Mwanza Region, Tanzania, and include many practical considerations. Important experiences in developing and implementing STD control using a syndromic approach, gained in the early 1990s, are integrated here.

HIV testing at district level is essential for prevention and care. Chapter 15 not only describes how to set up a sound system of HIV testing at district level but also presents different ways to decrease its cost.

Health interventions must also aim at reducing medical-care related transmission, including injections and blood transfusion. Chapter 16 describes how improvements in injection and sterilization practices can almost eliminate this transmission route. Methods to minimize occupational risks to health workers are included. Considerations related to reducing the risk of HIV transmission during blood transfusions are presented in Chapter 17.

Part V: Consequences of the epidemic

Several ever-increasing consequences of the epidemic need to be anticipated. At a time when most African health care budgets are being slashed, care of AIDS patients is making new demands on already overburdened health systems. Part V covers home-based care, counselling, tuberculosis and the consequences of the adult AIDS epidemic for children.

Care and counselling are addressed in Chapter 18. This includes the burden of AIDS care on hospitals and ways to strengthen home-based care programmes as a means of alleviating pressure on hospitals. Counselling for HIV negative and positive patients and psycho-social care of AIDS patients are also discussed.

Interactions between HIV and tuberculosis (Chapter 19) present an enormous challenge to the fragile health systems of many districts. Collaboration between AIDS and tuberculosis control programmes may help to strengthen both the district response to this challenge and the tuberculosis control programmes as well.

Chapter 20 presents the consequences of the adult HIV/epidemic for children. This includes the problem of mother-to-child transmission; AIDS care for children; and those whose parents die, leaving them orphans.

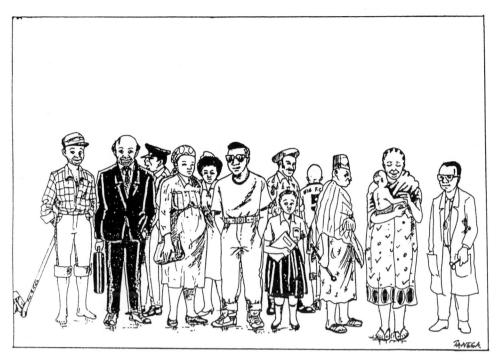

Who is most at risk of getting HIV/AIDS?

Part VI: Financing and sustainability

The final section (Part VI) addresses issues of financing and sustainability. Chapter 21 is an attempt to assess the economic costs of the components of an HIV prevention and AIDS care programme, and to relate these costs to the estimated effectiveness of interventions. This leads to the presentation of 'packages' of interventions and care that can be considered for use at district level, given different levels of resource availability.

Chapter 22 discusses the aspects of integration and sustainability of AIDS programmes. Sustainability may not immediately seem a priority when attacking a severe epidemic. However, it has now become obvious that the epidemic and its consequences will be with us for at least some decades. Due to the prolonged nature of the AIDS epidemic, it has become imperative to consider issues related to sustainability and integration.

Finally, the Appendix provides a list of addresses for selected sources of materials on HIV/AIDS, including many of the materials listed in the chapters under 'Further reading'.

We hope the collection of ideas and experiences found in these chapters of *HIV prevention and AIDS care in Africa: a district level approach,* being based on practical experience in dealing with these problems at district level, will stimulate discussion and planning, leading to the implementation of many new AIDS activities, projects and programmes in the districts of Africa.

Part one
Organization

1 Development of a comprehensive district HIV prevention and AIDS care programme

Japheth Ng'weshemi and John Bennett

- What steps can be used to develop a district AIDS programme?
- Should women be included in the planning group?
- Why is multisectoral involvement essential?
- Are donors the sole source of potential funding?
- What is the difference between a plan of operations and a plan of action?

The development of a district AIDS programme can be approached in many ways. This chapter contains recommendations based on what has been done in Mwanza, and our assessment of that experience. The approach suggested is a blend of top–down (starting from the district level) and bottom–up (coming from the community level). This chapter assumes a decision has been made to develop programmes at district level.

As discussed in Chapter 18, it is to the advantage of the community to have a comprehensive HIV/AIDS programme with HIV prevention and AIDS care included. For each of these two major components there are several objectives, each requiring different strategies and activities if they are to be achieved effectively and efficiently. The overview of steps given here can be used to implement such a programme, taking into consideration the resources that are apt to be available to an average district in Africa. The process described is initiated at district level, where district authorities will need to take a series of steps to define a programme and its components that are in line with national policy. These steps include a situation analysis, the development of a plan of operations and a plan of action, implementation of the activities and interventions, and monitoring and evaluation.

National policy and districts

Most African countries have a national policy document on AIDS. Typically, guidelines will have been established on how to translate this into the reality of a district. The district is usually a geographically defined administrative unit including a population of about 100,000-500,000 people. The district health management team generally coordinates a network of health facilities with a referral hierarchy: one or more district hospitals, a number of health centres, and more numerous clinics and dispensaries; terminology varies across countries. Staffing, including the ratio of staff to population, depends on nationally established norms and resources. Most countries have established district health systems that attempt to bring together and utilize all organizations, facilities and resources that can contribute to health. The importance of non-governmental organizations, private health units and practitioners, traditional healers and other sectors to the district will already be clear. If there is a district council, a district development committee and/or an intersectoral subcommittee for primary health care (PHC), it will facilitate the coordination of such resources for health.

The process of decentralization in Tanzania is probably relevant to many other countries as well, and may serve as an illustration. Mainland Tanzania is divided into 20 regions and 113 districts. The administrative levels in use are national, regional, district, ward, village, *kitongoji* (subvillage), and *balozi* (usually 10 households with a local leader who is connected to the political structures of the country). In 1992 the implementation of the national AIDS control strategy began with a workshop at national level, where principal secretaries and regional directors were briefed on the use of a multisectoral planning process. Regional and district AIDS programme coordinators were appointed. Regional medical officers and regional AIDS programme coordinators briefed their regional PHC committee members and their district medical officers and district coordinators, preparing them to plan workshops within the districts. These officers and coordinators in turn worked on situation analyses and carried out planning in cooperation with the district PHC committee. They did their best to include women, co-opting representatives of non-government organizations (NGOs) and other important stakeholders. This provided districts with baseline data, intervention packages and a year's workplan and budget; these were sent via the regions to national level, to be incorporated in a national workplan and budget.

This is an idealized scheme; it was often not followed exactly, due to local facilitating or constraining factors. Some districts had more donor-funded projects and NGOs; others were affected by poverty, drought, civil or international conflicts. Regions also differ with respect to more or less effective management, and in some districts only certain projects might take off, or this might happen only in limited areas. However, in all districts the aim is to repeat small successes on a larger scale, moving from these small successes to district and then to regional coverage. The enthusiasm of the people involved is the key to success. Thus, communication among villages and among districts becomes an important part of the effort to improve the national programme.

Broad involvement throughout the process

Multisectoral commitment

AIDS is a disease; therefore AIDS care and prevention of infections could primarily be seen as concerns of health programmes. Similarly, it could be mistakenly argued that reducing HIV transmission and AIDS care should be left largely to the health sector. As suggested in the Introduction, however, there are stronger arguments on the side of multisectoral involvement as an essential element. First, the PHC strategy, in the 1978 Declaration of Alma Ata, endorsed by all nations is very relevant to AIDS programmes; multisectoral involvement is a key element in this strategy. Second, the promotion of safe sexual behaviour (e.g. reducing the number of sexual partners and condom use) is recognized as the central intervention needed to reduce HIV (and STD) transmission. Changing sexual behaviour cannot be seen as a concern of the health sector alone. It cuts across many sectors, notably those involving youth, women and communities. Third, the magnitude of the AIDS epidemic in many districts in comparison to resources available for health is such that the needed interventions will not be possible unless support and staff from all sectors can be mobilized to carry out activities. Fourth, the consequences of AIDS – including increased morbidity and mortality among the part of the population that would normally be the most economically productive – is apt to affect all layers of society. Therefore, the planning of an AIDS programme needs to involve the community, including a variety of sectors, especially education, community development and planning, from the outset.

The community

As a part of decentralization, AIDS concerns need to be actively understood in communities. The need for community commitment and incorporation into local culture and organizations has become increasingly clear; further, the arguments for broad involvement given above also apply to communities. The best way to achieve this commitment is to involve community representatives early, during planning phases. This helps to ensure that the activities carried out later will fit the community and become known within it.

Steps in the development of a district programme

Subsequent chapters cover aspects of the development of a comprehensive programme in more detail. This chapter presents an overview of a way to approach planning, organizing and administrative aspects. A series of steps that can be used to develop an overall plan of operations for a period of 3–5 years will be described.

Step 1. Situation analysis

Situation analysis is a very important initial stage in the development of a programme. The results of this analysis provide a basis for further work, including a description of the magnitude of the HIV/AIDS/STD problem, the knowledge, attitude, and sexual practices of the population, the location and nature of high-transmission areas, and the current state of interventions and care, resources and so forth.

Box 1. A planning group in Magu District, Tanzania

The AIDS programme in Magu District was initially developed under the PHC committee, which is a subcommittee of the district development committee. The PHC committee includes representatives from a number of sectors, under the chairmanship of the district commissioner. The district medical officer serves as the secretary. This body, however, turned out to be too large to plan and oversee implementation of an AIDS programme. It was difficult to meet regularly, especially since the chairman and secretary had little time to attend.

Therefore, the PHC committee decided to establish a smaller action-oriented committee: the district AIDS action team. The members are the district planning officer (chair), district AIDS control coordinator (secretary), department heads of relevant sectors (health, education and community development), and representatives from NGOs. Members are nominated because of their positions in the government or NGOs; unfortunately this means that only one-fifth of the members are women.

A planning group should be formed, made up of staff from district level government sectors, NGOs, and community-based organizations. Special efforts should be made to assure that the community is well represented, and that the group includes representative women. If possible, those whose cooperation will be needed during implementation should be included in some way. Their series of meetings, including the situation analysis and planning, should be led by a competent manager who is well aware of gender issues, as well as those related to modern-day youth. Further initiative, assistance and support, including expert advice or guidance and other resources, may come from the regional/provincial or national levels, as well as donors or NGOs (Box 1).

The question of how such a group will organize itself is important. Usually members would like to meet and share experiences, resources and perhaps even some activities such as joint workshops, seminars or scientific conferences. Who will take the initiative and elaborate procedures for convening meetings tends to be the question. As pointed out in Box 1, the district medical officer may be very busy with urgent daily issues as well as seminars, workshops and other meetings, both within the district and elsewhere. This is a dilemma, because such a planning group is essential in the district; ideally, the district medical officer would coordinate it and facilitate communication, with the idea of promoting a desire to share resources among all those concerned with the AIDS epidemic the district is facing. Subcommittees may be needed to carry out specific tasks, as in Box 1, is one possibility. It is then essential to find ways to keep the group as a whole – including the district medical officer, whose support is vital – informed, involved and committed to the resulting plans!

The development of this intersectoral planning group, which can gather data to be used in a situation analysis and analyse it with a view to developing a plan of operations for a programme, is an important step. Not only does it bring together representatives from groups that are essential to implementation of any plans, but also the data collected in the situation analysis is vital. It enables the group to see the size of the problem in comparison to existing resources or lack of them, and to assess the effects of existing services and interventions. This stage clarifies the looming threat of AIDS as well as the potentially insidious increase in the hidden prevalence of HIV infections. The need for a considered approach to a division of resources between prevention and care should become apparent. Further, using questions such as those listed in Chapter 5 helps to assure that planning takes both women's concerns and the local situation with respect to gender into account. This gives the resulting programmes a boost on the way to success, because the information collected makes it easier to design activities that are well suited to the target groups and the area.

As discussed in the following chapter, some of the basic information required for the situation analysis will be readily available from various sectors, including NGOs and community-based organizations. Additional information is collected as needed to determine the extent of HIV infection and AIDS consequences, and the factors facilitating HIV spread. Maps may be drawn during a workshop to identify high-transmission areas. Throughout, it is important to take gender issues into account; a failure to do so may serve to block effective prevention and care.

The multisectoral planning group then analyses the data with a view to developing a plan of operations. Analysis of the data helps to indicate the strengths, weaknesses, opportunities and constraints and to identify priorities among problems. It also puts these in the context of historical origins, national policy and organizational structure, and resources.

Step 2. Development of a programme plan of operations
Process. Planning is a process that can be tackled in several ways. One good example of the process is given in Box 2. Another possibility is outlined below.

- A smaller core planning group or planning team can be formed, made up of some members from the whole planning group that helped in drawing up the situation analysis. For example, the core group might include managers of AIDS-related NGOs in the district, the district medical/health officer, district AIDS programme coordinator, district education officer, district community development officer, regional AIDS programme coordinator, district nursing officer and district finance and administration officer.
- Reference material must be available and consulted, including the national AIDS plan and examples of other national, regional or district plans could be obtained. The national AIDS plan for South Africa, for example, provides great detail regarding objectives, strategies, interventions, key players and the budget (1). Project or mission reports as well as research results with relevant information on the area should also be sought out.

The planning team's job is to work out aims and objectives, plus strategies and activities or interventions that will help to achieve these objectives; further, a budget to cover the

Box 2. A district AIDS planning workshop programme from Ghana

In Ghana a district AIDS planning guide was developed and presented as a five-day workshop for key players and resource persons. The workshop programme includes problem-solving procedures, objectives and strategies, setting priorities for and deciding on activities, supervision, job descriptions and budgets.

Day 1   Identification of AIDS strategies and their facets: STD care, prevention of HIV transmission (IEC), a continuum of comprehensive AIDS care and support, providing a safe blood supply, HIV surveillance and case reporting, and promoting community involvement in prevention and care. The content of major activities related to these issues is presented and ways of solving problems health planners commonly face are discussed.

Day 2   Situation analysis and priority setting. The guide presents an example of an objective way to set priorities.

Day 3   Setting objectives and selecting strategies by making a health systems matrix; a format for a district AIDS action plan is introduced.

Day 4   Planning for supervision, including supervisory checklists and job descriptions.

Day 5   Designing a budget, including determining the resources needed, cost/quantity/quality, sources for funding and the format table.

---

costs and defined ways of monitoring and evaluating the programme will need to be established.

Aims. Programme planning starts with the definition of aims, indicating what needs to be achieved. Aims are less specific than objectives; they are the 'higher order' goals to which a programme is expected to contribute. Typically the primary aims of an AIDS programme are to reduce HIV transmission and promote AIDS care. Where heterosexual transmission is the main route for HIV transmission the aim may be worded as 'to achieve behaviour change, so as to prevent HIV transmission in the short or long term.' The aims of AIDS care might be 'to alleviate suffering and prolong and improve the quality of life for those affected by AIDS.'

Objectives. Within these broad aims a whole set of objectives can be developed. Object-ives are much more specific than aims. They describe the desired effect or impact of a programme, and are thus essential – not only when designing a programme, but also for monitoring and evaluation, where the question is 'did we achieve our objectives.'

When objectives can be quantified and given a timeframe, monitoring and evaluation become easier. Thus – under the aim of reducing HIV transmission – an ideal objective might be 'to decrease HIV incidence from 1% per year to 0.5%'. However, it is typically not possible to use such an objective; measuring HIV incidence is very costly and difficult. Objectives that cannot be measured at all are not helpful! It is thus essential to define objectives clearly, and to look for less direct ways – indicators – to determine what a programme has done. The extent to which objectives are measurable depends on whether good, simple and low cost indicators are available. If we have no such indicators it is better to choose less specific overall objectives – for example, 'to reduce HIV transmission among adolescents'. Each of these broad objectives can then be broken down into a set of more specific objectives for which indicators are available (e.g. 'increased knowledge and changed attitudes of adolescents'). Specific objectives related to prevention might include, for example, those related to behaviour change, such as partner change and frequency of condom use; and blood transfusion, STD control and safety during medical procedures. Objectives related to care might relate to control of opportunistic infections (including tuberculosis), decreases in emotional and social consequences, improvements in the quality of life, diminished stigma and discrimination.

Chapter 6 (Monitoring and evaluation) gives details on several types of indicators, including input, output, process, effect and impact indicators.

Strategies. A strategy states what approach or resources will be used to achieve objectives. One important general strategy, for example, might be to put the bulk of resources into the intervention or set of interventions that is expected to be the most cost-effective. The more limited the resources, the more important such targeting becomes. Such a strategy might lead, for example, to specifically targeting vulnerable groups that are thought to have the highest rate of infection, and/or high-transmission areas. An overall strategy might also specify a major commitment to the use of education to achieve behaviour change. Another sort of strategy involves the overall approach of the programme. Examples include a decision to work with the community in a participatory way, to decentralize decision making, or to work toward collaboration and perhaps integration with other health services.

Apart from these broad, general strategies, more specific strategies are also necessary. These might include:
- using peer health educators;
- training for health workers;
- increasing social mobilization and involvement of groups and organizations in the community;
- setting up networks to involve all sectors and NGOs;
- basing approaches, activities, and content of education on research findings where possible;
- implementing effective monitoring and supervision to ensure that activities proceed well;
- improving management by means of training, plus use of a health information and management system.

Activities. To achieve the desired objectives, activities need to be designed, using the strategies that have been chosen. To tackle the broad aim of reducing HIV transmission, a wide range of activities will be needed. The focused interventions listed below are consistent with the health care reform measures recommended by the World Bank (2).

Promotion of safer sexual behaviour, for example, might entail activities in schools, high-transmission areas, and communities. Other examples of activities include instituting epidemiological surveillance, to keep track of trends in HIV infections and the consequences of AIDS; organizing and conducting health education in accord with a main strategy on behaviour change; strengthening programmes to control STDs, including treatment as well as the promotion of distribution and use of condoms; targeting young people for education about reproductive health and prevention of HIV infection; reducing unnecessary transfusions and improving the safety of blood transfusions; strengthening programmes to control tuberculosis; and increasing socioeconomic opportunities for women.

With respect to the aim of improving AIDS care, activities might include improving medical care in health facilities, working for better home-based care and counselling, organizing care for people with HIV infection who are not helped by family networks, and socioeconomic support to families, communities or institutions.

Strategies related to the overall approach of the programme guide the way in which activities are planned and carried out. In the following chapters many suggestions are made regarding the importance of working with the community in a participatory way, of taking gender into account and of beginning this early on, during planning phases. The importance of working toward collaboration and perhaps integration with other health services is also frequently mentioned. That is, activities should be integrated not only into an overall AIDS programme strategy, but also linked with other health interventions. Integrated services might include training for educators, peer education, community outreach, condom distribution, improved STD services, drama/music activities, activities directed at better recognition of gender differences, support for people with AIDS, monitoring and evaluation. Integration with other health programmes is typically strongest in the field of reproductive health (including e.g. family planning, antenatal and delivery care).

It is useful to make a summary table of objectives, strategies, activities, target group and collaborating sectors, such as the example shown in Box 3.

Finance, expenditure and budgeting. Each of the activities planned will create costs in terms of personnel, training, equipment, supplies, buildings and their maintenance, travel and time. These costs will be worked out as a part of the plan of action, but it is necessary to begin thinking very carefully about cost effectiveness and cost efficiency early in the planning stage. The choice of strategies is essential here, since these can either increase or decrease costs.

If the government budget is meager, sources of finance will have to be established. How can the budget be supplemented? Proposals to potential donors, NGO cooperation, cost sharing and cost recovery from the community (e.g. charging for condoms) have to be considered. Raising local funds is essential. For instance, the District Council or similar bodies should be asked to set money and other resources aside for the AIDS programme. If health sector reform measures have been taken, the district health sector will have increased authority and resources. The private sector may also contribute;

Box 3. Planning summary: examples of ways to address the aim of 'reducing HIV transmission'

Objectives	Strategies	Activities and target groups	Partners
Reduce HIV/STD	Use of peer educators	Training for barworkers, truck drivers and fishermen	District team, bar owners, village leaders
Reduce transmission in high transmission areas	Establishing and empowering village support committee	Setting up condom distribution via clinics, shops, peer educators	Target groups
		Identifying areas of high HIV/STD prevalence and their community leaders	District team, clinical facilities, AIDS coordinator
		Training community leaders	
Build support for HIV/AIDS/STD education in primary schools	Participatory approach involving teachers, schools, parents, district education sector	Training primary school teachers, parents, pupils and peer educators	Regional and district education office
Increase knowledge and change attitudes of adolescents		Identifying and training student guardians in whom girls can confide and who can counsel	District AIDS programme
Help to protect female students		Ensuring safe blood supply	Teachers
			Parents
			Pupils
Reduce medical care associated HIV transmmission	Cooperation among health services to improve:	Training health workers	District AIDS programme
	all blood transfusion practices	Improving supervision	Health staff in health units
	sterilization and injection practices	Distribution of protocols to clinics	Committees checking blood transfusion
		Setting up clinic committees	Community groups
		Reducing demand for injections in community	District Health Management Team supervisors

communities too can raise considerable funds if they consider HIV prevention and/or AIDS care a priority for their community. In Magu District, Tanzania, communities have increasingly contributed to the cost of things like AIDS campaigns in their villages. Campaigns are then used to generate further funds: for example, a fee is charged for watching video shows (on AIDS related topics; see Chapter 7 on Community level interventions).

In making a budget, projected expenditures must be blocked out for each activity, as well as for broad categories such as:
- personnel costs
- consultants (if any)
- maintenance of buildings
- equipment/vehicles/insurance
- communications
- supplies
- office expenses
- drugs
- education and training
- workshops
- educational material
- conferences.

Priorities. The planning team should consider where most of the effort will be put, especially in the initial phases. The idea is to achieve as much as possible in a short time: success breeds success. It is often better to start with areas in which there is already good cooperation and a good management structure, and some evidence that implementation and sustainability will not be thwarted by conflict and inertia. High-transmission areas with easy access, to avoid transportation and communication problems, could be a practical priority in many districts – or perhaps a ward with a good development or PHC committee.

The situation analysis and the resulting priorities may suggest that it is necessary to reallocate staff or other resources such as drugs because of the uneven distribution of AIDS within a district. Records of health facilities can be used to assess the workload due to AIDS and other conditions and how these are changing over time. The results of this assessment can be compared between facilities and related to staff and drug allocation by the district. Changes can then be made in staffing or drug kits if required (4).

Time frame and evaluation. In this first stage of developing an overall plan of operation for a period of 3–5 years, it is advisable to establish a logical time frame that indicates when each new component will begin, when evaluations are to be done and when new areas are to be addressed.

During this early stage monitoring and evaluation are key considerations: in addition to the time frame, a methodology should be established and indicators must be developed to appraise the achievement of objectives. As noted above, clarity of objectives is essential to later assessment of improvement or success, since evaluation and monitoring centre on the degree to which objectives have been achieved. (See also Chapter 6.)

Step 3. Plan of action

The broad plan serves as a framework for the development of a specific plan of action covering a shorter time period, e.g. one year. The plan of action begins from the objectives and strategies, activities, time frame, resources and ideas on monitoring and evaluation in the broad plan. However, it provides far more, in that the activities to be carried out must be stated and explored in detail.

For each major activity to be initiated in the first year the plan of action should clearly state the objective the activity is meant to meet – that is, the part of the problem it should resolve. In considering possible activities, use should be made of the situation analysis (including gender aspects); discussions should include target groups and strategies, possible constraints, the gender dimension of the situation, tactics needed to achieve sustainability, time frame and performance indicators that can be used to measure output. A planning summary (such as in Box 3) can be used to outline all of the activities that fall under one objective.

The action plan should also specify the details that will be necessary to achieve implementation. This includes the way key players, as well as resources from other sectors, NGOs and community-based organizations will be integrated and coordinated. That is, it must describe clearly who will do what, when, where, how and with what resources.

- 'Who' states name or organization, partnerships and responsibilities
- 'What' clearly states the specific action to be taken, e.g. peer health educator training in schools
- 'When' involves a detailed time frame, with dates
- 'Where' lists the villages, bars, schools, halls and so forth identified where activities will take place
- 'How' details strategies, mechanisms and processes
- 'What resources' indicates staff, other human resources and funds allocated, equipment and vehicles to be used.

Budget. As a part of a one-year action plan, a budget for each activity must be worked out in detail. For example, each workshop that will take place for training purposes should have its own budget (including allowances, facilitators, refreshments, training room, transport, training materials, resource materials and so forth).

Training. The plan of action should indicate the range of training that will be carried out, beginning with training of trainers, including tutors and facilitators. Training will be needed in relation to HIV/AIDS, STDs, tuberculosis, counselling and health education skills; those involved will be school teachers, community leaders, peer health educators, health staff and managers, field workers and information systems staff. Before training can take place, suitable health learning materials will have to be developed or otherwise obtained. Materials developed elsewhere will need to be pretested for suitability. The costs involved will also need to be included in budgets.

Research. In a comprehensive district programme there is always a need for research. This is not just a nicety: given better baseline information and/or better knowledge of the local situation or of trends occurring as the action plan progresses, it will be possible to better understand what is happening, and often to use resources more effectively. What is needed might be epidemiological research, health systems research or research on behaviours; any of these usually require academic rigour if the results are to be optimally useful. When extra resources will be required, they can be sought outside the district, perhaps from a university, a donor or an NGO. Any research proposal should include both clearance with respect to ethical aspects from district authorities and a plan for dissemination of results. Limited investigations such as those involved in checking the adequacy of STD treatment (low key operations research) can be included in implementation without requesting district clearance.

Step 4. Implementation

Organization and management. Implementation requires good management and administration. This in turn requires adequate organization across the district. Managers may need to be trained or given on-the-job training and increased motivation, for example by attending workshops or taking part in exchange visits to other programmes. Organization and management includes clearly defined job descriptions and work procedures to ensure properly defined responsibilities, lines of authority and account-ability plus staff remuneration.

The preceding steps regarding clear definition of objectives and budget are essential to achieving proper management and administration.

Supervision and quality of care. To keep a programme going and at the same time stay focused on the objectives, it is very important to have routines that follow written protocols. Problems arise, routines slip, punctuality becomes more elastic, and supplies leak away. To maintain quality of care and ensure that all components are operating as intended, a comprehensive district programme requires clearly defined supervision procedures, including the frequency with which supervision will be carried out. Super-visors will need instruments such as checklists, protocols and guidelines for standard performance, which should also be in the hands of the staff and available in all relevant offices. Supervisors who have had training and know they have the backing of manage-ment can inspire support, reinforce training and work with staff in solving problems. Maintaining morale is as important to their role in improving the quality of the work as the controls they carry out.

Community participation and social mobilization. The broad group of activities related to communication and mobilization for development is an essential part of the imple-mentation process. It requires ongoing involvement of committees, villages, govern-ment and NGOs. The discussion below is given according to the three components identified by McKee (3):

- *Advocacy*: organizing the available information into presentations that can be communicated through various interpersonal and media channels. The aim is to gain acceptance from the relevant political and social leadership, to help prepare the society to accept and support a development programme such as one to combat HIV/AIDS. An advocacy component is also a vital part of working through district and regional coordinators to obtain adequate funds and support from regional and national resources. Advocacy is also needed to gain political support within the district and village governments. The initial advocacy programme must raise the level of awareness of the dimensions of the problem; later, in coordination with the community persuasive presentations about what can be done will be needed.

- *Social mobilization*: increasing people's awareness, knowledge and ability to organize for self-reliance. Social mobilization goes beyond advocacy, which encourages acceptance and a positive attitude, and encourages people to take an active role themselves. That is, it helps people to become motivated and to understand their rights and duties, and thus to begin to demand satisfaction of their needs. When people understand that they have many interests in common with others, they will also be motivated to work together.

  Successful social mobilization requires the cooperation of all groups and organizations that have been identified as relevant. These might include committees in villages and organizations made up of women, youth and workers. They will need to be sensitized and involved, as will churches, NGOs and other sectors including government agencies. Those working toward mobilization need to understand people's existing ideas and beliefs before they can encourage behavioural change.

- *Programme communication*: whether for advocacy, mobilization or during implementation of activities, communication covers a wide range, beginning with identifying and targeting specific groups or audiences. The communication strategies chosen need to fit the specific target group being addressed. This might include messages or training programmes using various mass media and/or interpersonal channels, both traditional and non-traditional. Concepts and techniques outlined in later chapters can be used: for example, remember that lectures are less effective as a means of convincing people than other methods (perhaps a film or role play, with discussion), and that peers often understand better than outsiders what will be the most convincing. No matter what techniques are used, communities should participate fully in this process.

These aspects are covered in more detail in Chapter 7, on community level interventions, and in Chapters 9 and 10, on gender issues and youth. Such activities always take longer than first planned: they must be done at the people's pace, not that of the plan of action. This must be allowed for – and requires more funds as a consequence. However, if done properly, the time spent has a multiplier effect on potential for sustainability.

Supply. A comprehensive programme requires a wide variety of supplies. Each objective and its activities must be scrutinized before the programme begins for supply elements: vehicles, spare parts, drugs, laboratory tests and supplies, condoms, gloves, records, office supplies, books, videos and other health learning materials. Ordering, checking, supervision, supply control, distribution and storage all have to be planned. Although this is often overlooked, a big programme will have an important logistic component. Often it is necessary to establish channels with the suppliers both within and outside the district or country, depending on the type of supplies.

Step 5. Monitoring and evaluation
A programme develops over time; the initial steps in developing a plan are followed by years of developing activities and involving communities. Many aspects must be monitored, including the inputs, the indicators of achievement of targets and all the processes involved.

The monitoring process keeps the programme on course, ensures that no elements lag behind, so that the potential for synergy – activities reinforcing each other, giving results greater than the sum of the parts would suggest – is realized. To publicize successes and keep motivation high, as well as letting people know where more effort is needed, feedback from monitoring must be provided both to workers and to the communities involved. A simple quarterly or monthly newsletter can do this, if time and resources are available.

Evaluation might take either of two forms. A mid-term assessment looks at aspects such as community response and acceptance whether a functioning network, district-wide organization and activities in all high-transmission areas have been established, dropout rates of peer health educators, adequacy of supplies, linkage with regional and national programmes, and accessibility of condoms and numbers distributed, plus a quality of care assessment for STD and tuberculosis management.

A full evaluation is done only after 3–5 years, when it is feasible to expect some achievement of objectives. Such an evaluation can assess change in behaviour and the prevalence of HIV can be measured. Hopefully other results too will be tangible: the incidence of STDs should have dropped. HIV-positive individuals should have a better quality of life. Condom use will have become a way of life for those unable to maintain abstinence or faithfulness. However, an evaluation to assess these factors in detail is costly, requiring expertise from higher levels of the national programme and consult-ants. The average district will have to be content with a positive assessment of achieve-ment of its objectives, evidence that the necessary processes are in place, and a good account of what its money purchased. A very good process indicator is the extent to which communities are actively involved and contributing to AIDS programme activities.

Conclusion

The district is the key operational unit for the implementation of health and develop-ment programmes in most African countries. Therefore, the district should also be the key player in the development of implementation of a district programme. This should be a joint effort involving the communities and supported by regional and national levels. The district AIDS programme coordinator has a key role in coordinating the

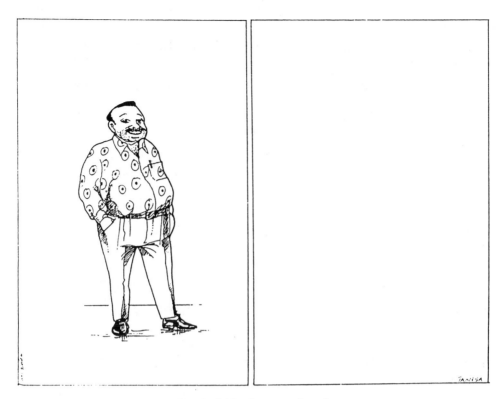

Mr X is HIV infected. What will he look like five years later?

many components of the programme and ensuring that prevention is given the necessary prominence. To be successful, HIV/AIDS programmes need to be multisectoral, including district planning, education, community development and other sectors, and making maximum effort to involve NGOs and community-based organizations.

Further reading

District AIDS Planning Guide, Ghana (undated).

Thorne M, Sapirie S, Rejeb H. *District team problem solving: guidelines for material and child health, family planning and other public health services.* WHO/MCH–FP/MEP/93.2. Geneva, 1993.

Cassels A, Janovsky K. *Strengthening health management in district and provinces.* WHO, Geneva, 1995.

Creese A, Parker D. *Cost analysis in primary health care. A training manual for programme managers.* WHO, Geneva, 1994.

References

1. NACOSA. *A national AIDS plan for South Africa 1994–1995*. National NACOSA secretariat, Sunnyside, July 1994.

2. World Bank. *World Development Report 1993*. New York, Oxford University Press, 1993.

3. McKee N. *Social mobilisation and social marketing in developing communities. Lessons for communicators*. Southbound, Penang, Malaysia, 1992.

4. Sandiford P, Kanga GJ, Ahmed AM. The management of health services in Tanzania: a plea for health sector reform. *International Journal of Health Planning and Management* 1994, 9: 295–308.

Part two
Defining and monitoring the epidemic

2 Situation analysis for a district HIV/AIDS programme

Ties Boerma and Marc Urassa

> - Who should be involved in a district situation analysis?
> - How can the number of HIV infected persons be estimated?
> - What can a map of bars and guest houses tell us?
> - What are the human resources in the district?

The AIDS epidemic has spread into most districts of Africa. As outlined in Chapter 1, to plan and implement relevant activities and effectively monitor the epidemic, it is necessary to conduct a situation analysis. The aim of this analysis is to gather, analyse and synthesize information that will provide a picture of the problem, including its size and the resources available to combat it. Even if information about the district itself is limited, it should be possible to carry out a situation analysis, using what is available plus information from other districts and carefully made assumptions. Second, the situation analysis is important as a process that involves different sectors, NGOs, community representatives and others: this process can make a vital contribution to mobilizing people and organizations for the HIV/AIDS programme. After briefly considering the process, this chapter describes each of the elements that should be included in a situation analysis for a district.

Process and contents

A district situation analysis should be designed and carried out by a group of people who represent different sectors and a variety of social layers within the population. As mentioned above and described in the previous chapter, choosing and organizing this group and paying attention not only to the information collected but also to the process that takes place is essential. Sectors that need to be well-represented include health, education, community development, information and planning. Community representatives and NGOs should be included, and women need to be well represented (at least one-third of the group members).

Participatory approaches have major advantages for a situation analysis: they can both increase the commitment of the participants to the results (and later plans) and help to make the information collected more complete. Each of those involved with the analysis sees only a selected group of cases. Therefore community members, agency representatives and health workers may considerably underestimate the magnitude of the problem. Joint calculations of the number of HIV-infected people and future AIDS patients in the district and community show that almost all participants considerably underestimate the size of the epidemic. Also to identify high-transmission areas, having different groups of participants (e.g. women and men, or youth and older men) draw maps to show the location of these areas (and then comparing their maps) has been very useful and revealing to participants. The approach can be used at both the district and community level (see Chapter 8). Attention to gender will be needed to assure that the situation analysis is relevant for women; see Chapter 5 for specific issues that will need to be considered.

A district situation analysis includes the following elements:
- *Population data*: the number of people living in the district and their distribution by age group and sex; these can be estimated from the latest census.

- *HIV and other STDs*: survey data and sentinel surveillance data are the best sources of data for estimating the prevalence of HIV infection and other STDs. If such data are not available for the district, regional data can be used, or data from a district elsewhere in the country that has similar features.

- *Potential high-transmission areas*: a simple analysis of the geographical distribution of the population and their economic activities can identify priority areas for inter- ventions. This includes identifying and mapping:
  - presence of urban centres
  - transport routes and roadside villages
  - centres with a high level of economic activity, including markets
  - settlements with guest houses, beer halls, bars, hotels, night clubs.

- *AIDS consequences*: given the estimated HIV prevalence and projected population numbers, the number of AIDS patients and AIDS deaths can be estimated. This also extends to child deaths and orphans. Data from the tuberculosis control programme should also be included (see Chapter 19). Further, if mortality is very high, severe economic disruption may occur that will affect the agricultural sector (1). Therefore information from this sector can also be useful.

- *District resources:* personnel, financing and equipment that, if mobilized, can be used to help reduce HIV transmission and cope with the consequences of the epi- demic. Schools, health services, NGOs and government structures at the peripheral and central levels of the district are all possibilities. Community-based organiza- tions, including churches and social clubs, are another resource, as are the private sector and the local information channels.

Each of these elements will be considered in turn in the sections below. For each of these, new information may need to be collected (see also Chapters 3, 4 and 5). On the other hand, creative use of 'secondary information' – material that is already available, perhaps in a census or government agency, a community-based organization, a research document or NGO project plan – is a quicker and a less expensive way of obtaining what is needed. Details are addressed in other chapters (3, 4, 5).

Population

For planning purposes, it is important to know how many people live in the district. If HIV prevalence is known or can be estimated, then it will be possible to calculate about how many people have been infected with HIV, how many more may become infected in the next few years, and how many AIDS patients and deaths can be expected. Population data can also be used to estimate the number of children infected with HIV by mother-to-child transmission and the increase in the number of orphans due to AIDS mortality among parents.

The national population census provides data by age and sex for each district. For the purpose of an HIV/AIDS situation analysis it is sufficient to use four age groups (0–4, 5–14 years, 15–49 years and 50 years and over). To estimate the population in the current year, it will be necessary to make a projection from the population numbers found in the census. For instance, in Tanzania the last census was conducted in 1988, while we needed to know the population size in 1994. The 1988 census report provided data on district population growth rates in the period 1978–1988. These rates can be used to make a projection: between 1978 and 1988, the population growth rate was (on average) 3% each year. If we assume the average rate remained the same in the following years, we can estimate the number of people in the district in 1994 by increasing the population by 3% for each year that has passed.

Magnitude of the HIV/STD/AIDS problem

To what extent is HIV infection a problem? The magnitude of the problem can be estimated from data collected in surveys or from sentinel surveillance (see Chapter 3 on Epidemiological methods). Sentinel surveillance data are mostly collected from antenatal women, or sometimes blood donors. In other cases, HIV prevalence rates are known for specific groups in which prevalence is higher than the general population, such as bar workers, patients with STD complaints or tuberculosis patients.

In interpreting the relevance of such data for the general population it is always necessary to consider how representative the data are. That is, to what extent is the population group on which the data are based similar to the general population. For example, antenatal women are often a good source of data for estimating the level of HIV infection in the population: although this may give a slight underestimate of the true prevalence among women, they are more representative than other groups who come for health care, such as patients with STDs. Data from blood donors can also provide an estimate of HIV prevalence in the population (2). However, if donors are relatives of a patient, prevalence tends to be somewhat higher than in the general population. Recent changes, however, including the awareness of donors (self selection) and the practices of blood transfusion services (deferring donors who have high scores with respect to risk; see Chapter 17) have made blood donor data unsuitable for use in estimating HIV prevalence in the general population.

How many AIDS patients and AIDS deaths can a district expect during the next decade? If we make some assumptions it becomes possible to estimate the number of people who are HIV-infected, the number of AIDS cases and the coming number of adult deaths in a district. We can also estimate the extent to which mortality rates will be increased due to HIV infection.

The following calculations are based on a district with an HIV prevalence of 7% among adults 15–49 years (7% of adults are HIV-infected) and an HIV incidence of 1% per year among adults (1% of adults become HIV-infected each year). The situation is assumed to be stable, and mortality is about equal to HIV incidence.

- If we do not know the total number of adults but do know the total number of people, we can estimate the number of adults 15–49 years by assuming that they make up about 40% of the population. *For example, if the total district population is 312,500, then there are about 125,000 adults aged 15–49.*
- Given the total number of adults 15–49, and figures for (or an estimate of) the HIV infection rate, we can estimate how many adults are HIV-infected. *If 7% are HIV-infected, then 125,000 times 7% = 8,750 adults 15–49 in the district are HIV-infected* (see also Box 1).
- If we estimate incidence, the number of newly infected adults can be calculated (for example, at 1%, 1 new case per 100 non-infected persons per year). *If we take the number of already-infected adults (calculated above) and subtract it from the total population (125,000 minus 8,750 = 116,250) and then multiply by 1%, the result gives us an estimate of the number of newly infected adults: 1,163 per year.*
- Given census data on adult mortality rates and estimates of the number of cases of AIDS, we can make calculations that give an idea of the potential increase in adult mortality caused by deaths from AIDS. *If the adult mortality rate is known or assumed to have been 5 per 1,000 adults (15–49) per year prior to the AIDS epidemic, in a population of 125,000 adults this corresponds with 5/1000 times 125,000 = 625 adults deaths per year. If we simplify the analysis by assuming that every person with HIV dies exactly seven years after becoming infected, after seven years all 1,163 adults who became infected in the year of the example will die. In other words, in that seventh year adult mortality will almost triple, going from 625 deaths to 1,788 deaths per year.*
- It is also possible to estimate the number of children born with HIV infection. For instance, in a district with 312,500 people and a crude birth rate of 4% (40 newborns per 1,000 population), there will be about 12,500 births every year. If HIV prevalence is 7% among pregnant women, then about 875 of the women who give birth will be HIV-infected (7/100 times 12,500 = 875). If transmission from mother

Box 1. Raising awareness among health workers

Calculations like those in the text can also be carried out for the population in the catchment area of a dispensary/rural clinic or health centre. For instance, in a catchment area population of 5,000, there will be about 2,000 adults 15–49. Among them, if prevalence is 5%, we can expect about 100 HIV-infected adults. With a catchment population of 10,000 there will be about twice as many HIV-infected persons: 200 out of 4,000 adults.

During the first day of a one-week training on HIV/AIDS in Magu and Mwanza Districts, Tanzania, health workers were asked to estimate the number of HIV-infected adults and children in their catchment areas. Subsequently, health workers went step-by-step through the above calculations of the numbers of HIV-infected persons in these catchment areas. In this case the trainers had 'hard data' on HIV prevalence in several urban and rural communities. Often the resulting numbers were more than ten times higher than what the health workers had expected.

to child is about 25% (that is, about one in four HIV-infected mothers transmits the virus to her child, mostly at the time of delivery) then one-fourth of 875 = 219 newborn babies will be infected with HIV. This is slightly less than 2% of all births. (See also Chapter 20 on consequences for children.)

Just as for HIV/AIDS, estimates can be made for the occurrence of other STDs. These include genital ulcer syndromes (syphilis, chancroid and so forth) and genital discharge syndromes (gonorrhoea, chlamydia, etc.). Such data can be obtained from population-based surveys and surveillance. Here too, it is important to keep in mind how representative the sample is of the general population before making generalizations from the data. Syphilis data are perhaps the easiest data to obtain, and the most reliable at present since serological tests are available. Active syphilis is defined on the basis of positive RPR and TPHA tests (for details, see Chapter 3 on epidemiological methods).

High-transmission areas

If at all possible, prevention and control activities should cover the whole district. However, to make the best use of resources it is important to pay special attention to areas where commercial sex and multiple partnerships are likely to be more common, increasing the likelihood of HIV transmission. Such behaviours are thought to be more common in urban areas, villages along transport routes and areas with more adult males than females, high mobility and/or high levels of economic activity.

The identification of high-transmission areas, as mentioned above, is best done as a participatory process, carried out or guided by the district planning team. A mapping technique was successfully applied in Magu District, Tanzania. In this case the team it-

Box 2. Listing the largest settlements

This table shows the 10 largest towns or settlements of Magu District in Tanzania, listed in order of their population as shown in the 1988 census. The total district population at the time was 311,385 (2).

Name of town/settlement	Population
Nyigogo (Magu) - urban	10,492
Mwananyili - urban	8,043
Kisesa - urban	6,752
Mahaha	6,127
Kahangara	5,661
Lamadi	5,392
Chamgasa	4,926
Kijireshi	4,585
Chabula	4,584
Mkula	4,544
TOTAL 10 largest settlements	61,106

As the list shows, this district is predominantly rural. Only 20% of the total population of the district live in the 10 largest settlements. Furthermore, the largest settlements are relatively small. Only Magu town had a population exceeding 10,000 in 1988.

self was split into different groups according to age and sex. (This could also be done in other ways, e.g. by sector.) Each group mapped its own perception of high-transmission areas. Then a plenary presentation and discussion took place to reach a consensus. The result is shown in Box 2. The same procedure has also been successfully used to help communities identify high-risk areas and behaviours in the community. This sort of process is very useful, not only in reaching consensus but in helping participants to understand that women and men, young and old, 'outsiders' and community members may have very different (and equally valid) views of the situation, all of which can contribute to a solution.

Simple demographic and socioeconomic data on the district can also assist in identifying high-transmission areas. With regard to *urbanization* two issues are important for a situation analysis. First, are there any towns in the district? The definition of a town varies from country to country, but generally this refers to a settlement with a population that exceeds 10,000. Second, it is important to establish the extent to which the district as a whole is urbanized. Ranking the ten largest settlements by their respective

Map 2. Potential high-transmission areas in Magu District, Tanzania

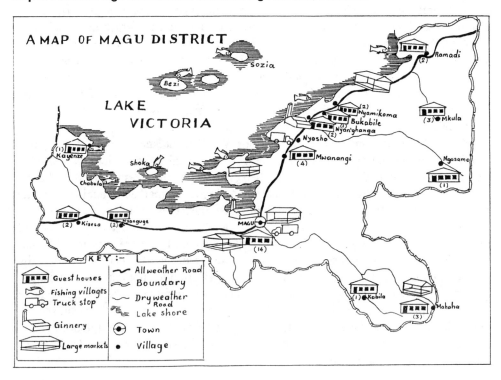

population sizes, based on the last census as in Map 1, is helpful in determining areas on which the HIV/AIDS programme should focus.

That is, in addition to size, rapid growth and other changes may signal the presence of areas where the programme is especially needed. Information from local people and other historical evidence may provide information about which areas/towns are growing most rapidly ('growth points'). The introduction of any industry, mine, army/police barracks and so forth immediately heralds immigration for economic reasons. Changes in other activities such as smuggling across borders also indicate trends in population movement. This can make border towns an important focus.

Among the various points a situation analysis needs to describe, *major roads* are important: it has been shown that commercial sex tends to be more common along highways and that frequent travel is associated with multiple partners, resulting in higher risks of HIV infection. A major road through a district is usually part of a long-distance highway, on which trucks and commercial vehicles (buses, taxis, etc.) are common. Truck stops, where truckers spend the night or stop frequently, tend to be high-transmission areas (as are railway stations, if a district has a railway passing through). Trading centres are also located along major roads. The magnitude of the problem is apt to be less in roadside villages with no truck stops, although there it will still be greater than in villages that are far from a road. A situation analysis needs to describe main roads, truck stops and roadside villages, in accord with their respective population sizes.

Some areas with many migrant labourers or high levels of *economic activity* may also be called high-transmission areas. For instance, a mine will attract many male workers; this is an incentive for commercial sex activities. Fishermen are generally young, mobile men with easy access to cash. Here, too, commercial sex may be common. Places such as factories and cotton ginneries, with concentrations of workers, may also – but not necessarily – lead to higher levels of sexual activity. However, it is also important to list these in the analysis, since they may provide a focus for interventions.

Marketplaces are important for two reasons. Whether markets are daily, weekly or monthly, they are an important meeting place where sexual activity with non-marital partners may be more frequent than elsewhere. Many men have cash at hand, and trans-actions involving sex are easier in the busy environment of a market. In addition, market-places are a potentially important place to bring IEC messages on HIV/AIDS to the public.

The number of *guesthouses and hotels* can often be used as indicators of the level of mobility, economic activity and sexual activity in an area. Therefore, it is useful to map the spatial distribution of guesthouses in the district, as in Map 1. Beer/local brew halls can also be mapped. This is more difficult, since they are often not registered and also tend to shift locations, but with the participation of community members it can be done. In fact, any place where alcohol is available and used is a potential high-transmission area. Alcohol abuse and casual sex often occur together and, with the influence of alcohol, sex without protective measures or irresponsible sexual behaviour (such as rape) is likely to be more frequent.

In most districts, the level of activity in all of these places may be affected by the season, by holidays or by other times of increased movement and economic activity. The sale of the cotton crop, the Christian and Islamic holidays when urban workers return to their rural homes, the market days at the end of the month when more alcohol is consumed – all are times when increased action may be needed. Planning could allow for increases in interventions before or during these periods. (Is it a coincidence that World AIDS day takes place on December 1st?)

Resources and potential for interventions

The process of identifying district resources should also be carried out by the multi-sectoral planning group as a participatory exercise, in collaboration with communities. When the magnitude of the problem has been established and high-transmission areas have been mapped, the various sectors involved can begin to identify resources that can be used to help in HIV prevention and AIDS care. In addition, communities can contri-bute to the assessment by carrying out a self-assessment of community resources that can contribute to the HIV/AIDS programme. For example, in Mwanza, in a district situ-ation analysis three communities were approached and have helped the district identify community resources available for HIV prevention and AIDS care.

Schools

How many schools and how many pupils (especially in the higher classes of primary school and in secondary schools) are there in the district? These data are important because these pupils are a key intervention population, for whom activities may need to be planned. Many will have started to engage in sexual intercourse or will do so in the near future, and are thus exposed to the risk of HIV infection.

As a part of the situation analysis, for each school, it should be ascertained whether an HIV/AIDS curriculum has been implemented, whether teachers have been trained, and whether HIV/AIDS control activities are occurring (for instance, a parent–teacher committee active in this area). An assessment of the quality of HIV/AIDS education and the extent to which it is integrated into, for example, family life education is also needed.

Health facilities and health staff

How many health facilities and health staff are there in the district? Health facilities play a key role in combatting the consequences of the AIDS epidemic and are also an important vehicle for health education (IEC activities). All health staff will need to be trained in the various aspects of HIV/AIDS and the resulting activities (see Chapter 12 on training). It is necessary to assess staff training needs related to STD management, IEC on HIV prevention and sexual health, medical aspects of HIV/AIDS, and home-based care and counselling. Brief assessments of the adequacy of the supply of drugs (particularly antibiotics for STD treatment; see Chapter 14 on STD control), the supply of drugs for complaints common in AIDS patients, the availability of safe blood for transfusion (see Chapter 17 on blood transfusion), and the availability of injection and sterilization equipment (see Chapter 16 on reducing medical care transmission) are also part of a situation analysis.

Because of the desirability of conserving resources by integration or at least collaboration among programmes, as mentioned in Chapter 1, health facilities of the government or NGOs and private health facilities need to be included. A situation analysis should include a listing of all facilities, covering staffing by cadre, existence and state of primary health care programmes. It is important to include any special vertical programmes, in particular those related to tuberculosis control or reproductive health, such as family planning and maternity care.

For any health services that may become part of a programme directed at HIV/AIDS, it is important to assess the level of knowledge and attitude of health workers in this area. Health workers can only become a resource for HIV/AIDS programmes if they are well informed and have a positive attitude toward education related to safe sexual behaviour, STDs and AIDS patients.

Other resources

What district structures are available for planning and implementing an HIV prevention and AIDS care programme, and what resources do they have available? These will include the district council, district development committee, district health management team, intersectoral teams such as primary health care committees, departments of community development and education, and others.

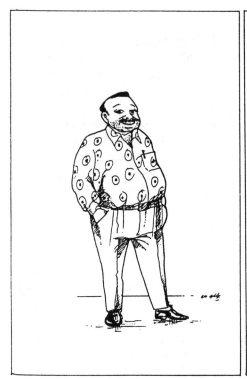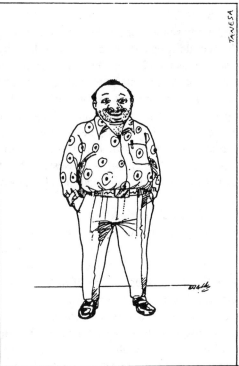

Mr X five years later.

A listing should also be made of the organizations and structures at community level. This should include village committees, women's groups, youth groups and so forth. Government structures at all levels too can play a key role in the programme. This includes dissemination of messages, influencing behaviour, and assisting communities, families or individuals in coping with the consequences of the epidemic. The existence of national or regional radio programmes in the languages relevant for the district should be noted, as well as whether any printed materials are being distributed.

NGOs can play an important role in an HIV/AIDS programme. They may have long-standing programmes in certain areas, on which these programmes can build; some may already be specifically focusing on the problem of HIV/AIDS. Incorporating HIV/AIDS activities in these existing programmes may be the most sustainable option. A mapping exercise that shows the distribution of activities and coverage of the various locally relevant NGOs can provide some evidence of the network that is potentially available.

The private sector is another resource. Businesses can institute helpful policies in the workplace, and they can be asked for donations. Churches and social clubs can also help disseminate messages and support local committees, health education and AIDS care activities. Local media such as newspapers and radio are modern and quite useful resources. While traditional communications media, entertainment and dissemination of messages are often overlooked, they can be very effective. For instance, in Tanzania *ngonjera* is a common and attractive way to act out scenes from real life; this is done in the form of two or more persons alternately reciting a poem.

Because their use is such an important intervention in controlling the spread of HIV and STDs, condoms are another important resource. In a situation analysis data from surveys can be used to obtain a rough idea of the current use of condoms. For instance, data from a national Demographic and Health Survey (DHS) will usually include figures on condom use by age and sex.

Condom availability should also be included. Data may be available on how many condoms have been distributed and where. A small survey of shops, health facilities and guesthouses can also provide important data on condom availability (and use). Such a survey could also indicate potential new distribution sites or agencies, e.g. truck repair or petrol stations.

Conclusion

A district situation analysis provides a basis for developing a realistic and workable district HIV/AIDS programme. A simple analysis of the population distribution and economy of the district will supply the essential information required to identify high-transmission areas. In addition, the situation analysis summarizes the key resources that are available in the district. The information collected can be used to make an action plan, as outlined in Chapter 1; this indicates which of these resources will need to be mobilized to stage a broad multisectoral and multi-level attack on the AIDS epidemic and its consequences.

Further reading and resources

Christian Medical Board of Tanzania et al. *Participatory Action Research on AIDS and the Community as a Source of Care and Healing*. Geneva, World Council of Churches, 1993.

Ssembatya J et al. Using participatory rural appraisal to assess community HIV risk factors: experiences from rural Uganda. *PLA Notes* 23, June 1995, pp. 62–65.

World Health Organization Global Programme on AIDS. *A Guide to Reporting on the Rapid Assessment Process*. Geneva, 1994.

The *Stepping Stones Training Package* consists of a 240-page manual and 70-minute workshop video in the English and Luganda languages. The package was designed to help trainers and community members organize a series of workshop sessions for peer groups of 10–20 people in which women and men of all ages explore their social, sexual and psychological needs, analyse the communication blocks they face and practise different ways of addressing their relationships. Single sets of the package cost 47.50 British pounds; a set of four manuals and one video can be ordered for GBP 85.00. Order from: TALC, P.O. Box 49, St Albans, Herts AL1 4AX, United Kingdom.

Facts about AIDS/*Sviripo maererano ne* AIDS (Zimbabwe, Shona/English, ca. 20 minutes, VHS PAL) is a video that gives information about HIV/AIDS by following a rural group which sets out to discover what their community knows about AIDS and what information people want. The group includes widows, a sex worker, a traditional healer, a youth drama group and village elders. Analogies are used; immunity is explained, for example, using the comparison of a fence which protects growing food. Order from: UNICEF Zimbabwe, AIDS Section, P.O. Box 1250, Harare, Zimbabwe.

References

1. Barnett T, Blaikie P. AIDS *in Africa: its present and future impact.* London, Belhaven Press, 1992.

2. Bureau of Statistics. *National Population Census 1988.* Mwanza Region report. Dar es Salaam (undated).

3. Barongo LR, Borgdorff MW, Mosha FF et al. The epidemiology of HIV-1 infection in urban areas, roadside settlements and rural villages in Mwanza Region, Tanzania. AIDS 1992, 6: 1521–1528.

3 Epidemiological methods

Jim Todd and Longin Barongo

- What is the difference between HIV prevalence and incidence?
- How can risk factors be determined?
- What simple method can be used to estimate HIV prevalence in a district?
- How can a KAP study help us understand the HIV epidemic?
- What is the meaning of 99% sensitivity and 99% specificity of an HIV or other test?

Clinical science is the process of diagnosing and treating disease in individual patients. Epidemiology is a public health science which studies the effect and patterns of disease within the community. In clinical medicine, there are many different techniques that doctors and health workers can use to help individual patients recover and cope with their disease. Similarly, there are many epidemiological techniques that doctors and public health officials can use in their daily work to help communities cope with the HIV/AIDS epidemic.

Collecting epidemiological data involves making use of the signs and symptoms observed in clinical treatment of HIV and STD patients. It may also involve the use of sophisticated laboratory tests for HIV and STDs. Epidemiology must also involve the communities in which we work, by listening to people within the community, gathering data from the health centre and conducting small surveys within communities. The HIV epidemic is changing fast. Small, clearly defined studies are the most helpful: epidemiological studies must take place within a defined time period. If data are collected in a scientific and systematic way, epidemiology can help us to:

- observe the natural history of a disease, in this case HIV and STDs;
- identify the causes and determinants of these diseases;
- observe the social consequences of these diseases on the community and its people;
- help to design and implement effective interventions to halt the spread of HIV, AIDS and STDs.

Small epidemiological studies are possible at district level and need not be costly. This chapter is intended to present some simple epidemiological techniques health workers and planners can use at district level. These techniques can be especially useful both in conducting studies within the district and in putting together information from other studies to learn how HIV and AIDS affect the district. It is important for health workers in districts to be able to use the results of epidemiological studies in their everyday work.

Epidemiological terminology

Epidemiological research is based on the assumption that disease does not occur at random. It assumes there are both preventative and causative factors which can be identified. Epidemiology includes the study of the distribution of disease within a population, and the distribution of demographic characteristics of the disease. Many training manuals have been written to help in developing research proposals and assessing health service needs (see 'Further reading', Wingo et al.). First, however, some terms should be briefly defined.

Frequency	Quantifies the occurrence of a disease. The frequency of a disease can be presented in absolute numbers. For example: 150 AIDS patients died in the district hospital last year.
Rate	The rate is a measure of the frequency of the disease within a specified population. For example, the 150 AIDS patients who died in the district hospital last year can be related to the total number of AIDS patients admitted to this hospital in the same year. Say 600 patients were admitted. These facts can be used to calculate a mortality rate for AIDS patients who were admitted to the district hospital last year: $150 \div 600 = 25\%$.
Ratio	A ratio is an expression of the relationship between a numerator and denominator, independent of the population base from which these are derived. For example, a mortality rate ratio can express the relationship between the mortality rates of AIDS patients and other patients admitted to the district hospital.
Distribution	Comparing the frequency with which a disease occurs among different sub-groups shows its 'distribution' in a population. Considering such patterns of disease helps make it possible to identify factors that may cause or prevent the disease. This can lead to strategies to combat it.
Descriptive studies	'Descriptive' studies can be case studies of individual patients or cross-sectional studies involving many thousands of people. Descriptive studies are attempts to gain a better understanding of the way a disease progresses, and to generate hypotheses about the routes of transmission, etc. They are often carried out with very little knowledge of the causes of the disease: they simply describe its facets and try to correlate population

	characteristics with the occurrence of the disease.
Analytical studies	Analytic studies are used to investigate and test hypotheses as well as to establish causal links between disease and environmental and social factors. The main types of analytic studies include cohort studies and case-control studies, as well as the evaluation of interventions.
Cross-sectional study	A study in which a sample of the population is surveyed at one particular time. This provides a simple picture or description of the characteristics of the population, including the frequency of the disease under study and risk factors of interest.
Cohort studies	A study of one sample of people, who are followed over a period of time. These dynamic studies can tell us how disease patterns change over time, and help identify causes of disease.
Eligible population	The 'eligible' population includes all persons at risk of the disease. The transmission of HIV is predominately through sexual contact, so the eligible population is often taken to be sexually active adults. Some studies define this as persons aged between 15 and 49 years of age. Such definitions are important because the results of study can only be generalized to similar populations.
Random sample	In most studies, it is impossible to survey every person in the population. Thus, a sample of the population will be drawn and surveyed, preferably at random – that is, in a way that ensures that all members of the population have an equal chance of being chosen. This procedure increases the likelihood that the results of the survey will be applicable to the whole population. In situations where there is no list of the population to be sampled, or people are widely dispersed, cluster sampling can be used to obtain a 'random' sample. A cluster could be a household, a village or any group of individuals who can be easily identified and enumerated, so that a selection can be made. (See Kirkwood, in 'Further reading' regarding sampling.)
Outcome measures	In any epidemiological study, outcome measurements need to be defined carefully before the study starts: these are the variables that will be monitored and used in evaluating results. Examples of possible outcomes are: death, HIV infection, clinical AIDS, a reported STD episode, or a laboratory-confirmed STD.

AIDS is a clinical disease: it has been defined by WHO, based on various signs and symptoms (see Box 1). It is very difficult to diagnose AIDS outside of major hospitals, and so in many epidemiological studies it is not a useful outcome measurement. HIV infection can be measured more objectively, as this is usually based on the results of a

Box 1. AIDS clinical case definition for use in surveillance

In an adult, AIDS is defined by the presence of at least two major and one minor symptom (1).

Major symptoms
- weight loss greater than 10% of body weight
- chronic diarrhoea for more than one month
- fever lasting for more than one month

Minor symptoms
- persistent cough for more than one month
- generalized pruritic dermatitis
- recurrent herpes zoster
- oral or pharyngeal candidiasis
- generalized lymphadenopathy
- chronic or persistent herpes simplex

The presence of either Kaposi's sarcoma or cryptococcal meningitis alone is sufficient to diagnosis AIDS.

laboratory test of blood or saliva (examples of HIV tests are given in Chapter 15). In many studies HIV infection is used as an outcome measure, indicating the magnitude of the AIDS problem in communities. Small blood samples are taken from a representative sample of people; these are used to estimate the prevalence of HIV in their communities.

The prevalence rate (a snapshot of HIV in the community)

The prevalence rate, or point prevalence, reflects the proportion of the population that has a disease such as HIV at a given moment in time. The prevalence rate is usually obtained by measurements of a random sample, as described above. If the sample is representative, the results can be used as an estimate of the prevalence rate for the whole population being studied.

A definition of prevalence

$$\text{Prevalence rate} = \frac{\textit{Number with the disease in the random sample}}{\textit{Total number in the random sample}} \times 100\%$$

Box 2. HIV prevalence by age, residence and sex

Overall prevalence in urban areas is higher than for roadside settlements, and both are higher than in rural villages. Prevalence in females is highest in the younger age groups, but for males peak prevalence occurs at 35 to 44 years (2).

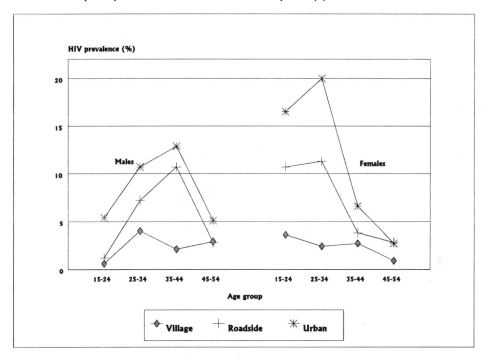

How do we interpret an HIV prevalence rate? If a study shows an overall prevalence of 10% among the adult population, this implies that out of every 100 eligible adults, 10 are likely to be HIV infected. Thus in a district with a population of 125,000 adults (total population 300,000) there will be about 12,500 HIV positive adults. Note that if the study defined the eligible population as adults, and therefore sampled only this group, the results will only show the prevalence for adults. They will provide no information about the prevalence of HIV among other groups such as children.

The prevalence rate in a district is often useful in gaining an understanding of the size and scope of a problem, and its demands on health resources. The main drawback to the use of prevalence data is that it does not differentiate between people who acquired HIV recently and those who have been seropositive for a number of months or years. Also, it is wise to break down data on prevalence: there can be great differences in prevalence rates, for example between sexes, for different age groups or in different areas. Box 2 presents a graph from a regional survey of Mwanza which illustrates these differences.

Box 3. Assessment of STD prevalence

A cross-sectional study of a sample including 12,534 adults conducted in 1992–1993 in Mwanza Region found the following prevalence of STDs, using the laboratory tests described above (3).

	Males	Females
Ever had a genital discharge	28%	8%
Ever had a genital ulcer	15%	6%
Past serological syphilis (TPHA +)	15%	16%
Active syphilis (TPHA + and RPR +)	10%	9%
N. gonorrhoea/C. trachomatis	2.8%	N/A

The serological tests for syphilis indicate a similar, and high, prevalence for men and women, but answers to the question about previous STDs show that reported prevalence is much lower among women. The longer the time period over which people are asked to remember, the less reliable their answers will be.

The prevalence of other, traditional STDs can be measured using the same methodology. In a random sample of people from the eligible sexually active population, STDs can be measured in several ways. Tests for syphilis such as RPR (rapid plasma reagin) or TPHA (treponema pallidum haem agglutination) can be carried out in the laboratory. Specimens for the culture of *Neisseria gonorrhoea* and for an antigen test for *Chlamydia* can be taken by cervical or urethral swab during physical examinations (see Chapter 13 and 14). Patients can be asked to recall symptoms of STDs, such as genital ulcers (GUS) and genital discharge (GDS) and their treatment-seeking behaviour on such occasions (see Box 3).

Sentinel surveillance – multiple pictures of the prevalence rate

Drawing a random sample from a population at one point in time will give us the prevalence rate of the disease at that time. Repeating the study methodology on a fresh random sample from the same population at a difference time will give a new prevalence rate. Collecting repeated samples from the same population is called 'sentinel surveillance' for the disease, and gives a good measure of changes in prevalence over time. In many countries, special 'sentinel surveillance' programmes for HIV have been set up, to provide a series of pictures of the HIV prevalence rate at regular intervals. A selected group of people attending various clinics for other reasons is tested anonymously. Examples include women attending an antenatal clinic or people asked to give a blood donation for a relative. The assumption is that these people represent a random sample of the population being studied. If prevalence is seen to be increasing (or decreasing) in this group, it is apt to be changing in the same way throughout the community. Thus testing serves as a 'sentinel' – it warns of what is happening. Although the assumption that the group tested is a random sample may not always be true, sentinel surveillance has often provided a useful picture of the degree of HIV prevalence in various countries and over prolonged time periods.

Women attending antenatal clinics usually provide a good sample of the sexually active population, for obvious reasons. In sentinel surveillance of those attending antenatal clinics, the same number of women are anonymously tested for HIV and syphilis, usually at intervals of three months or one year. At each interval, a different set of women is tested, but the selection and testing is done in exactly the same way. For accuracy, at least 300 women should be anonymously tested at the same clinic on each occasion. Therefore the most feasible plan may be to conduct annual sentinel surveillance at the largest antenatal clinic at district level. Box 4, however, gives an example of the results of quarterly sentinel surveillance among women attending an antenatal clinic in Mwanza, Tanzania.

Sentinel surveillance can give a useful indication of changes in the prevalence of HIV infection within a community. Sentinel surveillance is a useful way of monitoring HIV infection trends over time, but it does not really enable us to see the progression of the disease. If prevalence rises over a defined time period in the group being monitored, it suggests that more people are becoming infected with HIV than are dying from this disease. Prevalence stabilizes when new infections approximately equal the number of deaths. However, sentinel surveillance cannot tell us the number of new infections, nor the number of people who have already died of HIV.

In many districts sentinel surveillance of those attending antenatal clinics includes monitoring the prevalence of serological syphilis, using the RPR test. This is a cheap and easy way to measure the prevalence of syphilis in a population and to see the trends over time. In the town of Mwanza the prevalence of syphilis, as measured by the RPR test, has been stable at about 7.5% for the past 5 years. Sentinel surveillance can also be used to evaluate the effect of an intervention against syphilis in a given population: the disease is easy and cheap to treat; if screening and treatment are available the prevalence of syphilis recorded in the sentinel surveillance data should decrease in the district.

The incidence rate: new cases of the disease

The first measure of the dynamics of the HIV epidemic is based on the number of new cases of the disease; these are called the incident cases. The proportion of incident cases found in a population over a given period of time can be used to calculate the incidence rate.

Box 4. HIV seroprevalence among antenatal women in Mwanza, Tanzania, 1988–1994

This graph shows the results of quarterly sentinel surveillance of HIV prevalence among 300 pregnant women attending a large urban antenatal clinic in Mwanza. In the town of Mwanza over the past five years, prevalence of HIV infection among those attending antenatal clinics has stabilized at around 12%. Some women will have died of AIDS during this time, but other women will have recently acquired the disease. Other women may appear two or more times in the graph, if they attend for subsequent pregnancies.

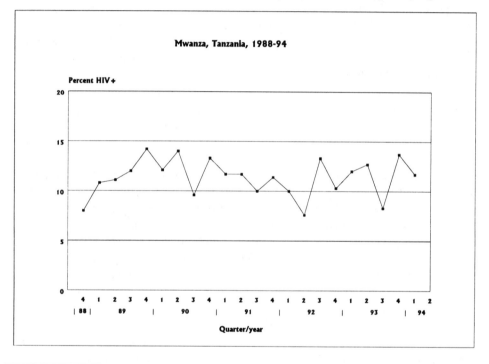

Definition of incidence

Incidence rate = $\dfrac{\textit{Number of new cases of the disease in the sample}}{\textit{Total number in sample x time in period observed}}$ x 100%

To measure the rate of incidence of HIV, we need to follow people over time. To do this we establish a cohort of people in the community who are free of the disease (HIV negative). Only those who are HIV negative at the beginning of the study can be monitored to establish an HIV incidence rate. We then follow those same individuals over a defined period of time, perhaps months or years. When a repeat HIV test is performed, the incident cases are those who have seroconverted from HIV negative to HIV positive during that time period. Such *cohort studies* are costly because all participants must be tested twice or more for HIV and tracked over prolonged periods of time, which can be time consuming and expensive.

What is the meaning of the incidence rate? An incidence rate of 1% per year indicates that for every 1,000 persons who are HIV negative, ten contract HIV after one year; in the next year another ten people will become HIV positive, and so on each year. In a large rural study in Mwanza Region, the observed incidence rate among a cohort of 4,500 people followed for two years was 0.93% per year, but where STD treatment was integrated into the health centres, the observed incidence rate in a similar cohort was only 0.58% per year (4).

The relationship between prevalence and incidence is dependant on the duration of infection. In the early stage of an epidemic, such as HIV/AIDS, incidence is proportional to prevalence and the epidemic grows very fast. As the epidemic proceeds, the incidence rate may remain high, but the prevalence rate may seem stable, because people who first contracted HIV may then be dying of AIDS and associated diseases. In the later stages of the HIV epidemic, behaviour changes or other interventions may lower the HIV incidence rate, but the HIV prevalence will remain high for several years to come.

AIDS, and in general HIV, eventually lead to death. Thus, for the HIV prevalence to be stable there must be as many new (incident) cases as there are people with HIV who die. If the prevalence is stable at 10% and the average life expectancy after acquiring HIV is ten years, the incidence rate must be about 10% divided by 10, or 1% per year. Thus, in a town of 20,000 adults and a stable HIV prevalence of 5%, the annual incidence rate is about 0.5% and there are about 100 new cases of HIV every year.

Interventions against HIV are intended to reduce the incidence of new cases. Once HIV has been contracted there is no known cure. The only way to stop the epidemic is to help unaffected, HIV-negative people to avoid acquiring HIV and becoming new incident cases. Incidence rates in people who engage in high-risk behaviour, such as having multiple partners without the use of condoms, and who have or have had STDs, can be 50 or 100 times as high as rates in people who stick with one sexual partner. Research has shown that 50% of HIV incident cases occur under the age of 25 years: youth often practise high-risk sexual behaviours. Thus, it is vital to develop a set of effective interventions targeted at young people.

Clinical epidemiology and health information systems

Valuable epidemiological data are contained in the routine health records kept at hospitals, health centres and dispensaries. Clinical records provide the basis for understanding the progress of the HIV/AIDS epidemic. Even if HIV testing is not routine, many other measures can be taken in a district health centre to show the progress of HIV/AIDS. Clinical records are summarized in data sent to regional and national health authorities. Mortality records are one such example. However, data often go to district administration without being incorporated in the health information system in a meaningful way. HIV often leads to premature death among adults aged 15–49 years. An HIV prevalence of 4% in the adult population has been shown to lead to a 35% increase in adult mortality and an HIV prevalence of 8% to a 60% increase in mortality (5). Many of these terminal cases exhibit some signs and symptoms of HIV/AIDS infection, but often records do not show HIV or AIDS as the cause of death. Nevertheless, the effect of HIV on overall mortality in a district may be quite dramatic.

Additional difficulties for record keeping arise because few district hospitals or rural health centres can make a definitive diagnosis of AIDS. Although chronic wasting and other symptoms are often reported, diagnosis can be difficult. In rural areas people with advanced HIV disease often cannot get to health facilities and are not seen by health workers.

On the other hand, other diseases associated with HIV infected individuals do require notification of health authorities: tuberculosis is one example. Records in Magu District, Tanzania show that new cases of pulmonary tuberculosis rose from 142 in 1984 to 295 in 1993, reflecting an early effect of HIV at the community level. Other rare diseases, such as Kaposi's sarcoma, are exclusively seen in conjunction with HIV infection. Health centres and hospitals may routinely report herpes zoster, oral candidiasis and other chronic complaints which are more common among HIV infected people. Even if HIV/AIDS cannot be assessed directly, monitoring these diseases may help to assess the effect of HIV on a community's health needs.

Information about such opportunistic infections and their treatment can help many people living with HIV to have longer and more productive lives. Most opportunistic infections can be treated, or alleviated, with drugs and proper care, but it is essential to plan and prepare for these in advance. Proper diet, good treatment and self-esteem can help people with HIV continue to live active and useful lives.

In rural districts, clinical AIDS may be uncommon, but HIV related morbidity is seen frequently, even though it is often not recognized. It is essential for district hospitals to monitor the syndromes associated with HIV infection and to assess the trends in such syndromes over time. An increase in HIV prevalence will also increase demands on health services, putting an extra burden on district health resources. Thus monitoring these trends can help to predict demands.

Laboratory epidemiology

The prevalence and incidence of any disease can only be established if there are reliable tests for that disease. These may be clinical signs or symptoms, but the definitive test is usually laboratory-based. Definitive laboratory tests are called the 'gold standard', and are usually expensive and difficult to perform: for HIV the gold standard is a 'Western blot' test. At the district level, ELISA-based tests are both sensitive and specific, and are much cheaper and easier to perform (see Chapters 15 and 17).

The degree of sensitivity of a test is the degree to which it correctly identifies actual positive cases, as defined below; specificity indicates the degree to which actual negatives are correctly identified. This can be seen in Table 1.

Table 1. Actual disease status (as determined by the 'gold standard')

Test result	Negative	Positive	
Negative	True negative (A)	False negative (B)	All test negatives (A+B)
Positive	False positive (C)	True positive (D)	All test positives (C+D)
	All true negatives (A+C)	All true positives (B+D)	

Sensitivity and specificity can then be defined as shown below:

$$\text{Sensitivity} = \frac{\textit{True positives (D)}}{\textit{All true positives (B + D)}}$$

$$\text{Specificity} = \frac{\textit{True negatives (A)}}{\textit{All true negatives (A + C)}}$$

The positive predictive value (PPV) and the negative predictive value (NPV) of tests can be similarly defined. The PPV is the proportion of all test positives which are truly positive. The NPV is the proportion of all test negatives which are truly negative (see 'Further reading', Armatige and Berry, Chapter 15).

For syphilis, the test most commonly used in developing countries is the rapid plasma reagin (RPR) test. The RPR test has high sensitivity, in that it identifies most actual cases of syphilis. Treatment protocols based on the RPR test therefore can effectively treat most people infected with syphilis (see Chapters 13 and 14). However, the RPR test may also give positive results for some people who do not have syphilis. Thus it is not very specific: the number of 'false positives' is great enough that the positive predictive value RPR test may be as low as 50%, depending on the true prevalence of syphilis in the population. The sensitivity and specificity of other simple laboratory tests for STDs and other infections is either much lower still, or is not well established. A simple leucocyte esterase dipstick test has been suggested for detecting urethritis in men as the sensitivity is high; however the specificity may be only 30%. Wet mounts for the detection of *Candida albicans* may be quite specific, but they may miss over half of infected cases, i.e., their sensitivity is less than 50%.

Knowledge, attitudes and practices: KAP studies

At present, medical treatment for HIV/AIDS is expensive and not very effective. HIV/AIDS is a disease with many social taboos and moral overtones. There are also complex social and cultural reasons for the spread of infection. In such a situation it is not enough to conduct epidemiological surveys that concentrate on medical or laboratory results alone. We also need to know about the knowledge, attitude and practices (KAP) of the community. These attitudes and practices can be vital to containing the disease and building lasting structures in communities.

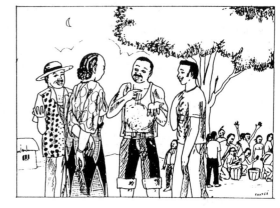

Risk behaviour: Chagulaga, a cultural event of the Sukuma people, in which a woman has the privilege to choose any man. The game makes promiscuous behaviour more acceptable to the society.

KAP studies do not require laboratory testing and sampling, unless carried out in conjunction with a prevalence or incidence study. However, they do require special skills in asking the right questions in the right way. Several methods may be used. One method is to survey a large number of people, asking simple questions about normal events in their lives. This approach is similar to the use of a questionnaire in a cross-sectional study. For example, within a survey, people might be asked whether they have ever had an STD; questions could also be asked about their knowledge of routes of HIV transmission. These quantifiable answers may give some insight into patterns of illness and AIDS awareness and possibly help in planning and evaluating future interventions.

Another method is to question a small number of people more intensively about their knowledge and attitudes. This may take the form of open-ended questions in questionnaires or a *focus group discussion* could take place. In either case people are encouraged to express themselves freely, and the responses are later coded and analysed. A third approach is a study which goes further, concentrating on one or two individuals. In-depth discussions may be held with these people or they may be observed for a period of time. In both cases the individuals are chosen on the basis of certain qualities, such as leadership or membership in a particular group (see also Chapters 4 and 9 and references 7 and 8).

KAP studies which concentrate on a small number of people may not be representative of the community as a whole but can provide valuable insight into the mechanism of HIV transmission if they are well analysed. For example, sub-groups can be examined and compared to each other. Subsequent studies can then look at the applicability of the findings in the wider community. However, despite the fact that KAP studies may not be representative of the whole population, KAP studies have played an important role in understanding the HIV/AIDS epidemic with respect to identifying core groups and those that are highly vulnerable.

Core groups

The concept of 'core groups', groups with a high level of transmission of HIV, has been central to understanding the HIV epidemic. Details of the core group concept and the use of this approach are described in Chapter 14. From an epidemiological point of view successful interventions among core groups not only prevent new infections among core groups (such as prostitutes) and their sexual partners, but also prevent the spread of the virus among other layers of the population not directly associated with the core groups (e.g. wives whose husbands have sex with prostitutes).

Epidemiology of HIV/AIDS in children

In Africa, evidence shows that if a mother is HIV positive, 25% to 35% of her children will also be HIV positive. It is difficult to measure this at birth using ELISA-based HIV tests, because maternal antibodies for HIV – as all antibodies – easily cross the placenta. Thus, either the virus must be measured directly, using the polymerase chain reaction, tissue culture or antigen detection, or a waiting period of 18 months must be applied. After that time, maternal antibodies will have dissipated and the child's own antibodies can be measured.

While antibodies are easily transmitted, it is not easy for the HIV virus itself to cross the placenta. Studies have also shown that transmission from mother to child is increased if the mother is simultaneously experiencing other immunological challenges, such as malaria infection or vitamin A deficiency. However, the virus may also be transmitted in the birth canal at the time of delivery, through the mixing of maternal blood with the baby's blood. Interventions to reduce the mother-to-child transmission of HIV should include care for expectant mothers and the provision of safe delivery methods. A baby can also be infected by its mother during breastfeeding: the HIV virus may be secreted in the breast milk, but this should not stop HIV-positive mothers from breastfeeding their babies.

The consequences for children born to HIV-positive mothers are serious. For those born with HIV, infections of infancy and childhood quickly devastate the immune system. A large proportion of HIV-positive children die before reaching 12 months of age. Those who are free of HIV but whose mother is infected often become orphans when the mother dies. The number of orphans in Tanzania was estimated to be 700,000 in 1994 and will approach two million by the year 2000. This puts the extended family under considerable stress and may make the vicious cycle of poverty, exploitation and degradation inescapable for many families (Chapter 20 is also relevant to these discussions).

Undertaking an epidemiological study

An epidemiological study needs to be carefully designed. Even a small study requires serious consideration of the reasons for the study, the expected implications of the results, how the study will be conducted and how it will be funded, just as in designing a research proposal.

To begin, both the problem and the questions the study will address need to be identified. A survey of the literature should reveal whether any other studies have been done on the same topic. This literature search may present relevant ideas, or even fully answer the proposed questions, and hence make the new study unnecessary. If the study is to be carried out, it must be clearly defined and simply presented, including the reasons for undertaking such a study in one particular district rather than elsewhere.

The design of the study is important. Can the question be answered by a simple survey, or is a lengthy follow-up period necessary for a cohort? Is the objective to describe the situation in one particular district, through a simple descriptive study, or to find explanatory factors using an analytic study design? Will the study be part of the evaluation of an intervention? Does ethical clearance need to be obtained for the study from regional or national authorities?

Methodology is the next consideration. The following parameters should be defined: the eligible population, the sample size required, the outcome measurement of principle interest. How are the variables to be collected, has the questionnaire been tested? The data will need to be collected and analysed, either manually or using a computer-based programme. Most methodological problems can be overcome by consulting a professional in that field or relevant textbooks on the subject (see 'Further reading', Smith and Morrow). Practical guidance on undertaking an epidemiological study can be obtained from WHO and CDC publications (see 'Further reading', Smith and Morrow).

Finally, any study must analyse the data, prepare the results and present its conclusions clearly and simply. This presentation of conclusions might include:

Maps	Maps can show the area where the study took place, helping to identify the population to which the results are applicable. Geographical features which help to explain the results can also be shown.
Tables	Tables showing frequencies and percentages should be kept simple. Do not try to present too much in one table: this can be confusing. For example, results should be shown separately for each sex. The risk factors examined and the extent to which these factors are present should be adequately explained.
Graphs	Line graphs can show trends over time. Bar graphs or pie charts can be used to present the data for various subgroups. Graphs and charts give readers a visual overview of results; this helps to make results more interesting, in both written and oral presentations.
Statistics	Many statistical techniques can be used to help explore the data. Simple techniques should be used first, to get a good understanding of the data before attempting more complex techniques. These should be used sparingly; the help of an experienced statistician is needed in making the related decisions.

Box 5. Risk factors associated with HIV infection

Demographic characteristics:	age and sex, circumcision status, mobility (travel to large towns), work (gold miners, fishermen, truck drivers), marital status (divorced, widowed, single).
Behavioural characteristics:	use of condoms, number of sexual partners, type of sexual partners.
Medical characteristics:	prior history of STDs (genital ulcer or discharge), blood transfusions, injections with unclean needles.

Comparing groups – risk factors

Epidemiology cannot establish the biological mechanism underlying a disease. We cannot tell why one person gets HIV and another does not. What epidemiology can do is to examine associations between HIV/AIDS and other diseases, and between HIV/AIDS and risk factors. We can use the fact that areas have different characteristics (young people coming to urban centres to look for work, or not), and ethnic groups have different cultural customs (prevalence of circumcision varies). The prevalence of other STDs also varies. Epidemiologists look at these local differences in comparison to the incidence of HIV infection, to determine whether there seem to be associations between the two.

Studies have shown that religion, ethnicity and education may be associated with higher HIV infection. These and other risk factors may operate through particular behavioural characteristics. We can try to measure the associations between such risk factors and HIV infection by including a simple questionnaire with an HIV survey or sentinel surveillance. Simple but relevant questions, combined with HIV test results, can be used to obtain the HIV prevalence in relation to the level at which a particular risk factor is present or absent. This can help to discover the behaviour that is behind the relationship observed between these risk factors and HIV infection. Some of the general characteristics that have been shown to be risk factors are given in Box 5.

More detailed analysis can be used to obtain an estimate of *relative risk (RR)*. The RR quantifies a comparison between two groups within a community with respect to their prevalence of HIV. If desired, a crude RR can be given, or the RR can be adjusted for the presence of other known HIV infection risks (see 'Further reading', Armitage and Berry, Kirkwood).

One way to investigate HIV risk factors is to carry out a *cross-sectional study*. However, such studies can be large and expensive. An alternative way to investigate HIV risk factors is a *case-control study*. In such a study, HIV positive cases are matched, on the basis of particular characteristics, with an equal number of HIV negative cases. These negative cases serve as a control group. This method makes it possible to collect useful information while carrying out far fewer interviews. Because there are fewer interviews, more detailed questions can be asked. However, in a case-control study it is not possible to calculate HIV prevalence for specific groups or risk factors: that is, the

RR cannot be obtained. Instead, an odds ratio (OR) is calculated to quantify the increased risk of HIV infection. However, the OR can then be used to estimate the RR, or vice versa. The two measures can be similar, but are calculated slightly differently, as can be seen in the data taken from a regional cross-sectional study in Mwanza (6) (See Table 2).

Table 2. Presence of active syphilis (based on TPHA and RPR tests)

Males only	Negative	Positive (%)	Total
Occupation			
Farmer	1212	127 (9.5%)	1339
Other	613	43 (6.5%)	656
Total	1825	170 (8.5%)	1995

The prevalence of syphilis is seen to be 9.5% for the group of farmers and 6.5% for other occupations. By comparing other occupations to farmers, we can calculate the relative risk: 6.5%/9.5% = 0.68. In making this calculation, it is assumed that the data was collected from a random sample of the total population.

Calculating odds ratios, on the other hand, does not require making any assumptions about the total population. It is only necessary to assume that syphilis positives and negatives have been chosen on the basis of the same characteristics (but not necessarily from a random sample from the total population). To obtain an odds ratio, first the odds of syphilis must be calculated for each of the two groups by dividing the number of syphilis positives by the number of syphilis negatives. This gives 0.105 (127/1212) for farmers and 0.701 (43/613) for other occupations. A comparison of other occupations with farmers (0.701/0.105) then yields an odds ratio of 0.67.

Conclusions

Epidemiological methods can help us to understand the development of the HIV/AIDS epidemic. These methods have constraints, including the need to sample from the population, and the difficulties of both laboratory testing and preparation of a useful questionnaire. Nevertheless, we can examine overall HIV prevalence in a community or district, which can help to assess the size of the problem it faces.

A sentinel surveillance system can be used to monitor trends in HIV prevalence. Incidence of HIV is far more difficult to measure, requiring the establishment of a cohort, who will be followed over time. However, lowering HIV incidence is the only way to stop the epidemic, and measuring the incidence of HIV is a way to measure the effectiveness of interventions.

Finally, it is important to determine the association between risk factors and HIV infection within the community. This enables interventions to be targeted on specific groups who are at increased risk of acquiring the infection. Behaviour changes may be difficult but can be achieved in small groups.

The purpose of this chapter is not to go into great detail about how to conduct studies at the district level, but to point out that small epidemiological studies are possible at district level and need not be costly. We would like to encourage those interested in developing a study proposal to do so, making use of the many manuals and other aids that can help in this process.

Further reading

Armitage P, Berry G. *Statistical methods in medical research*. Second edition. Oxford (OX2 0EL, UK), Blackwell Scientific Publications, 1987.

Kirkwood B. *Essentials of medical statistics*. Oxford (OX2 0EL, UK), Blackwell Scientific Publications, 1988.

Smith PG, Morrow RH (eds.). *Methods for field trials of interventions against tropical diseases – a toolbox*. UNDP/World Bank/WHO Special Programme for Research and Training in Tropical Diseases, Oxford University Press, (Oxford OX2 6DP, UK), 1991.

Rose G, Barker DJP. *Epidemiology for the uninitiated*. British Medical Journal, (Tavistick Square. London WC1H 9JR), 1986.

Rothman KJ. *Modern epidemiology*. Boston, Massachusetts 02108, Little, Brown and Company (for the more advanced student).

Wingo P, Higgins J, Rubin G, Zahniser S (eds.). *An epidemiological approach to reproductive health*. WHO Special Programme of Research, 1994.

References

1. World Health Organization. WHO case definitions for AIDS surveillance in adults and adolescents. *WHO Weekly Epidemiological Record* 1994, 69: 273–275.

2. Barongo LR, Borgdorff MW, Mosha FF et al. The epidemiology of HIV-1 infection in urban areas, roadside settlements and rural villages in Mwanza region, Tanzania. *AIDS* 1992, 6: 1521–1528.

3. Grosskurth H, Mosha F, Todd J et al. A community trial of the impact of improved STD treatment on the HIV epidemic in rural Tanzania: 2. Baseline survey results. *AIDS* 1995, 9: 927–934.

4. Grosskurth H, Mosha F, Todd J et al. Impact of improved treatment of sexually transmitted diseases on HIV infection in rural Tanzania: randomised controlled trial. *Lancet* 1995, 346: 530–536.

5. Mulder D, Nunn A, Wagner H et al. HIV-1 incidence and HIV-1 associated mortality in a rural Ugandan population cohort. *AIDS* 1994, 8: 87–92.

6. Newell J, Senkoro K, Mosha F et al. A population-based study of syphilis and sexually transmitted disease syndromes in North-western Tanzania. 2. Risk factors and health seeking behaviour. *Genitourinary Medicine* 1993, 69: 421–425.

7. WHO. Qualitative research methods: teaching materials from a TDR workshop. *Resource papers for social and economic research in tropical diseases,* no. 3. Kikawawila study group. UNDP Special Programme for Research and Training in Tropical Disease (TDR – Geneva), 1994.

8. Helitzer, AD, Makhambra M, Wangel AM. Obtaining sensitive information: the need for more than focus groups. *Reproductive Health Matters* 1994, 3: 75–82.

4 Anthropological research on AIDS

Robert Pool

- What kind of problems are encountered in a social science study of AIDS?
- How can a delicate, hidden topic such as sex be studied?
- How useful are 'rapid' social science methods for studying AIDS-related topics?
- What is a language-centred approach to the study of social behaviour and attitudes?
- What is the difference between a narrative interview and a life history?

AIDS is a social disease: its transmission is related to certain identifiable forms of social behaviour, and right at the centre of that behaviour is sex. In the absence of a medical cure for AIDS or a vaccine to prevent HIV, radical changes in behaviour seem to be the only way of preventing the spread of AIDS. Here there are two options: reducing the number of sexual partners and increasing the use of condoms. The major thrust of AIDS-related social science research must therefore be aimed at charting forms of sexual risk behaviour and understanding related attitudes. However, sexual behaviour does not occur in a vacuum; it is important to know and understand the social, cultural and economic context of that behaviour. In addition, a thorough understanding of people's knowledge of – and ideas about – AIDS, and the relation between these ideas and more general causal models is also essential.

The important issues in AIDS-related social research are therefore:

- sexual behaviour and related attitudes
- knowledge and perceptions of AIDS
- local etiologies and treatment-seeking behaviour
- social organization, customs and norms
- underlying socioeconomic factors
- coping with AIDS and its consequences.

In what follows various anthropological methods relevant to studying the AIDS-related topics mentioned above will be described. In the final section two examples of multi-instrument research will be briefly presented.

Anthropological research

Although anthropologists have traditionally studied social organization, local customs, economic organization and illness, sexual behaviour and attitudes have been largely ignored. This reluctance to study sex is partly a result of the fact that it has been, until recently, difficult to publish studies on sex, and partly because of the sheer difficulty of studying the topic in a socially acceptable manner. You usually cannot observe it, and it is often not socially acceptable to question people about it. Be that as it may, anthropology is the obvious choice when it comes to studying sexual behaviour in its socio-cultural context, as well as knowledge, attitudes and beliefs related to AIDS.

Participant observation has been the basic anthropological research technique (1). Traditionally this meant that the researcher joined the group he or she was to study – usually another culture – and participated in their activities. He was always around to observe what they were doing, and having done this for an extended period of time, often several years, was able to form a picture of their culture and develop an understanding of what they were doing and why. Although much academic anthropological research is still in this form, the demands of policy makers and the pressure to solve urgent social problems have led to more emphasis being placed on rapid, short-term research techniques, some of them traditionally anthropological, some derived from other disciplines, others newly developed to study a specific problem. This has led to a blurring of the boundaries between different disciplines.

Participant observation is still at the core of anthropological research. This is an informal research method which boils down to a combination of observing what people do and listening to what they say. The basic fact of participant observation seems to be simply that the researcher is *there*, tagging along, looking, listening, poking his nose in wherever he can and asking questions. The usefulness of this approach is based on the assumption that much relevant and interesting information, particularly regarding topics which are delicate, taboo or hidden, is more likely to surface in informal contexts than in a formal interview setting; and to get that information you have to be there.

Although observation is emphasized in the name of this method, speaking is, perhaps, more central to participant observation. How otherwise can we study such phenomena as traditional religion, etiology, witchcraft beliefs or attitudes about AIDS, which are largely embodied in spoken discourse? And how can we study activities which are observable (and unspoken) but (nonetheless) hidden from the researcher, such as sexual behaviour or illegal abortions. Participant observation is therefore not simply a rather unsystematic basis for quantitative methods, but often the only way to adequately study certain social phenomena.

Social knowledge

It is not only the fact that a culture or a certain aspect of a culture is inaccessible, or that a social phenomenon is delicate, taboo or hidden, that justifies the use of anthropological methods, but also the very nature of social processes generally and the way in which social knowledge is generated and exchanged.

One of the most important objections to participant observation is that the data it produces may be biased. To prevent this it is argued that the researcher should try to exclude his own views and preconceptions in order not to 'contaminate' the model of what the people being studied are doing. But this implies that it is possible to simply turn off our culture-bound way of seeing and interpreting. Another important objection focuses on the problem of 'informant accuracy' – the fact that different informants may say different things about the same topic.

These problems are, however, only apparent. They are based on untenable assumptions about the nature of social processes, social knowledge, everyday communication, our attempts to study these and our resulting scientific knowledge of them. Everyday social life is both less systematic and less rational than has been assumed in some social-science models. Human communication is always open to different, sometimes contradictory, interpretations. People can give different answers to the same question, depending on the situation, what was said before, who is present and what mood they are in. An individual can simultaneously employ different, even mutually contradictory, explanations or interpretations of the same phenomenon without being aware of any contradiction.

The central concept here is that of *discourse*. A discourse is a more or less consistent way of speaking about a certain topic; it also embodies a world view and various assumptions. It has become clear that in everyday life people may make use of different, sometimes contradictory discourses with regard to the same topic. In the example shown in Box 1 villagers simultaneously make use of a biomedically inspired discourse of concern and a discourse of indifference without being aware of the apparent contradiction. Neither represents what the person 'really' believes, as this depends on the situation.

Box I. Discourses and AIDS

People in the fishing villages in Magu District, Tanzania, make use of two discrete discourses when talking about and interpreting AIDS and their risk of getting it. When they discuss health threats to the village or illness, generally they tend not to mention AIDS at all. There is much complaint about poor sanitation, dirty water, diarrhoea, stomach ailments and so on, and STDs are considered to be the most important illness, especially by the fishermen (perhaps reflecting their high prevalence). However, when they are asked specifically about AIDS, the same villagers suddenly express a great deal of concern and may even claim that AIDS is the most important health threat facing them. In this 'discourse of concern' villagers switch over to the language and priorities of the health care providers and the AIDS educators. These differences also coincide, to a certain extent, with the methodology used: in focus group discussions villagers are more likely to express concern about AIDS than in individual in-depth interviews.

In interpreting the results of social scientific research and the presentation of findings, these multiple interpretations must be taken into account. The degree of certainty is, of course, relative. Some forms of knowledge are highly systematized, such as some kinds of technical and medical knowledge; practical activities based on that knowledge are systematic and predictable. In many fields knowledge is formalized and written down: in case of doubt one can always look it up. In other domains less systematic social knowledge plays a greater role and actions are determined to a far greater extent by factors such as situation, mood, personality, implicit communication. In such cases it is sometimes difficult for those involved to explain why they acted as they did, or to make the rules governing their actions fully explicit (for example, the interactions of people at a party). Finally, some kinds of knowledge are still in the process of being formed and are therefore perhaps even more chaotic (e.g. attitudes to a new disease such as AIDS).

The important point here is that a research method is not a neutral instrument that generates objective knowledge. The researcher always influences the reality he studies: recording conversations, or simply the presence of a researcher or a tape recorder, influence what people say, how they say it and how they act. Because it is impossible to ask all possible questions or record all impressions the researcher must make a selection. The traditional distinction between data and interpretation is untenable because the decision as to what will count as data is already the result of interpretation. This applies to all methods, and perhaps even more so in the case of quantitative methods that are generally considered to be more objective.

Finally, the methods researchers choose, the phenomena they decide are important and need studying, and their interpretation of the findings also depend on the theoretical orientation of the researchers. For example, if a researcher subscribes to a theoretical approach that claims social behaviour is determined largely by economic factors, he is more likely to focus on the economic activities of women as a possible determining factor in their participation in transactional sex. If, however, he subscribes to a theoretical model which places primacy on the determining role of culture, he is more apt to focus on attitudes toward sexual relationships and the meaning of exchanging money for sex. It is therefore well to take some time to reflect on the underlying and often only half conscious theoretical choices that have been made.

Specific research tools

There are no ready-made research instruments which can be applied to all situations and all social phenomena. Methods must be adapted to the situation and what it is you want to know, and this requires some creativity and willingness to innovate. Although the relatively unsystematic scanning of the environment provided by participant observation is the basis for most anthropological research, multiple research instruments are generally used.

Participant observation

This has been discussed above. Here we need to note that real participant observation, in the sense of long-term residence in the group being studied, is often impossible or impracticable, either because it is too time-consuming or, as in the case of many AIDS-related topics, because it is practically and ethically unacceptable (see Box 2).

Box 2. Participant observation and sex research

When studying female bar workers, participant observation, although theoretically possible (female researchers could have got jobs as bar workers, male researchers could have acted as clients), was, for obvious reasons, never an acceptable option. Participant observation therefore remained limited to what was acceptable: visiting bars and observing the behaviour of bar workers and their clients, to the extent that this was public and visible. In the Gambia, researchers got as close as possible to observing the sexual behaviour of prostitutes and their clients by posting researchers outside bedroom doors and interviewing clients immediately afterward (2).

Field journals

During participant observation, however limited, all relevant observations, impressions, etc. should be noted in a field journal. Notes should be as detailed as possible, and they should describe situations rather than interpret them. For example, you should note 'Agnes shouted at Joyce and banged her fist on the table,' rather than 'Agnes was angry with Joyce'. These notes provide background for the information provided by the more formal methods. Journal notes should be as specific as possible. In more formalized research settings such as interviews there are a number of important aspects that should always be noted and used alongside the interview texts when these are being interpreted. These are referred to as the components of communicative events:

1. Type of event (joke, story, lecture, interview).
2. Topic: what are those involved talking about?
3. Purpose or function: why are they talking to each other?
4. Setting: location, time, season, physical aspects of the situation (inside or outside, type of room and so forth).
5. Participants: age, sex, ethnicity, social status, or other relevant categories, relationships to each other, etc.
6. Message form: which languages are being spoken, are people speaking formally or informally, etc.
7. Message content: what is being communicated? (That is, they may be communicating something different to what they are saying explicitly. For example, someone may be talking politely but at the same time convey anger by the use of gestures and formal language).

8. Turn taking: do they take turns or talk at the same time? Who determines turn-taking?
9. Rules for interaction: are there any rules for turn-taking? Should youth defer to elders or women to men? Are there greetings, handshakes, and the like?
10. Norms of interpretation: what common knowledge, relevant cultural assumptions, shared understandings, etc. influence how people interpret the situation and what is being said (3, 9)?

Tape recording

Where possible all verbal interaction (interviews, focus group discussions, informal conversations, etc.) should be tape recorded. Depending on the goal of the research, the approach and the time available, these tapes may be transcribed verbatim and analysed in detail, or they may simply serve as a background for working out interview notes. It is always useful to have the recordings to fall back on, especially given the fact that note-taking is always selective and factors that do not seem relevant during an interview may turn out to be crucial later on. Ideally, interviews should be taped so that the interviewer can concentrate on what is being said and how it is being said, and have time to note down the components listed above, impressions, body language, and so forth, as well as noting questions that arise during the interview, rather than concentrating only on writing down as much as possible of what the informant is saying.

Interviews

Fieldwork requires more than what can be observed and heard first hand; there are a number of more formal methods that may also be used. The basic formal tool of anthropological research is the interview (see Box 3).

Interviews can be of various kinds, but the most important is the open, in-depth, key informant interview. Key informants, as the name implies, are an important source of information and insight and their selection is crucial to the success of research. For the kinds of topics that anthropologists usually study, a few good key informant interviews are often worth more than large numbers of superficial interviews, even if these are carried out with a more representative sample. There are no fixed rules as to who suitable key informants are and how to select them: recruiting suitable key informants usually depends on the researcher's insight and knowledge of people. Community leaders or those with a higher than average degree of formal education do not necessarily make the best key informants. Indeed, it may be better to avoid such obvious choices in favour of ordinary, well-informed, intelligent citizens. The number of key informants and whether they are male or female, young or old, will depend on the topic and the scope of the research.

Once key informants have been selected interviews can begin. There are three stages (3, 4):

- *Outline interviews* are held with a few key informants and are intended to provide a general outline of the topic to be studied. These interviews are informal and open, and informants are encouraged to express what they think are the important issues relating to the research topic, giving their interpretations. Outline interviews should also generate relevant topics and research questions which have not occurred to the researcher (who is often an outsider). On the basis of these interviews a general outline of the phenomenon to be studied can be drawn up, in collaboration with the key informants, and further, more specific questions developed.

- *Detailed interviews* form the second phase. After a general outline has been extracted from the first round of interviews a number of general themes can be identified and more specific questions developed. With these the researcher goes back to interview the original key informants, as well as newly recruited key informants. In this stage the researcher can also interview ordinary informants. Key informants differ from ordinary informants in that the researcher continually returns to them in a process of cumulative dialogue, whereas interviews with others may be one-time affairs that simply provide more breadth of coverage.

- *Follow-up interviews* constitute the third phase of the interview process and are intended to gather additional information or fill in gaps left after the previous phase. These interviews may continue indefinitely and be spread over many rounds, depending on the topic, the length of time needed to cover it sufficiently, and the time constraints. In this phase both key informants and ordinary informants are consulted.

Box 3. Interviews with bar workers

In research on bar workers an initial series of interviews were carried out, which explored various topics in a general way: the nature of bar work, income, relationships with men, knowledge of AIDS and STDs, condom use, etc. Analysis of these interviews led on to a second phase of interviews, some with the same informants, some with new ones. (Because of the mobility of bar workers it was not always easy to return to the same key informants.) These interviews focused on obtaining more elaborate information about certain aspects of sexual relationships that had emerged from the first round. These included the characteristics of male partners, exchange in sexual relationships and the distinction that women made between regular and casual partners. A third round of follow-up interviews, which also included single women who did not work in bars, focused on attitudes to marriage, divorce and the sexual double standard that allows male promiscuity while expecting women to remain faithful to a single partner.

Narratives
Narratives, although basically also a form of interview, are different in that the emphasis is on the informant telling a story about some relevant aspect of his/her life, rather than being questioned about a topic that the researcher has predefined as

important. This distinction is relative, as key informants also contribute to defining relevant research topics and researchers can elicit narratives on topics that they think are important, but in broad terms the distinction holds. In interviews there is a continual interaction between researcher and informant, whereas in a narrative the informant may speak almost exclusively.

Narrative interviews are particularly suitable for getting information on a specific event in the life of an informant. 'Tell me the story of your marriage and how it ended in divorce?' or 'Tell me about how your first relationship developed?' or 'Describe what happened the last time you went to a traditional healer for treatment' would be typical questions leading to a narrative exposition of a specific event. Narrative interviews can also be used to gather general information on a certain type of event. 'Tell me how marriages typically end up in divorce' or 'How do first sexual relationships between people typically develop?' or 'Describe what happens when you visit a traditional healer for treatment' are typical questions. The narrative approach is also suitable for studying such AIDS-related topics as sexual relations, coping, development of the disease, family reactions and so forth.

Life histories

Life histories are similar to narrative interviews, but instead of focusing on a specific event or type of event they cover a person's whole life, or at least a significant part of it. Life histories are particularly suitable for obtaining information on social change (or how people perceive social change). For example, in the fishing villages of Magu District the spread of AIDS and the high incidence of STDs is often said to be a consequence of the erosion of traditional restrictive norms relating to premarital and extramarital sexual relationships, resulting from recent rapid socioeconomic change. While this popular explanation sounds plausible, in the absence of documented history there is no real evidence of the nature and extent of changes in sexual behaviour and related norms. Here oral histories, although they can never be definite evidence of past behaviour and norms (because, like all narratives, they are reconstructions: expressions of how people today interpret the past they once experienced directly), can give us some impression of the direction of change, particularly if there is agreement among different people's stories. Oral histories can also give us a picture of how particular women end up in prostitution, how marriages break up and what strategies women subsequently employ to survive, or the devastating effect of infertility on the lives of women in a society that places so much emphasis on bearing children.

Ordinary conversation

Formal eliciting situations such as interviews are not the only verbal source of information. Informal conversations and discussions can also be rich sources of information and understanding, and may even be more suitable in the case of topics that are socially problematic, taboo or restricted in some way. There is, however, no clear line to be drawn between spontaneous conversation and more informal interview settings. Informal conversation or discussions may simply be overheard by a researcher who happens to be there, or they can be consciously provoked and steered by the skilful researcher (see Box 4).

Box 4. Informal discussion as research

During performance workshops carried out as part of a study of sexual relations among primary school pupils in Magu District, pupils often used the Swahili words *kupenda* and *mapenzi*. At first it seemed they were using these terms in more or less the same way as the term 'love' is used in English in that context, i.e. to refer to romantic love. However, further analysis of the use of *kupenda/mapenzi* in discussions among pupils seemed to suggest that the terms referred simply to sex. During analysis of these findings at the office, discussions developed between the researchers about what exactly the pupils meant by the words *kupenda/mapenzi*, and what these words meant in their own lives and relationships. These discussions were recorded and proved to be a rich source of data on attitudes to sexual relationships.

Questionnaires

At the opposite end of the qualitative–quantitative spectrum are formal questionnaires and surveys. The intention here is not to go into the details of survey research (Chapter 3 gives more information) but to point out the use of simple, customized questionnaires as part of a broader, multi-instrument approach. Such questionnaires could be integrated into the third phase of interviewing discussed above, to further broaden the scope of coverage and representativeness. For example, in the third phase of interviews in fishing villages, short, specific questionnaires were used to gather information on treatment preferences for STDs, knowledge of STD symptoms, knowledge of AIDS and perceptions of health threats.

Role plays and performance

Sometimes research needs to be done on forms of interaction that are not easily observed. In such cases role plays or performances, in which respondents enact that behaviour, can complement interview data and lead to new insights, particularly when performances are not simply repetitive miming but contain an element of reflection on what is being enacted (5) (see the school research example below).

Focus group discussions

Focus group discussions are basically key informant interviews applied simultaneously to a group of informants (6,7,8). Focus group discussions generally involve 8–10 participants who discuss a predetermined topic; a moderator ensures that the discussants keep to the subject. Focus group discussions have the advantage of being quick and relatively cost-effective. They are also said to be more representative, although in the case of delicate or taboo topics, this may mean they are representative of the socially accepted norm. In group discussions individual attitudes can be tested by presenting them to the group, but because of group pressure, individual ideas/variation may also remain hidden. Clearly informal group discussions, group interviews and focus group discussions are all parts of one continuum.

Box 5. Peer research among bar workers

As part of an evaluation of interventions among bar workers in urban Mwanza, bar workers who had been working as peer health educators were asked to interview fellow bar workers on various topics concerning AIDS-related interventions, including sexual behaviour, sexual techniques and condom use. From these interviews it became clear that unprotected anal sex was more important than had been thought. When interviewed by researchers, bar workers had always denied engaging in anal sex, but they could hardly deny it when questioned by colleagues who knew from their own experience that it was not uncommon.

Peer research
When topics are difficult for an outside researcher to study because they are part of a group sub-culture that is not easily accessible, it can be fruitful to use peer researchers: people from the group itself, who are already participating in the behaviour or activities that are the object of study and who are recruited to study those activities from the inside (see Box 5).

Ranking, classification and semantic differential
Various simple non-oral techniques can be used to find out how people rank and classify various aspects of their environment. For example, to find out how people classify diseases, terms related to illness can be written on separate cards. Informants are then asked to sort the cards into categories. Or, if knowledge is needed about the extent to which local illness terms coincide with their biomedical equivalents, inform-ants can be asked to sort cards containing descriptions of symptoms into syndromes. The same technique can be used to classify people's perceptions of the symptoms of AIDS, or to rank risk factors or means of prevention.

Similarly, in what is called a semantic differential test, informants judge various concepts or statements against a series of evaluative scales (good–bad, fair–unfair, big–small, very good–reasonably good–average–poor–bad–terrible). This is a relatively quick and easy way to get the opinion of a large number of informants on such matters as attitudes to AIDS patients, sexual promiscuity, condoms, monogamy or perceptions of the chance of becoming infected (10).

Non-verbal techniques
In addition to general observation, it is sometimes useful to study less conscious and overt expressive bodily behaviour more systematically (see Box 6). 'Proxemics' focuses on the symbolic use of space (such as closeness or keeping one's distance), while 'kinesics' focuses on the details of body movement (bowing, walking away, etc.) (10).

Box 6. Non-verbal techniques in a performance workshop

During performance workshops held with school pupils to study sexual relationships, an understanding of seduction behaviour was facilitated by relating body movement and positioning (as recorded on video) to what pupils were actually saying during the filmed encounter. For example, a boy and a girl are talking under a tree. The boy insists that the girl has sex with him. The girl keeps refusing and saying she wants to go home. She turns to walk away but he grabs her hand, though not firmly. At first she does not attempt to pull free and the dialogue continues. When she does pull free she walks away, saying she has had enough and is going home. But she stops after a couple of metres, turns and comes back to let the boy grab her hand again. This sequence of movements, which is repeated over and over, clearly suggests that the girl is interested, her body language and use of space contradicting her more explicit verbal denials.

Triangulation and reliability

Although earlier in this chapter emphasis was placed on the naturalness of indeterminacy and contradiction in people's everyday discourse and the necessity of accepting this as a normal characteristic of our social research data, this by no means implies that 'anything goes' in social research. While absolute certainty is unattainable, it is possible to obtain reasonably accurate information, and there are criteria to use to distinguish reliable from less reliable information. It will be clear from the discussion of specific methods above that social scientists have an arsenal of methods and techniques at their disposal, and various methods can be used together: the findings from one method can be used to cross-check the reliability of the findings from another. In social research, this cross-checking is called triangulation (see Box 7).

Various methods may also be combined, when each one is suitable for obtaining data of a specific kind. The proper use of such multi-round, multi-instrument research can generate large amounts of rich data in a relatively short period of time.

Rapid, multi-instrument research: some applications

Since the middle of 1993 TANESA has been carrying out anthropological research (as part of a larger, multi-disciplinary effort) to study various AIDS-related factors in various communities in Mwanza Region. One of our target groups has been primary school children, while another focus has been the fishing villages along the Lake Victoria shoreline. In what follows two examples of the application of multi-instrument research are briefly described.

Box 7. Triangulation

In 1991 the project in Mwanza began a cohort study in a large urban textile factory and by late 1994 approximately 2,500 workers and their spouses had been enrolled. A clinic was set up in the factory and participants were asked to make follow-up visits every four months. During these visits a physical examination and lab tests were carried out and each participant completed a standardized questionnaire. In addition to free treatment for the cohort, interventions in the factory included distribution of condoms, health education, training of peer educators and so forth. Analysis of the questionnaires showed a marked reduction in the number of sexual partners. Many men claimed to have become monogamous since hearing of AIDS. Because project interventions had focused on the desirability of reducing the number of sexual partners, it seemed likely that a social desirability factor was involved. This was contradicted, however, by the fact that there was a less significant increase in reported condom use, another focus of project interventions. In late 1995 these issues were followed up by selecting a small group of workers for further, individual in-depth interviews. This group included a number of workers with self-reported genital discharge during the last four months and a number who had seroconverted. In addition, interviews were held with a number of spouses about their husbands' sexual behaviour. These interviews, which were recorded and transcribed verbatim and analysed in some detail, showed that the reports of about three-quarters of the men were consistent with all other sources (questionnaire and in-depth interview, spouse, and biomedical data) (11).

Primary school pupils
After initial reconnaissance of the schools in one division of Magu District it was decided that a small survey would be a suitable and relatively cost-effective way of gathering baseline data. Six schools were selected and questionnaires were distributed to all pupils in the two highest classes of each school (n=213). The questions were open-ended and covered, apart from background information about each pupil, most of the relevant AIDS-related topics: knowledge of AIDS symptoms and modes of transmission, risk perception, prevention, sexual behaviour and condoms. The survey provided adequate information on all topics except sexual behaviour and condom use (12).

An attempt was then made to fill this gap by conducting a number of semi-structured interviews (n=35) with individual pupils. These interviews, some of which were recorded, also provided information about pupils' knowledge of AIDS, risk perception and prevention, in addition to new information on the socioeconomic situation of school pupils, but once again no information on sexual behaviour was forthcoming. As in the questionnaire, most pupils denied being involved in sexual relations, in spite of the fact that it was common knowledge that many school pupils were involved in such relations.

These methods thus appeared to be inadequate for producing reliable information on adolescent sexual behaviour and attitudes. Short of actual participation in the sub-culture of school pupils, which was obviously ruled out by age differences, it was felt that the only way of gaining access to pupils' experience of seduction and sexual encounters was to study their discourse: how they talked about such matters. A methodology was needed that would generate stretches of discourse in which young people discussed their sexual behaviour and attitudes freely and spontaneously. Given that the researchers could not gain access to such spontaneous discourse, it was decided to experiment with a performance approach, in which pupils would develop scripts based on significant episodes in adolescent relationships and then enact these in a way that was meaningful to them. They would then discuss the results among themselves and with the researchers.

Ideally we needed researchers who were young enough to be acceptable to primary school pupils as peers, but old and experienced enough to take the initiative, make creative use of opportunities that presented themselves and critically reflect on what was happening. Recruiting primary school pupils who conformed to these requirements was not easy, and in the end two ex-pupils who had recently participated in a secondary school AIDS programme run by Kuleana, a local NGO, were recruited. Together with one of the TANESA sociologists Kuleana recruited the ex-pupils and organized three performance workshops.

The performances were recorded on video and played back to the group for comment and discussion. All discussions were tape-recorded and transcribed. Although discussions among pupils did get underway after some initial hesitation, the most fruitful discussions were in fact the more focused sessions facilitated by the 'peer researchers'. The dialogues from the videotaped performances and the tape-recorded discussions were transcribed and subjected to a rudimentary discourse analysis with help from the *Ethnograph* software program. Simple proxemic and kinesic analysis also played a role in the interpretation of the videotapes.

In spite of their limitations, the performances did create a relaxed and informal atmosphere which facilitated the open discussion of issues that would otherwise have remained hidden, and the participants agreed that the performances were an accurate representation of their reality.

In the primary school study the use of multiple instruments therefore produced a comprehensive picture of all relevant AIDS-related topics. The survey generated a picture of pupils' knowledge of AIDS symptoms and modes of transmission, risk perception and prevention; the in-depth interviews filled out this picture and provided additional information on their socioeconomic background. The performance workshops, which were themselves multi-instrument (combining the narrative development of scripts, performances, informal discussions and focus group discussions, as well as making use of simple discourse analysis, proxemics and kinesics) provided the necessary information on sexual behaviour and related attitudes, and showed that this approach can be used to provide detailed information on sexual matters in certain groups with relatively little investment of effort and time, and using local staff with only minimal training.

Fishing villages

Phase I. After discussions with district authorities a number of reconnaissance visits were made to all fishing villages along the Magu shoreline, and a number of villages were selected for further study.

Phase II. An epidemiological/demographic survey was carried out in four of the villages to gather data on HIV and STD prevalence, risk factors, sexual behaviour and so forth. Simultaneously, a number of focus group discussions and an initial series of key informant interviews were broadly directed at all the topics considered relevant: perceptions of health threats and ideas about illness generally, social mobility, economic activities, fishing, beliefs relating to AIDS, etc.

Phase III. Based on an analysis of the first phase of key informant interviews a series of more specific, open-ended questionnaires were developed, each focusing on a topic that had emerged from the initial interviews. With these the researchers returned to the villages to conduct a second round of interviews. The topics included sexual behaviour and social mobility, and questions focused more directly on AIDS-related factors such as number of partners, condom use and acceptability. This second series of in-depth interviews coincided with a number of smaller surveys on knowledge of STDs, treatment-seeking for STDs and social mobility. These were partly based on the results of the epidemiological survey, which had since been made available.

Phase IV. From the second series of in-depth interviews the importance of the transactional component in sexual relationships and the distinction between regular and casual partners emerged. An analysis of these interviews led to the realization that important contextual information was still missing. This resulted in a third series of in-depth interviews concentrating on topics such as how people define different categories of sexual partner; the precise nature of, and attitudes about, the double standard (according to which it is considered normal for men to be promiscuous and have extramarital relationships whereas the same behaviour is unacceptable for women); and the exact role of exchange in sexual relationships. The results of the small surveys in phase III also led to a larger survey on social mobility and an in-depth study of the role of traditional healers in the treatment of STDs.

Throughout the whole research process participant observation also played a role. Many of the researchers were present in the villages for extended periods during both the quantitative and qualitative research, and the team of social scientists also stayed in guesthouses in the villages for the specific purpose of observing village life, and particularly night life, from nearby.

Here, the combination of quantitative and qualitative methods, including surveys, in-depth interviews of key informants, focus group discussions and participant observation have provided a comprehensive picture of all relevant AIDS-related factors in the fishing villages.

Conclusion

AIDS is a social disease. Research on sexual behaviour is required to develop meaningful and effective interventions, and anthropological research can make an important contribution. A wide range of anthropological methods are available for the study of sexual behaviour and AIDS. Some are fairly complex and require anthropological expertise; other methods are less complicated and can be utilized by district teams. Perhaps one of the most important lessons learned after several years of research in Tanzania is that rigid adherence to a single method such as focus groups is not likely to be useful. Studying sexual behaviour and AIDS is complex and requires a creative approach employing a variety of methods.

Further reading

Adolescent Health Programme. *The narrative research method: studying behaviour patterns of young people – by young people. A guide to its use.* Geneva, WHO, 1993.

Boulton M, ed. *Challenge and innovation: methodological advances in social research on HIV/AIDS.* London, Taylor & Francis, 1994.

Briggs CL. *Learning how to ask. A sociolinguistic appraisal of the role of the interview in social science research.* Cambridge, Cambridge University Press, 1986.

Dawson S, Manderson L, Tallo VL. *A manual for the use of focus groups.* Boston, INFDC, 1993.

Morgan DL (ed.). *Successful focus groups. Advancing the state of the art.* London, Sage, 1993.

Pelto PJ, Pelto GH. *Anthropological research. The structure of enquiry.* (2nd edition) Cambridge, Cambridge University Press, 1978.

Spradley JP. *Participant observation.* New York, Holt Rinehart and Winston, 1979.

Spradley JP. *The ethnographic interview.* New York, Holt Rinehart and Winston, 1979.

Standing H. AIDS, Conceptual and methodological issues in researching sexual behaviour in Sub-Saharan Africa. *Social Science and Medicine* 1992, 34: 475–483.

Stewart DW, Shamdasani PN. *Focus Groups. Theory and Practice.* London, Sage, 1990.

AIDS Health Promotion Exchange issue no. 1 on 'Out-of-school youth: a need for NGO and governmental collaboration'. Amsterdam, Royal Tropical Institute, 1994.

References

1. Spradley JP. *Participant observation.* New York, Holt Rinehart and Winston, 1979.

2. Pickering H. Prostitutes and their clients: a Gambian survey. *Social Science and Medicine* 1992, 34: 75–88.

3. Briggs CL. *Learning how to ask. A sociolinguistic appraisal of the role of the interview in social science research.* Cambridge, Cambridge University Press, 1986.

4. Spradley JP. *The ethnographic interview*. New York, Holt Rinehart and Winston, 1979.

5. Nnko S, Pool R. The discourse of sex among primary school pupils in Magu district, Tanzania. *TANESA Working Paper,* no. 3. Mwanza, 1995.

6. Dawson S, Manderson L, Tallo VL. The focus group manual. *Methods for social research in tropical diseases*, no. 1. UNDP/World Bank/WHO, 1992.

7. Morgan DL (ed.). *Successful focus groups. Advancing the state of the art*. London, Sage, 1993.

8. Stewart DW, Shamdasani PN. *Focus groups. Theory and practice*. London, Sage, 1990.

9. Saville-Troike M. *The ethnography of communication*. Oxford, Blackwell, 1982.

10. Pelto PJ, Pelto GH. *Anthropological research. The structure of enquiry*. (2nd edition.) Cambridge, Cambridge University Press, 1978.

11. Pool R, Boerma JT, Maswe M et al. Changes in male sexual behaviour in response to the AIDS epidemic. 2. Validation of reported changes. *TANESA Working Paper,* no. 7. Mwanza, 1995.

12. Nnko S, Wa Shija R, Chiduo B et al. Perceptions of AIDS and risk among primary school pupils in Magu district, Tanzania. *TANESA Internal Report Series,* no. 3. Mwanza, 1995.

13. Standing H. AIDS: Conceptual and Methodological Issues in Researching Sexual behaviour in Sub-Saharan Africa. *Social Science and Medicine* 1992, 34: 475–483.

5 Gender and HIV/AIDS/STDs

Zaida Mgalla, Lilian Wambura and Maria de Bruyn

- What does being a man or woman have to do with the HIV/AIDS epidemic?
- How do sexual 'double standards' affect the spread of HIV/AIDS?
- How is female literacy connected with HIV/AIDS?
- Why does HIV/AIDS cause extra problems for widows?
- Who carries the burden of AIDS-related care?

Why talk about gender? As HIV/AIDS and sexually transmitted diseases (STDs) take a greater hold on communities, it becomes clear that the epidemic affects women and men differently. For this reason, it is important for programmes to incorporate a gender perspective into their work.

What is gender? 'Sex' indicates whether a person is biologically male or female. 'Gender', on the other hand, refers to common, shared ideas and norms in the community concerning women and men, rather than to biological attributes. The ideas are what people think are 'typically' feminine and masculine *characteristics* and *abilities* (for example, intelligence, emotional stability, management capacity, leadership qualities). The norms include expectations about how women and men should *behave* in various situations (for example, as parents, during sexual encounters and in decision-making within relationships). These ideas and expectations are learned from and taught by family members, friends, opinion leaders, religious and cultural institutions, schools, the workplace and the media (1). Gender ideas and norms reflect and influence the roles which women and men take on in daily life as well as their social status, economic and political power. Roles, status and power in their turn affect individuals' risks of infection and communities' abilities to cope with HIV/AIDS and STDs.

We distinguish between 'sex' and 'gender' for an important reason. If people believe that female and male characteristics, abilities and behaviours are based on sex or biology, they will see them as unchangeable or permanent. If they understand that these characteristics, abilities and behaviours are determined socially – by ideas and expectations – they can learn that it is possible to make changes in female and male roles, social status and the distribution of power.

A 'situation analysis' from a gender perspective asks how HIV/AIDS and STDs affect women and men differently and why. A district level situation analysis can be based on a list of questions designed to assess the importance of gender issues for the HIV/AIDS epidemic, concerning demographic, epidemiological, medical, sociocultural and economic issues.

In this chapter we will give examples of questions that should be considered in such an analysis, each followed by descriptions of some of the gender issues that may emerge. These issues need to be addressed in HIV prevention and AIDS care programmes. Questions that may be asked from a health perspective are followed by those related to cultural and socioeconomic aspects. In the conclusion, assessing gender sensitivity is briefly addressed.

Gender-based situation analyses: the health perspective

Are women biologically at greater risk of HIV infection?

Women may be at greater risk of HIV infection than men because of physiological factors. They are more exposed to the virus during sex because of the large mucosal surface in the vagina. Semen (which has a higher concentration of the virus than vaginal fluids) stays in the vagina a relatively long time. In addition, women are more likely to have asymptomatic STDs. More than half of gonorrhoea and chlamydial infections in women, for example, are thought to be asymptomatic. As a consequence, women may have an STD for a long time before receiving treatment. STDs, especially genital ulcer diseases, can facilitate HIV transmission (2): studies in the Mwanza Region of Tanzania have shown the importance of STD control for HIV transmission (see Chapters 13 and 14).

Despite women's greater vulnerability, in most countries HIV prevalence among adult men and women is about the same. The main reason for the lack of difference is probably that, even though women are more likely to become infected during a sexual encounter, men generally have sex more often (more sexual partners and contacts with commercial sex workers) (3).

How common are certain high-risk sexual practices?

In some cultures, women may use herbs or other agents to dry out and tighten the vagina because it is believed that men prefer 'dry sex' or because they think that female vaginal fluids are unclean. The substances used can erode the vaginal mucous membranes and cause inflammation, which may facilitate HIV transmission, although evidence is not conclusive. 'Dry sex' may also refer to the situation where men do not allow women time to become aroused, producing natural vaginal fluids before sex. The practice of dry sex may also reduce willingness to use condoms with lubricants as well as vaginal microbicides, thus increasing the risk of virus transmission for both women and men (4, 5). Heavy rubbing of the genitals ('rough sex') may also cause sores in the mucous membrane.

Anal intercourse is very risky because it may lead to bleeding and lesions, again facilitating entry of the virus. Couples practise anal sex to preserve virginity, prevent pregnancy, increase sexual (male) pleasure or vary their sexual life. Though many people deny practising anal sex, sex workers report that clients request it.

Are women and men infected at equal ages?

Women are generally infected at an earlier age than men, partly because they tend to have sexual contacts with men 5–15 years older. Some reasons for this age difference are discussed in the section 'The cultural perspective' (see below). A relatively simple way to find out whether women in a given area are infected earlier than men is to analyse the ages of male and female hospital admissions (see Box 1).

Box 1. Hospital admission data on age and sex

From August to December 1994, the Bugando Medical Centre in Mwanza, Tanzania, admitted 478 women and 581 men to the medical and tuberculosis wards. The mean age of those admitted was 27.7 years for women and 28.8 years for men. The women diagnosed as having AIDS were on average 29.3 years old, while the men with AIDS averaged 32.6 years.

The difference between the sexes became more pronounced when the ages of those who died in hospital were analysed. Women with AIDS who died were on average 27.8 years and men with AIDS who died averaged 33.8 years. These data suggest that overall the women were about six years younger than the men when infected, if it is assumed that average survival time is the same for both sexes.

Is circumcision practised?

The geographical overlap between areas with high HIV prevalence and those with low levels of male circumcision has stimulated a lively debate about the protective role of circumcision in men. Male circumcision appears to be related to a lower incidence of STDs; it therefore most likely also lessens circumcised men's risk of contracting HIV (6). Male circumcision is no longer strictly limited to specific ethnic groups or religions (see Box 2).

Circumcision in women, on the other hand, may place them at greater risk of infection. The opening to the vagina may be made very small, leading to tearing and bleeding during sexual intercourse. This in turn may lead couples to practise riskier anal sex instead. If extensive bleeding is associated with circumcision – for example, just after the procedure or after delivery of a child, a woman may require a blood transfusion; if HIV testing of blood donors is not yet a routine procedure or a steady supply of HIV tests is unavailable, this may involve contaminated blood. Both women and men run risks if the instruments used to perform circumcisions have been contaminated with blood from an already infected person.

Box 2. Changing circumcision practices

The indigenous population of Mwanza Region in Tanzania is made up of the Sukuma people, who did not traditionally practise male circumcision. Today, however, 32% of the male population aged 15–49 years in the region is circumcised, a development that cannot be explained by immigration alone. It is not uncommon to find circumcised Sukuma men (13% of all rural men, including both Christians and Muslims). Living in a town or even a roadside village apparently increases the chances of being circumcised: 59% of urban men are circumcised, 28% of the men living in roadside villages and 14% of rural men. Also, boys who have attended secondary schools (73%) are more often circumcised than boys with less education.

Does infertility increase risks for women?

A possible consequence of STDs is infertility. In most African societies, great value is placed on parenthood, especially for women, whose status is heavily dependent on their being mothers. When a couple fails to have children, this can lead to marital breakdown. Infertile women may have sex with multiple partners in an effort to become pregnant; this in turn increases their risk of HIV/STD infection. A study in Northwest Tanzania has indicated that infertility may be indirectly associated with HIV infection. Compared to fertile women, infertile women suffered more marital breakups; they also had a markedly higher prevalence of HIV: 6.6% versus 18.2%, respectively (7).

Is the course of the disease different in women and men?

Women living with AIDS generally have the same symptoms as men – with the exception of Kaposi's sarcoma, which is more common in male patients. However, women may suffer additional reproductive health problems such as chronic vaginitis, pelvic inflammatory disease and cervical cancer (8, 9). Fertility is not affected, nor is there evidence that pregnancy hastens the development of AIDS in HIV infected women. However, HIV-positive women may have a higher risk of spontaneous abortions, stillbirths and post-operative complications after caesarean sections (10). Women may also make less use of medical services than men or postpone this until they are more seriously ill; this makes treatment more difficult and expensive.

The cultural perspective

What are the sexual norms and expectations?

Some cultural norms include a double standard which gives men freedom to be more sexually active while restricting female sexuality. This does not mean that only men have multiple sexual partners or that women do not have sexual needs and desires. What it does mean is that different norms are applied to women and men, with men having greater decision-making power regarding sexual and reproductive health matters (see Box 3).

Box 3. Decision-making power and sexual health

If a man with an STD goes for treatment, he may inform his partner and tell her to get treatment as well. Women, however, have no power to force their male partners to be examined and seek treatment. A woman in Tanzania said: 'My husband forced me to take a course of 30 tablets of tetracycline. When I asked him why, he just told me to take the tablets and ask no questions. Later I realized he had infected me with gonorrhoea.'

In many communities, it is more or less taken for granted that men need to have sex regularly (even if unmarried) and that they should be dominant, deciding when, how and with whom they will have sex. On the other hand, women are expected to remain faithful, do what their partners want and not question their partners' behaviour. This does not mean that women have no possibilities for negotiation, but these possibilities are limited, even more so if they are married (11–13).

The result of these expectations regarding male and female behaviour is that the ability to engage in protective behaviours is reduced. Men may feel pressured to 'prove their masculinity' by being dominant and having many sexual partners; they may fear ridicule from their friends if they remain faithful to one woman. Women may feel unable to discuss matters such as faithfulness, condom use and sexual practices with their husbands and boyfriends because they may be accused of unfaithfulness, be beaten or perhaps abandoned.

Due to cultural influences, both women and men may resist women taking a more assertive approach to sex. Men interviewed in Mwanza Region, for example, said they would not tolerate it if their wives refused to have sex with them. However, although women are not expected to take an active role in decisions concerning sex, they *are* held responsible for the consequences. For example, girls who become pregnant usually must leave school, while the boys who fathered the children can continue their education, even though several countries have laws prohibiting dismissal of schoolgirls for reasons of pregnancy. Unwanted pregnancies are another sad consequence of women's limited possibilities to use contraception, such as condoms. Women may use various methods to induce abortion (such as swallowing detergent), endangering their lives (14).

Age differences between sexual partners influence how strongly sexual norms are applied. In most of Africa, men are considerably older than the women they marry. A study in Tanzania showed that the median age at first marriage of men was 25 years, compared to 18 years for women (15). In Kenya, the age difference between spouses was more than ten years for 24% of couples (16), while in Senegal the mean age difference between spouses was 14 years (17).

Age differences between sexual partners are considered one of the driving forces behind the HIV/AIDS epidemic in Africa (18). Younger women have less decision-making power at the household, community and higher levels, including in matters related to sex and protecting themselves against infection. Moreover, it has been observed in various African countries that men increasingly seek younger women for sex because they believe that younger girls will be free from infection. The immaturity of the genital system of young girls puts them at higher risk of contracting HIV than other women and men (19). Also, the sexual history of these men is likely to be longer and they may already be infected themselves.

Two cultural practices that can contribute to the large age gap between spouses – polygamy (having multiple spouses) and payment of bride wealth – may need to be included in a situation analysis.

Is polygamy common?
In many parts of Africa polygamy is still common, although the practice has declined considerably in the last decades. Demographic and health surveys in 17 African countries show that about one-third of married women are co-wives (20). For example, in Tanzania 28% of women are in a polygamous union, in Uganda 34%, in Kenya 23% and in Zambia 18%. In most West African countries, more than one-third of women are co-wives. In Togo this is as high as 52%.

There is no evidence that polygamy in itself is a risk factor for HIV infection. However, the system of polygamy may influence societal norms about sexual relationships. Also, to support multiple wives, men need to marry at a considerably older age than women; this results in a prolonged period during which premarital sexual activities are predominant.

What are the customs concerning bride wealth and bride price?
In many African societies, a man (or his family) must accumulate a considerable amount of wealth (cash, cattle or other assets) before he can marry. Strict respect for the rules of providing bride wealth in times of economic hardship results in delaying marriage until sufficient assets have been obtained (21). In this situation, men have a long period of premarital sexual activity and the age gap between potential spouses may become even wider. However, in some areas (especially urban), the system of bride wealth may be weakening rapidly.

What effect does losing a partner have?
The norms applied to married, single, divorced and widowed women may be different. Many societies in Africa may have less strict rules concerning the sexuality of women who are not married (see Box 4).

Divorce and its consequences may play an indirect role in putting some women at higher risk of HIV/STD infection (22). In societies with matrilineal descent, children belong to the mother's family or clan and property passes from her brother to her son. In the case of divorce, the woman can be assured of some support from her family so she does not have to resort to desperate measures to ensure an income. In societies with patrilineal descent, property passes from the husband to his own relatives and children and divorced women are not able to keep many resources. This may favour marital stability, although women's lack of access to land and other assets may also decrease their motivation to stay in an unsatisfactory marriage. In most of Africa, women remarry fairly quickly after divorce but some may end up in commercial sex work to survive.

Box 4. Norms on female and male sexual behaviour

Research among men and women in Mwanza, Tanzania, showed that the restrictive norms on female sexuality only applied to married women. The double standard did not apply to single women. Men were unanimous in declaring that while they would not tolerate their wives having an extra-marital relationship, it is quite acceptable for non-marital partners to do so. This applies to their casual partners as well as women with whom they have long-term relationships.

The norms regulating widows' re-marriage and sexual behaviour may affect infection risks of both men and women (23). If widow inheritance is practised (as is the case among groups in Kenya, Uganda, Zambia and Zimbabwe, for example), sexual contacts between a recently widowed woman and one of her male in-laws are encouraged. If the woman has become a widow because her husband died of AIDS, she may be HIV-positive and transmit the virus to her in-law. If she is HIV-negative and her in-law already has the virus, he may infect her. It is possible for communities to change the rituals around widow inheritance so that they no longer involve sex. For example, in some communities, the male in-law 'symbolically' inherits the widow (for instance, passing a stick between her legs) and agrees to provide her with support.

Is sexual violence common?
It is now recognized that violence against women and girls is not uncommon. Alcohol abuse may be an important underlying factor for irresponsible and harmful sexual behaviour and violence. When this includes forced sex – incest and rape – the risk of HIV and STD transmission is high because condoms are not used and violence often leads to bleeding and wounds, making passage of viruses more likely. Although most victims of violence are female, some young boys may also be exposed. A study among 122 street children in Mwanza District, Tanzania, for example, showed that one girl and one boy had been infected with syphilis after being raped (24).

Are women more likely to be blamed and rejected?
The idea that people living with HIV/AIDS are 'immoral' – as well as unwarranted fears of casual infection (for example, through sharing eating utensils) – leads to stigmatization and discrimination directed at both infected women and men. Women, however, are more often blamed for spreading HIV/STDs than men. For example, men are warned to stay away from sex workers because they may be infected, but little is said about the chance that men may infect sex workers or their own regular partners. Among married couples, HIV infection is often first discovered in the woman, for example during

antenatal testing, and she is then accused of bringing AIDS into the family. Women are more often rejected and abandoned by their spouses and in-laws than vice versa.

The socioeconomic perspective

Do women and men have equal levels of education?
Educational level is an important indicator of social status and economic opportunities. Educated people are generally more able to obtain information and to translate it into action. For instance, a mother's educational level is one of the most important factors affecting her children's survival chances.

In general, women receive less schooling than men. This is not because they are less intelligent but because many families prefer to spend what money they have on the education of male children. Some households rely on female children's labour for agricultural and domestic tasks, even when financial support for their schooling could be made available. In addition, boys are expected to take over family responsibilities in the future, such as supporting their old parents. Girls are expected to marry, leave their parents and care for their husbands' children and their in-laws.

As a result, throughout Africa there are more illiterate women than men and fewer women with an education beyond primary school. For example, in Malawi 21% of adult men are illiterate compared to 47% of women. Only 4% of women have more than a primary level education while 14% of men have a secondary education or more. In Tanzania, 33% of women are illiterate and 5% have a secondary education or more; among men 20% are illiterate and 9% have a secondary or higher education.

Are economic opportunities the same for women and men?
Women's lower educational levels mean that they do not have as much access to well-paying or other jobs as men and are economically dependent on them. Women who are economically and socially dependent on men are in a poor position to insist on a larger share of household resources being allocated for their own and their children's needs and health. They also have less power to insist on their own wishes and rights, even with regard to protecting themselves against HIV/STDs.

When a spouse dies, women may be at a great disadvantage, partly for cultural and legal reasons. Among many tribes, male members of the deceased husband's family inherit the couple's property. Widows and children may suddenly find that their resources must be shared with male members of their clan; at worst, they may be harassed by in-laws who take their property and even evict them from their houses, thus making it very difficult to survive. Some women may even lose their children to their in-laws (see Box 5).

Box 5. Inheritance and widows

'I am not on good terms with my brothers-in-law. They took all properties left by my late husband, including my own. They took our big house and have put tenants in it for their own benefit. They allocated only one room for me and my five children. They did all this to me but they never contributed even a single shilling to build that house.'
woman in Ukerewe, Tanzania

Another very vivid testimony is the story of a widow shown in the video *Neria*, which was filmed in Zimbabwe. When Neria's husband dies, her brother-in-law helps himself to their car, bank book, furniture and house. He claims that tradition and law are on his side. When he then takes her children as well, Neria seeks justice, learning that law and tradition can also be on her side if she intelligently fights for her rights (see also 'Further reading and resources' at the end of this chapter).

When women – as well as street children of both sexes – find themselves in economic hardship, they may supplement their income by trading sex for money or goods. In this way they gain access to resources under male control. As one woman in Magu District, Tanzania, commented: 'I preferred to be a bar worker as the work does not require any special qualifications that would be needed for me to get the job.' Although unequal access to resources is a key reason for commercial sex, women also become sex workers for other reasons. For example, a study among sex workers in the Gambia showed that they also chose this type of work to avoid dull domestic jobs and the long hours required to run an informal business (25).

In many communities both women and men believe that women should receive something in return for granting sex to their partners (see Box 6). Female traders may do so to get (more or better) supplies while secondary school students exchange sexual favours for items such as pens or money for school fees. University students might also use this strategy; law lecturers at the University of Zambia gave extra marks to female students who slept with them (26).

Are there differences between men and women concerning coping and care?
Although 'women's work' often is not seen as having an economic value, women have heavy domestic workloads. One study in Rungwe, Tanzania, showed that on average women work ten hours daily, against only four hours for men (28). Women's work is spread out from morning to night and involves hard labour such as farming, cutting firewood, collecting water, picking vegetables and cooking several meals.

Box 6. Sex and material transactions

Boy: 'The girl's first interest is money. So if you fail to give her money then she will definitely be dissatisfied and unwilling.'
Boy: 'The girl does not only expect money from the schoolboy. She may need exercise books, so you tell her you will buy her books; she will need school fees and you may pay for her, but she may be afraid that her parents will ask her where she got the money. If it is pens then you may give them to her.'
Girl: 'She may accept him and be given money later.' (12)

Unemployed 18-year-old girl in Ghana: 'I entered into a sexual relationship because when I was 16 years old my mother refused to buy pants and other things for me. Whenever I asked her she would say: 'You're old enough; don't be asking me for such things.' So I took a partner who will be willing to provide these things.' (27)

Are there differences between men and women concerning coping and care?
Although 'women's work' often is not seen as having an economic value, women have heavy domestic workloads. One study in Rungwe, Tanzania, showed that on average women work ten hours daily, against only four hours for men (28). Women's work is spread out from morning to night and involves hard labour such as farming, cutting firewood, collecting water, picking vegetables and cooking several meals.

For such busy women, getting medical check-ups or attending antenatal clinics is not a priority; they may not see a health practitioner until they are seriously ill, so that treatment is delayed and perhaps more difficult and expensive in the end. For example, a coping study by the Bugando Medical Centre in Mwanza, Tanzania, found that both HIV-negative and HIV-positive women report far fewer symptoms than men.

Most people expect women to care for ill family members and older relatives, even if they are sick themselves. Men are not asked and usually do not volunteer to carry out household work, care for children or nurse the sick. When a household is affected by HIV/AIDS, the major portion of the caring burden therefore falls on women's shoulders. Because of women's care-provider role, they are also affected more by mother-to-child transmission of HIV. Besides the distress of seeing children suffer from opportunistic infections and dying quite young, HIV-positive women additionally must often care for very ill infants while they are ill themselves.

Do women and men have equal access to information?
Providing information alone is not sufficient to motivate people to change risk behaviours. Nonetheless, people need knowledge about the body, HIV/STD transmission and disease prevention to be able to change behaviour effectively. Many people have inadequate knowledge about reproductive biology and they may have mistaken ideas about biological processes. For example, one schoolboy who participated in discussions about adolescent sex in Magu District, Tanzania, remarked: 'It is not easy to

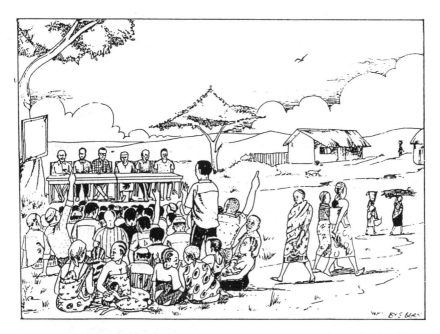

Gender and community action: a community meeting with men alone at the 'high table'. Women are barely participating; they lose interest and resume carrying out their many tasks.

make a girl pregnant because our seed is not ripe enough.'

Although some printed information is available, women often have less access to it than men, either because of lower literacy skills or insufficient time and opportunity to acquire it. Men also generally have greater access to information provided by radio and television. This problem could be overcome to some extent with good communication between sexual partners and between parents and children. However, discussion about sexual and reproductive health matters is often considered inappropriate or embarrassing. Men in Kenya who wanted to negotiate a monogamous relationship due to fear of HIV/AIDS, for example, found it difficult to discuss this with their wives because they had no experience with such dialogue (13).

Reluctance to talk about sexuality may also mean that teachers and health workers asked to provide information feel uncomfortable with this task. This especially decreases women's and girls' opportunities to obtain information.

Conclusion: assessing gender sensitivity

Gender sensitivity can be incorporated into all aspects of a district programme. Using questions like those discussed in this chapter in a situation analysis can help show differences in the epidemic's effects on women and men. Box 7 shows examples of factors which may place women and men at extra risk of HIV infection. The same type of analysis can be made regarding coping and care.

uations requiring blood transfusions, possibly with
ᴜᴜ blood (due to anaemia and complications related to pregnancy).
ᴍale–female transmission occurs more easily.
- Young women are less physically mature and older women's vaginal mucosa thin out; in both cases there is less of a barrier to entry of the virus.
- STDs in women are often less evident (the first symptoms are internal) so they receive treatment later; also, women may resist getting treated for fear of stigmatization.
- Self-treatments for vaginal complaints and to prepare for 'dry sex' can increase risk.
- The need for extra income can lead to unprotected sex with multiple partners.
- Women generally have less power than men in negotiating sexual relationships.
- There is a low availability of female-controlled barrier methods (microbicides, female condoms).

MEN
- Work may take men away from their regular partners for very long periods.
- Men are often influenced by societal beliefs which dictate that they must have sex regularly to avoid illness or impotency.
- Peer pressure (and/or sometimes parental pressure) encourages men and boys to engage in casual sex.
- Men are unfamiliar with and may therefore dislike condom use.
- Cultural customs encourage heavy drinking, which may cause men to forget their intentions to practise safer sex or stay faithful.
- Current gender roles prevent or discourage men from sharing decision-making about sex with their female partners.
- Social condemnation of homosexuality leads some men to have secret homosexual relationships but, at the same time, to marry due to social pressure.

A comprehensive HIV/STD prevention and AIDS care programme must consider gender issues in planning, implementation, monitoring and evaluation. A situation analysis should be conducted to raise awareness and analyse gender issues with policy-makers and implementing staff in the district. This could, for example, be done in workshops, using the type of questions outlined in this chapter.

When a gender perspective is integrated into a programme, ideas and norms concerning women and men as well as their actual roles, status and power are taken into account. Interventions are then based on this analysis; this helps to assure that risks of infection are reduced for women as well as men. In addition, both female and male community members can be encouraged to provide care and support. A checklist can serve as a useful starting point for programme staff, to assess their own sensitivity, plan a programme or assess how effectively implementation is being carried out (see Box 8).

Box 8. Checklist on gender sensitivity

	Yes	Some-what	No
Are women's groups involved in policy and programme development and decision-making?	❏	❏	❏
Do women and men share programme goals?	❏	❏	❏
Do you organize activities at locations and times convenient for both women and men?	❏	❏	❏
Do your programmes consider differences in access to resources and decision-making that affect both women's and men's abilities to protect themselves?	❏	❏	❏
Do you create situations in which women and men can talk freely about their opinions, feelings and needs?	❏	❏	❏
Do your prevention programmes:	❏	❏	❏
— challenge double standards regarding a) teenage sexuality, b) casual sex, and c) sex outside marriage?	❏	❏	❏
— address sexual abuse and violence?	❏	❏	❏
— address difficulties in condom use from both women's and men's perspectives?	❏	❏	❏
— teach both women and men how to use condoms?	❏	❏	❏
— promote easy access to condoms for women and men?	❏	❏	❏
Do your programmes explore and use the most appropriate information channels for different age and gender groups?	❏	❏	❏
Do your programmes call for gender-based sexual health education in school curricula?	❏	❏	❏
Do your programmes encourage couples, parents and/or children to discuss sexual health?	❏	❏	❏
Do your programmes address the need to motivate men to inform their wives if they are HIV-positive?	❏	❏	❏
Do your services:	❏	❏	❏
— ensure equal access by men and women, particularly for STD treatment?	❏	❏	❏
— make family planning services attractive and accessible to men?	❏	❏	❏
Do your programmes:	❏	❏	❏
— address inheritance laws and customs where these put women and children at a disadvantage?	❏	❏	❏
— ensure that girls' care roles and lack of money do not exclude them from school	❏	❏	❏
— encourage men to take on greater care roles in the family	❏	❏	❏

Further reading and resources

AIDS/STD Health Promotion Exchange issue no. 3 on 'Gender, sexual health and reproductive health promotion'. Amsterdam, Royal Tropical Institute, 1995.

AIDS Health Promotion Exchange issue no. 3 on 'Why women and HIV? It takes two to tango, safely'. Amsterdam, Royal Tropical Institute, 1992.

AIDS Health Promotion Exchange issue no. 4 on 'Men's responsibility and partnership in the prevention of AIDS'. Amsterdam, Royal Tropical Institute, 1991.

Facing the challenges of HIV/AIDS/STDs: a gender-based response. This is a resource pack including background information, educational tools and resources for training. It contains a set of eight activity cards with training guidelines to stimulate consideration of and discussion on gender issues. Published by the Royal Tropical Institute (KIT), P.O. Box 95001, 1090 HA Amsterdam, The Netherlands; Southern Africa AIDS Information Dissemination Service (SAfAIDS), 17 Beveridge Road, P.O. Box A509, Avondale, Harare, Zimbabwe; and World Health Organization, AIDS/HIV and STD Unit, 1211 Geneva 27, Switzerland (free of charge).

Neria, a full-length (103 minutes) feature film from Zimbabwe, tells the story of a woman's empowerment as she recognizes her rights following her husband's death. It is available in English, KiSwahili and Portuguese versions, both as a VHS PAL video and 35-mm film; the Portuguese version is also available as a 16-mm film. Cost is US$ 59; for further information contact: Development through Self-Reliance Inc., 9111 Guilford Road, Columbia, MD 21046, USA; or Media for Development Trust, P.O. Box 6755, Harare, Zimbabwe.

Reid E, Bailey M. Young women: silence, susceptibility and the HIV epidemic. *Issues Paper,* no. 12, New York, UNDP, 1993.

References

1. De Bruyn M et al. *Facing the challenges of HIV/AIDS/STDs: a gender-based response.* Amsterdam, KIT/SAfAIDS/WHO, 1995.

2. WHO/GPA. *Magnitude of sexually transmitted diseases worldwide.* Geneva, WHO/GPA, 1995.

3. Caldwell JC. Understanding the AIDS epidemic and reacting sensibly to it. *Social Science and Medicine,* 1995, 41: 299–302.

4. Dallabetta GA et al. Traditional vaginal agents: use and association with HIV infection in Malawian women. *AIDS,* 1995, 9/3: 293–297.

5. Sandala L et al. 'Dry sex' and HIV infection among women attending a sexually transmitted diseases clinic in Lusaka, Zambia. *AIDS,* 1995, 9(Suppl. 1): S61–S68.

6. Caldwell JC. Lack of male circumcision and AIDS in sub-Saharan Africa: resolving the conflict. *Health Transition Review,* 1995, 5: 113–117.

7. Favot I, Ngalula J, Gumodoka B et al. Female infertility as a risk factor for HIV infection: evidence from a hospital-based study in Tanzania. *TANESA Working Paper,* no. 5. Mwanza.

8. Shaker IL. AIDS in women continues to increase – may pass men within the decade. *Searchlight*, May/June 1993: 6–7.

9. Verkuyl DAA. Practising obstetrics and gynaecology in areas with a high prevalence of HIV infection. *Lancet*, 1995, 346: 293–296.

10. Semprini AE et al. The incidence of complications after caesarean section in 156 HIV-positive women. *AIDS*, 1995, 9: 913–917.

11. Strebel A. 'There's absolutely nothing I can do, just believe in God': South African women with AIDS. *Agenda*, 1992, 12: 50–62.

12. Nnko S, Pool R. School pupils and the discourse of sex in Magu District, Tanzania. *TANESA Working Paper*, no. 3. Mwanza, 1995.

13. Balmer DH et al. The negotiating strategies determining coitus in stable hetero-sexual relationships. *Health Transition Review*, 1995, 5: 85–95.

14. Klepp KI et al. AIDS and its consequences for families, health care and education in Arusha and Kilimanjaro, Tanzania. *Forum for Development Studies*, 1993, 1: 63–73.

15. Ngallaba SAM, Kapiga SH, Ruyobya I et al. *Tanzania Demographic and Health Survey 1991/92*. Bureau of Statistics, Dar es Salaam and Macro International Inc., Maryland, USA, 1993.

16. NCPD. *Kenya Demographic and Health Survey 1993*. National Council for Population and Development and Central Bureau Statistics, Dar es Salaam and Macro International Inc., Maryland, USA, 1994.

17. Ndiaye S, Diouf PD, Ayad M. *Enquête demographique et de santé au Sénégal (EDS II) 1992/93*. Ministry of Economics, Finance and Planning and Macro International Inc., Maryland, USA, 1994.

18. Garnett GP, Anderson RM. Factors controlling the spread of HIV in heterosexual communities in developing countries: patterns of mixing between different age and sexual activity classes. *Philosophical Transaction of the Royal Society of London. Series B*, 1993, 342: 137–159.

19. Reid E, Bailey M. Young women: silence, susceptibility and the HIV epidemic. *Issues Paper*, no. 12, New York, UNDP, 1993.

20. Westoff C, Blanc AK, Nyblade L. Marriage and entry into parenthood. *DHS Comparative Studies*, no. 10. Macro International Inc., Calverton, Maryland, USA, 1994.

21. Larson A. Social context of HIV transmission in Africa: historical and cultural bases of East and Central African sexual relations. *Rev. Inf. Dis.*, 1989, 11: 716–731.

22. Carael M. The impact of marriage on the risk of exposure to sexually transmitted diseases in Africa. In: Bledsoe C and Pison G (eds.). *Nuptiality in sub-Saharan Africa*. Oxford, Clarendon Press, 1994, pp. 255–273.

23. Palloni A, Lee YJ. Families, women and HIV/AIDS in Africa. CDE Working Paper 90–32. Madison, University of Wisconsin-Madison, 1990.

24. Rajani R, Kudrati M. *Streetchildren of Mwanza. A situation analysis*. Kuleana in association with UNICEF-Tanzania, Mwanza, 1994.

25. Pickering H, Wilkins HA. Do unmarried women in African towns have to sell sex, or is it a matter of choice? *Health Transition Review,* 1993, 3 (Suppl.): 17–28.

26. Kunda A. We've gone sex crazy. *New African* 1995, 327: 21.

27. Ankomah A, Ford N. Sexual exchange: understanding pre-marital heterosexual relationships in urban Ghana. In: P. Aggleton et al. *AIDS: foundations for the future*, London, Taylor & Francis, 1994, pp. 123–135.

28. Mbilinyi. Women's initiatives in the United Republic of Tanzania. A case study on co-operative organisations in Isange village of Rungwe District, Tanzania. (Unpublished report), 1987.

6 Monitoring and evaluation

Awene Gavyole, Ties Boerma and Dick Schapink

- Can communities evaluate their own programmes?
- Is reduction of HIV incidence a feasible success indicator?
- What are the differences between output and impact indicators?
- Can the stigma associated with AIDS be measured?
- What are the steps in setting up a monitoring system?

Monitoring and evaluation of HIV prevention and AIDS care programmes provide a way to see if programmes are achieving what is intended. Both monitoring and evaluation need to be planned into a programme from its beginning.

Programme *monitoring* follows the progress of ongoing activities with respect to achievement of objectives; this can be done by using indicators designed for the purpose. Are the planned activities being implemented according to the objectives and schedule? What is actually happening? The aim of monitoring is to identify problems early and suggest the action necessary for improvements in the implementation of the programme.

Evaluation can be considered both a learning tool and an action-oriented management tool. It is a process intended to determine, as systematically and objectively as possible, the relevance, effectiveness and impact of activities, seen in the light of their objectives. Is the planned approach achieving the stated objectives? Who has benefitted and how much? Evaluations are done at specific points in the lifecycle of a programme; they can improve both current activities and future planning, programming and decision making (1, 2).

Monitoring and evaluation is often a weak programme component, and AIDS programmes are no exception. Recording and reporting may be irregular and incomplete because staff have not been trained. If the purpose of the data collection is not clear and feedback is never given, staff may not be motivated to complete the arduous daily task of filling in forms. Inappropriate indicators and unmeasurable objectives may have been chosen. The role of monitoring and evaluation in the planning and implementation cycle may be obscure. Some examples of problems encountered in monitoring interventions within a truck stop project are shown in Box 1.

Box 1. Problems in project monitoring and evaluation

A fairly sophisticated monitoring and evaluation system was designed for a truck stop AIDS intervention project in Tanzania (see Chapter 8). Peer educators were supposed to collect, record and report information on truck drivers, other travellers and condom use. Two forms had to be completed on a monthly basis: one about distribution of health education materials and one to report activities. This information was gathered by project staff, who entered the data in the computer, analysed the data and gave feedback to the peer educators. Also, a diskette was sent to the national project coordination unit in Dar es Salaam with all data.

There were multiple constraints. The peer educators' reports were irregular and incomplete, and some did not understand the coding system. The field staff of the project had problems with the computers and neither used the data nor gave appropriate feedback to the peer educators. The national coordination unit received fewer diskettes than anticipated, had operational difficulties in making summaries and gave no feedback to field staff.

Evaluation of the situation made clear that the system was too complicated in relation to the inputs (training and supervision, qualified staff and computers) available to run a system with such elaborate data collection, analysis and feedback systems. Unless a major commitment can be made to monitoring and evaluation, the system needs be simple and limited in scope.

What needs to be monitored?

In planning, monitoring and evaluating programmes, baseline data on the spread of the HIV/AIDS epidemic are needed. This is a new disease, with an insidious and potentially devastating impact on health, social life and economy. We need to know how the virus spreads in the district, what the level and trends are in HIV prevalence, and what kinds of consequences need to be anticipated. However, monitoring these aspects of the epidemic appears to be beyond the resources of most districts. AIDS cases in the health facilities can be monitored, but since the incubation period of HIV is very long this does not provide up-to-date information. Estimates about its spread will therefore be necessary, based on inferences from regional or even national data.

Districts have launched (or will launch) interventions focused on reducing HIV transmission by various modes. Most important are HIV/AIDS educational activities (in schools, communities, high-transmission areas and so forth) intended to lead to behavioural change, including condom use. Other interventions include prevention of transmission through blood transfusion and injection and sterilization practices and those related to AIDS care. All of these call for monitoring and evaluation, which in this case must be carried out at district level.

Basic steps in a monitoring and evaluation system

Monitoring and evaluation should be an integral part of an AIDS programme. The design of a monitoring and evaluation system for an AIDS programme can be seen schematically as a number of successive steps (3, 4).

1 *Baseline data:* baseline data indicate the starting point – what the situation was before the programme began. Good baseline data thus provide a foundation for a credible monitoring and evaluation system, as well as giving a basis for planning. This data may come from a review of existing data (not necessarily limited to the district itself), a base-line survey and a participatory community needs assessment, focused on AIDS know--ledge and attitudes and sexual practices in the community. For example, in preparation for a monitoring system in relation to activities in schools, a survey might be conducted among school children, parents and teachers to assess knowledge, attitude, practices and risk perception in relation to sexual behaviour and STD/AIDS. Both questionnaires and qualitative methods can be used.

2 *Determine objectives:* as mentioned in Chapter 1, both overall objectives (related to the programme as a whole) and specific objectives related to activities should be considered. Objectives related to activities should be measurable; otherwise they will not provide a guide for monitoring and evaluation. Objectives should also be limited in scope, so that they can be reached within the stated time period. The overall objective of a school AIDS programme might be to increase knowledge and improve attitudes and risk perception among school children. The specific objectives of a particular activity might relate to improvement in the accuracy of their knowledge. A more ambitious objective would be to change sexual behaviour among school children. In this case, specific objectives might include a decrease in the self-reported number of sexual partners, postponement of first sexual intercourse, increased condom use, or a reduction in school-girl pregnancies.

3 *List activities and their relationship to overall strategy, and the tasks they will require:* for each of the objectives, activities to be carried out – and the strategies that will be used in doing so, as discussed in Chapter 1 – should be considered. For example, one strategy might be to focus on the use of peer educators. In setting up peer educator activities among school children, among the tasks involved will be selection, training and regular support for the peer educators.

4 *Select indicators and set targets:* for each of the objectives associated with an activity, 'indicators' (discussed further below) and targets are needed. Targets are quite literally something to aim at – what you expect to happen with respect to the activity. The

indicators provide a way of seeing how implementation and achievement are proceeding – is the activity on the way to the target or objective? – and eventually to show the extent to which an objective has been achieved. They should be realistic and practical. For a school programme, changes in the level of knowledge of AIDS prevention among pupils, the number of trained and active peer educators, and the number of schoolgirl pregnancies per year are examples of such indicators. Numerical targets can also be set, e.g. the target might be 'our target is to see that 100% of pupils in the highest three classes of the primary school know that HIV can be transmitted by sexual intercourse', or 'one year from now, we will have one trained and active peer educator for every 20 pupils'.

5 *Collect data:* costs and resources need to be taken into account in designing a monitoring and evaluation component. Indicators that focus on programme input and output are the least expensive to monitor; if it is necessary to cover indicators of programme effects (or, even more, impact), monitoring will be far more expensive (see below). There are many ways to collect data: a small survey may be needed to assess knowledge levels of pupils; assessing a supervision system of peer educators will require continuous assessment of the number of active peer educators; and to know the number of school-girl pregnancies, a reporting system can be set up. Qualitative information is also very important. For example, a few interviews with peer educators can produce a summary of the problems they meet in their work, and suggest *why* problems are occuring – e.g. the reasons behind a high drop-out rate.

6 *Analyse data:* regardless of whether quantitative or qualitative data are involved, data analysis often takes more time than anticipated. Analysis and report writing for even a small survey or perhaps five focus group discussions may take a few weeks. However, a successful monitoring system – one that serves to improve implementation – requires results on a regular basis. Thus programmes need to be designed so that collecting, analysing and giving feedback is built into the targets and procedures, and real efforts should be made to see that this becomes routine.

7 *Take action:* as the programme develops, monitoring and evaluation will suggest areas where improvement is needed. Sometimes a set of recommendations will be immediately apparent, and can be implemented to improve programme performance. They might be included in the routine feedback after the evaluation. On the other hand, this may provide a good opportunity to discuss the problem with those concerned and get them involved in working out their own solution. This participatory approach with staff makes monitoring and evaluation a positive experience, and is often the best way to assure motivation and implementation.

Indicators

Various levels of indicators – measures that help to assess the situation – can be distinguished.

Input	human resources used in carrying out an activity, such as staff labour and efforts; knowledge and skills put into the programme, e.g. administrative, medical, communications; equipment and materials such as facilities, medical supplies, gloves; condoms; and direct funding.
Output	products or coverage of activities, such as number of training sessions held, number of health staff trained in counselling, number of people reached by campaigns, number of adult STD patients treated using the syndromic approach, number of HIV tests performed, and so forth. Output indicators become more meaningful if an attempt is made to estimate coverage. For instance, reporting that 75% of the 400 total health workers in the district have attended a one week training course on counselling gives more information than just mentioning that 300 health workers have been trained. Furthermore, the quality of the output needs to be taken into account, if possible.
Process	Another area in which indicators are needed relates to *process* – the way the programme implements its activities in interaction with the target population and the extent of their involvement. Indicators generally require the collection of qualitative information on how activities are run, including participants' impressions on topics such as the extent of involvement of the community in a workshop, the relevance of workshop activities, the amount of resources (including time and labour) generated by the community, and/or the number of villages requesting assistance from the programme.
Effect	changes in awareness, knowledge, attitudes, behaviours (or reported behaviours) related to HIV/STD risks, preventive measures, condom use, medical care and/or counselling.
Impact	impact of activities on changes in the health status of a target population; for example, reduction in HIV/STD incidence and prevalence, or alleviation of the consequences of AIDS-associated morbidity and mortality at individual, family and community levels. However, in most cases it is not appropriate to choose the number of new HIV infections as an indicator of programme success, since measuring incidence is very difficult and costly. It is also not realistic to aim for a reduction in prevalence – even if programme interventions are successful and incidence decreases, it will takes a long time for HIV prevalence to decline (see Chapter 3 on Epidemiological methods).

Generally, as we move from programme inputs to impact in the list above, the measurement of indicators becomes more difficult and more costly. In some cases, a proxy indicator (that is, a related measure that is easier to obtain and can be expected to give an idea of changes in the more complicated indicator) can be used as an indirect measure of the topic of interest. For example, condom distribution and condom demand are easier to monitor than actual condom use. Prevalence or incidence of STDs that produce immediate symptoms (such as urethritis in men) can be used as a proxy for the occurrence of unprotected sexual intercourse with infected partners.

A set of ten indicators primarily intended for monitoring AIDS programmes at the national level have been developed by the Global Programme on AIDS of the World Health Organization (5, 6). One indicator refers to knowledge of preventive practices, two to condom availability, two to self-reported sexual behaviour, two to STD case management, and three to STD/HIV prevalence or incidence. These indicators need to be collected in a population-based survey or to be based on health facility data.

Who is involved in monitoring and evaluation?

At district level, the measurement of progress within an AIDS programme is the responsibility of staff involved in the implementation of the programme. This includes the district medical officer, AIDS programme coordinator, members of the district health management team, and staff of other sectors such as education and community development. As Box 1 makes clear, however, if monitoring and evaluation are to be effective, staff need to be trained and motivated. The reason for filling in forms must be clear and feedback must be given.

If external funding is obtained for AIDS-related activities, an external evaluation may be requested by the donor. Such evaluations are carried out by experts to satisfy standard requirements. Such evaluations are costly and should not be done frequently. More commonly, a small number of external evaluators is requested to work with a team of staff, community representatives and affiliated NGO members.

Participatory monitoring and evaluation in the community

Monitoring and evaluation can also be done cooperatively by the programme staff and the communities involved in programme activities (the target groups). Such efforts are called participatory monitoring and evaluation. They are planned and conducted by the programme staff and the target groups, working together (see Box 2). The process of involvement in monitoring or in an evaluation may be an eye-opener to all participants.

A participatory monitoring and/or evaluation system can be used to assess inputs, outputs and some effects of community level interventions. One of the most important aspects of such a system, however, is the opportunity it offers to use the process of monitoring and evaluation to generate and sustain a sense of ownership and commitment to the programme in the community. This can increase understanding between the community and the staff, and helps to ensure that the recommendations resulting from the evaluation will be implemented afterwards. With a minimal level of external facilitation, activities are planned by the target group, monitoring and evaluation questions are chosen with the target group, data are collected and analysed by the community, and recommendations for planning and implementation are drawn up by the community. However, such endeavours are not automatically problem-free. An example of a process-oriented monitoring system and the difficulties encountered during its implementation is presented in Box 3.

Box 2. A participatory evaluation with female bar workers

A participatory evaluation of a mobile STD clinic for bar workers was carried out in a peri-urban area of Mwanza, Tanzania. In addition to providing information about the mobile STD clinic, the evaluation had a process goal: to strengthen the sense of owner-ship of the programme by the target group, the female bar workers. A team including two project staff and four peer educators (representing the bar workers) was selected. They developed two questionnaires: one covered bar workers' views of the mobile clinic and the use of condoms. The other was related to the sexual practices of the bar workers, and was intended to assess the appropriateness of the interventions. The first questionnaire was developed by the project, the second by the six-member evaluation team.

In total, 47 bar workers were interviewed by their peers. Every second day, project staff and peer educators met to discuss problems and analyse the answers given by the respondents. The field work took one week. The final analysis was done by the facilitators, and included an analysis of the records of the mobile clinic. Conclusions were discussed with the full evaluation team, and subsequently with the whole team of peer educators (10). The information collected was used to develop new messages for health education and to improve utilization of the STD clinic.

One of the most interesting evaluation findings concerned sexual practices. For example, while it is generally difficult to obtain information on anal or oral intercourse, it appeared that the bar workers were much more open about these issues during interviews with their peers than with outsiders. This led to the development of new health education messages for bar workers and their sexual partners. In addition, the data on attitudes towards the mobile clinic, its staff and services, were sufficient to allow planning for changes in the operation of the mobile clinic.

What can be done at district level?

There are apt to be existing data sources districts can put to use; also, low-cost methods can be employed to gather data that can be used to monitor the input, output and effects of interventions. These three levels offer the most practical and effective indicators for use by districts. Some examples follow.

Input
- amount of resources received from central or regional governmental levels for AIDS control or STD control activities per year;
- amount of resources generated locally for AIDS and STD control activities;
- number of trained supervisors; availability of checklists, vehicles and field allowances;
- number of staff committed to HIV prevention and AIDS care activities;

Box 3. Participatory monitoring system

Igombe is a bustling fishing village along the southern shores of Lake Victoria in Mwanza District, Tanzania. A group of young unemployed women were trained to be peer educators as part of a broad community HIV/STD education programme. To develop monitoring indicators that could be used by the peer educators and by the programme, a three-day workshop was held with seven peer educators and two facilitators. The first half of the workshop was used to explain the goals of monitoring and to discuss behavioural change. The group then developed five indicators: observed sexual behavioural change (decreases in rate of partner change of peers), friends and relatives; self-reported behavioural change; demand for condoms; prevalence of STDs (discharge, ulcers); changes in number of young women in stable relationships. Unemployment, poverty, alcohol abuse and rape were also considered important contributing factors to the spread of AIDS, but were not chosen as indicators. The peer educators agreed to have monthly meetings to discuss their work; project staff met once every three months with the peer educators.

Six months later a brief evaluation was carried out. One peer educator had moved and one was ill with AIDS. Among the five remaining women three had been active and were able to report that they themselves had changed to a single partner, and several other women in the target group had changed as well. Notably, they mentioned that hasty sex outside bars was less common now. The other two peer educators said they too had changed but the others did not agree. Monitoring of activities was weak and records were not kept well. The peer educators said they needed more training and support to keep written records of their activities. This evaluation highlights the specific difficulties that are encountered in attempting to set up a participatory monitoring and evaluation system with groups such as young women involved in commercial sex. Their educational levels are generally low and their lives are very busy, filled with attempts to solve their own and sometimes their family's (parents, siblings, children) problems. In this context, peer educators expected the project to make the largest contribution to the monitoring of activities, rather than doing this themselves. Perhaps in these circumstances it is more feasible to aim at maximum community participation at the stage of indicator development, while the project or district staff have a more prominent role during data collection and analysis, including more frequent supervisory visits.

- number of times AIDS has been on district meeting agendas (e.g. of the district health management team or district PHC committee);
- number of condoms received in the district per calendar year.

Output
- number of training sessions held; number and type of participants; types of sessions on e.g. HIV prevention education, counselling, coping with AIDS;
- number of campaigns held and number of people reached by the campaigns;

- number of supervisory visits/trips made to health facilities;
- number of condoms distributed to bars and guesthouses, and to health facilities;
- number and per cent of establishments with condoms available throughout the year;
- per cent of schools with AIDS education programmes;
- per cent of villages with AIDS action committees;
- number of trained and active counsellors in the district;
- number of people counselled on HIV status;
- number of HIV tests done;
- per cent of clinics using syndromic approach to treat STDs;
- per cent of clinics with safe injection and sterilization practices;
- per cent of clinics and maternities with adequate supply of gloves;
- number of blood transfusions given and per cent screened for HIV, syphilis and hepatitis B.

Process
- amount of resources committed to the programme by district authorities;
- number of communities actively participating in and contributing to the programme.

Effect
- per cent of adults (15-49) knowing sexual transmission route of AIDS;
- per cent of adults knowing that a healthy person can carry HIV for at least five years;
- per cent of adults who say they have changed their sexual behaviour since they have heard of AIDS (e.g. have one sexual partner now, or fewer sexual partners nowadays);
- per cent of adults who consider condoms as an acceptable method of STD/HIV prevention.

The best indicators of programme effects would be changes in sexual behaviour – such as a decrease in the number of partners and increased use of condoms in high-risk encounters. Unfortunately, people's reporting of their own sexual behaviour is already subject to many biases; it is difficult to find out about the actual behaviour. People tend to report that they have changed, perhaps because they would like to change or because they think this is what the interviewer wants to hear (Box 4). In particular, if the interventions being implemented by the programme are sending out messages about the desirability of behavioural change, the answers to such questions may even become more remote from true behaviour.

Impact
- number of schoolgirl pregnancies;
- per cent of adults reporting an STD (e.g. genital ulcer or genital discharge) in the past two years;
- number of STD cases seen at health clinics.

Occasionally it will also be possible to assess impact, but this is less frequent.

A decrease in the number of school-girl pregnancies is an indicator of impact of the programme for which data may be relatively easy to get. Here too, though, a concerted effort will be needed to obtain complete and accurate data. Many girls may resort to abortion to terminate their pregnancies in an early stage; these may easily be missed in the statistics.

Both self-reported data on STDs and the number of STD cases seen at health facilities may rise as an HIV/STD programme begins, because of increased awareness of STDs and the need to go in for treatment. Such data should therefore be interpreted with caution.

Box 4. Behavioural change: real or reporting bias?

In a survey of four fishing villages in northwest Tanzania, 85% of adults aged 15–44 years reported they had changed their sexual behaviour since they heard about AIDS (7). Most said they had reduced the number of their sexual partners, and some said they were now using condoms. This was remarkable, since no interventions had been launched in the villages. Also, the prevalence of STDs was very high in these fishing villages. For instance, 20% reported having had a genital ulcer in the past year and 15% showed serological evidence of active syphilis. Other qualitative data from the same villages also indicated that changes had not taken place, or if at all, only on a very modest scale. The most likely explanation for the discrepancy is that people over-reported changes in their own sexual behaviour: perhaps change is now considered desirable by adult men and women, but few have been able to do this. Moreover, survey respondents often tend to report what they think interviewers would like to hear.

Attitudes to persons with HIV/AIDS are important. As the epidemic becomes more evident to the general population – because friends, family and peers are dying – attitudes may change over time. A less negative attitude and decrease in the stigma associated with AIDS could make behavioural change easier (see also Chapter 18). Although little experience has been gathered in measuring stigma, questions can be included in surveys to attempt to measure attitudes to persons with HIV/AIDS (5). Some sample questions on stigma are shown in Box 5. However, the results must be analysed carefully. Attitudes of care givers or potential care givers may differ from those who most likely will not have to care for an AIDS patient. Attitudes of women (who are often care givers) and men (generally not care givers) should be considered separately.

Several sources can be used to obtain data on the indicators listed earlier in the chapter. Most input and output indicators – for example, the number of condoms received in the district during a calendar year or the number of counsellors trained and active – can be derived from simple bookkeeping. Indicators of effects generally require a survey, which could be carried out either among a particular population (e.g. secondary school children) or in a random sample of the whole population. More detailed information on preparing and conducting surveys can be found in a World Health Organization manual

Box 5. Survey questions on stigma

1a	Would you be willing or not willing to take care of a female family member with AIDS?	Willing 1 Not willing 2 Do not know 3
1b	Would you be willing or not willing to take care of a male family member with AIDS?	Willing 1 Not willing 2 Do not know 3
2a	Should a woman who knows she is infected with HIV be entitled to keep this fact secret from her husband or should she tell him?	Entitled to keep secret 1 Should be revealed 2 Do not know 3
2b	Should a man who knows he is infected with HIV be entitled to keep this fact secret from his wife or should he tell her?	Entitled to keep secret 1 Should be revealed 2 Do not know 3
3	Should persons who know they are infected with HIV be entitled to keep this fact secret from the community where they live or should this information be revealed?	Entitled to keep secret 1 Should be revealed 2 Do not know 3
4	If you were to find out that you are infected with HIV, would you tell your friends or family?	Not tell anybody 1 Tell my friends 2 Tell my family 3 Tell friends and family 4 Do not know 5
5	Should persons with HIV who work with other people, such as in a factory or hospital, be allowed to continue their work or not?	Allowed 1 Not allowed 2 Do not know 3

on evaluating a national AIDS programme (5).

The health information system being used to collect routine data can be used to provide some data on the course of the epidemic in the district. Such data are collected in health facilities according to standard national procedures and are usually fed into a national health and management information system. Local analysis of levels and trends in the health facilities is an essential but often neglected component (3).

In most countries AIDS is a notifiable disease, but in Africa reporting of AIDS cases tends to be grossly inadequate. In part this is due to difficulties in making the diagnosis (for example, tests for HIV may not be available). This problem can be partially (but *only* partially) solved by using the WHO clinical case definition for AIDS (see Chapter 4 on epidemiological methods). For instance, in Rwandan health facilities the sensitivity of the clinical case definition was found to be only 33%, and in Mwanza only 27% (8, 9). In other words, using the clinical case definition alone, only one-fourth to one-third of HIV-positive patients were identified. Underreporting of AIDS may also be due to delayed or incomplete reporting to the central level. However, it is to the advantage of a district to monitor trends in AIDS admissions and deaths in both adult and paediatric wards of the hospital(s). This data does not only show the importance of AIDS for hospitals, but also may make it possible to see trends over time. Data from an urban hospital in Mwanza, Tanzania (9), where the population prevalence of HIV among adults is estimated at 10–14%, illustrates the importance of HIV infection:

- 44% were HIV infected;
- 30% of adult admissions 15–44 were diagnosed as having AIDS on the basis of the expanded WHO clinical case definition, which uses clinical signs and symptoms plus serological data (HIV antibodies);
- 14% of adult admissions who were found to be HIV-positive died during their stay in hospital, compared to 4% mortality among those who were HIV-negative.

Simply monitoring the number of hospital admissions diagnosed with AIDS each year provides some information on the epidemic and its impact on inpatient health services. If HIV testing facilities are available, the number of HIV-positive adult admissions and the per cent of total adult admissions who are HIV infected are useful indicators.

Monitoring trends in tuberculosis incidence can also be a way to obtain an idea of changes in the HIV epidemic. Tuberculosis in Africa is on the increase, due to the HIV epidemic. For example, in 1994 it was estimated that in Tanzania 40% of all new tuberculosis cases were attributable to HIV infection. If the district has a well-established tuberculosis control programme with a good monitoring system, then data on tuberculosis incidence should be included as a part of monitoring HIV. Examples are given in the chapter on tuberculosis (Chapter 19).

Surveillance of STDs is also important. STDs are a public health problem in themselves, as well as an important factor contributing to HIV transmission (see Chapters 13 and 14, on STDs). A sentinel surveillance system may be the best option for collecting such data at district level. In such a system, a few sites are selected here the incidence of STDs, genital ulcer syndromes and genital discharge syndromes, along with drug sensitivity and treatment patterns, will be monitored. The RPR test can be used to test pregnant women for syphilis at sentinel surveillance sites; results can also be used to monitor trends over time.

Conclusions

Monitoring and evaluation should be an integral part of an HIV prevention and AIDS care programme. No matter what methods are used, it is essential to begin with baseline data that are as good as possible, plus clear objectives, strategies and targets. This provides a foundation for the design of a monitoring and evaluation system that uses indicators to assess the programme. At district level, the primary focus is on input and output indicators, and on indicators related to process – those associated with community involvement in the programme. If additional resources are available small-scale surveys can be conducted to collect information on indicators covering the effects of the inter-

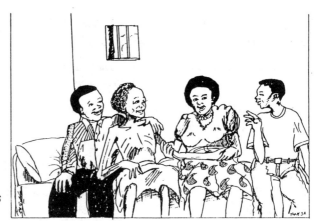

Home-based care: the family has no fear for the person with AIDS.

ventions among the sexually active population. Staff involvement in all phases of the monitoring and evaluation process, combined with proper feedback and discussion of the results, is an important way of motivating them to collect data and make use of it.

With respect to the community, participatory monitoring is a low-cost method, for which an important goal is to stimulate the involvement of the target group and enhance their sense of 'ownership' of and commitment to the programme, and thus help to ensure immediate use of the results from monitoring or evaluation. Target group involvement may also make it easier to collect more reliable data on a difficult topic such as sexual behaviour, where other methods often fail.

Further reading and resources

AIDS *Health Promotion Exchange*, issue no. 4 on 'Assessing prevention achievements and failures: the importance of monitoring and evaluation'. Amsterdam, Royal Tropical Institute, 1993.

AIDSTECH, *Tools for project evaluation: a guide for evaluating* AIDS *prevention interventions*. Research Triangle Park, Family Health International, 1992.

Boerma JT. *Health information for primary health care*. Nairobi, AMREF, 1991.

Feuerstein MT. *Partners in evaluation*. London, Macmillan, 1986. (Teaching aids at low cost – TALC, P.O. Box 49, St Albans, Hertfordshire AL1 4 AX, UK).

Folmer H et al. *Testing and evaluating manuals: making health learning materials more useful*. Amsterdam, Royal Tropical Institute, 1992.

Mertens T, Carael M, Sato P et al. Prevention indicators for evaluating the progress of national AIDS programmes. *AIDS* 1994, 8: 1359–1369.

Sohm ED. *Glossary of evaluation terms*. Joint Inspection Unit JIU/REP 78/5. Geneva, United Nations, 1978.

Vaughan JP, Walt G, Ross D. Evaluation of primary health care: approaches, comments and criticisms. *Tropical Doctor* 1984, 14: 56–60.

World Health Organization. *Evaluation of a national AIDS programme: a methods package. 1. Prevention of HIV infection.* WHO/GPA/TCO/SEF/94.1. Geneva, WHO.

World Health Organization. Monitoring of national AIDS prevention and control programmes: guiding principles. *WHO AIDS Series,* no. 4. Geneva.

References

1. Sohm ED. *Glossary of evaluation terms.* Joint Inspection Unit JIU/REP 78/5. Geneva, United Nations, 1978.

2. Vaughan JP, Walt G, Ross D. Evaluation of primary health care: approaches, comments and criticisms. *Tropical Doctor* 1984, 14: 56–60.

3. Boerma JT. *Health information for primary health care.* Nairobi, AMREF, 1991.

4. LeSar J, Mitchell MD, Northrup R, Harrisson PF. Monitoring and evaluation of child survival programmes. In: Cash R, Keusch GT, Lamstein J. *The UNICEF GOBI-FFF programme.* Beckenham, Croom-Helm, 1987, pp. 173–204.

5. World Health Organization. *Evaluation of a national AIDS programme: a methods package. 1. Prevention of HIV infection.* Geneva, WHO/GPA/TCO/SEF/94.1.

6. Mertens T, Carael M, Sato P et al. Prevention indicators for evaluating the progress of national AIDS programmes. *AIDS* 1994, 8: 1359–1369.

7. Barongo LR, Senkoro K. Boerma JT. HIV, STD and sexual behaviorin fishing villages, Magu District, Tanzania: report of an epidemiological survey. *TANESA Working Paper,* no. 2. Mwanza.

8. Harms G, Kleinfeldt V, Bugingo G et al. Recognition of AIDS by health personnel in rural South-Rwanda. *Tropical Medical Parasitology* 1994, 45: 36–38.

9. Kalluvya S, Ishengoma M, Mkumbo EN, et al. HIV/AIDS in the medical wards of an urban referral hospital, Tanzania. *TANESA Working Paper,* no. 9. Mwanza, 1996.

10. Van Cleeff MRA, Chum HJ. The proportion of tuberculosis cases in Tanzania attributable to human immunodeficiency virus. *International Journal of Epidemiology* 1995, 42: 637–641.

7 Community level interventions

Deo Luhamba, Dick Schapink and Wences Msuya

- What can communities do to reduce and prevent HIV transmission?
- How can communities be mobilized for action?
- How can a district's priority communities be chosen?
- How can local resources be mobilized?

The community has a major influence on the behaviour of individuals. If the HIV/AIDS epidemic is perceived as a community problem, rather than as the problem of particular individuals, it then becomes possible to discuss general issues that may lead to behavioural changes. Furthermore, involving communities can help to incorporate local knowledge and commitment, which are vital parts of successful interventions. A community approach is therefore an essential element of AIDS programmes.

The initial emphasis of HIV/AIDS education was on the general public (through mass media campaigns) and specific target groups who were thought to be practising high-risk behaviours. This emphasis created problems, since the community often responded by associating AIDS with specific groups, such as sex workers, fishermen and truck drivers. This led to the false perception that AIDS was a problem of 'others', which was reinforced in areas where only a few people were known to have AIDS or to have died from it. As the epidemic spread, however, it became clearer that all sexually active persons are at risk. Therefore, the emphasis shifted from 'high-risk groups' to 'high-transmission areas', that is, areas where the whole community is more vulnerable and therefore needs to be mobilized to limit the spread of HIV (see Box 1).

Analysis of gender relations and differences shows that many women cannot put the usual basic messages for HIV prevention (condom use, faithfulness and reducing the number of partners) into practice. Messages for women often fail to recognize the social pressures on men and boys: for example, the pressure to have many sexual partners and for boys to start having sex early. Married women may be faithful, but usually have no power to decide on condom use; therefore, they run the risk of HIV infection through the promiscuous behaviour of their husbands. Unmarried women lacking economic security may not be in a position to reduce their number of partners if they must depend on these partners' material support for survival.

Box 1. Shift in emphasis from the individual to the community level

- During the development of an intervention package for fishermen on the shores of Lake Victoria, Tanzania, it was soon realized that exclusively targeting of fishermen and their onshore fishing posts was actually a way of stigmatizing them. Peer health educators among the fishermen therefore decided to involve the wider community in their activities. The reaction of the village was positive: they in turn insisted that the programme be extended to include all sub-village communities.
- In Mwanza, Tanzania, peer educators among young women working in bars planned activities to influence their peers' behaviour. They found it necessary to talk to peers individually and in groups, and to discuss risk behaviours and consequences with influential elders and friends. Their colleagues' male sexual partners were also included, since the young women are very dependent on them regarding condom use. Furthermore, they stressed that improvement in the women's economic situation was necessary before behaviour could be changed. That is, two aspects of community support were essential for behavioural change: increased respect for the young women and support for improving their socioeconomic status.

Unless gender relations in the community change and economic security for women increases, women will continue to lack the ability to protect themselves. Both gender relations and economic security are issues to be addressed at community level (see also Chapter 9). Detailed knowledge about prevalent risk behaviours is often present within the community, along with an understanding of the reasons why this behaviour takes place. It therefore makes sense to fully involve communities in planning and implementing activities aimed at reducing the risk-taking behaviour. The full involvement of communities will increase the sense of ownership in the activities undertaken, and will make it possible to mobilize available resources for these activities.

This chapter describes the processes involved in beginning a community level approach for an HIV/AIDS intervention programme. It emphasizes the importance of a participatory process and the linkages to development issues, and outlines the techniques that can be used to ensure this.

Setting priorities among the communities within a district

An average district with a population of 300,000 includes many communities and a wide range of ways of life, norms and values. Communities may be located within towns or may share a basic economy (e.g. cotton farming, shopkeeping). In rural areas communities usually have a 'village basis', with a shared history, culture and administration, to which people recognize themselves as belonging. Communities are not necessarily homogeneous: internal conflicts and rifts may first require attention to resolving conflicts and strengthening community organization. Conflicts that may arise due to a lack of good leadership in a community will directly influence the response of the community to interventions.

Community interventions typically take considerable time and resources. Hence, it is difficult for a programme at district level to achieve district-wide coverage; it is necessary to make choices among areas, and interventions. Large-scale intervention programmes involving all of the communities in a district are generally not feasible: costs, including staffing and vehicles, are too high in relation to effectiveness. A situation analysis (see Chapter 2) can help planners to identify high-transmission areas, and can be used as a basis for decisions regarding the selection of communities and priorities. Criteria that can be used to identify these areas include:

- the number of guesthouses and bars in communities;
- the existence of permanent or occasional markets;
- bus or truck stops, and the number of buses and trucks that remain there overnight;
- the extent of economic activities;
- areas with more men than women.

This information can be analyzed by district planners and the district health management team, and be used to identify high-transmission areas (see Box 2).

Box 2. Identification of high-transmission areas

In Magu District, Tanzania, ten communities were selected as high-transmission areas. The choice of priority communities made by a multisectoral planning team was negotiated with and then approved by the district council, which is made up of ward representatives. (The ward is an administrative division; typically there are about 10,000 residents per ward.)

The high-transmission areas identified included roadside villages along the main bus route through the district, which also serve as truck stops and where many guest-houses are found; fishing villages with dynamic economic activity; villages with many social and economic activities, including markets and guesthouses.

Community interventions take place at the level of the behaviour-determining context, and are intended to generate action that will help to create a supportive environment for behaviour change among community members. Community-based action, however, requires much voluntary work and, if the intervention is to be sustainable, the financial resources needed for interventions should be mobilized locally to the greatest extent. This immediately necessitates a participatory approach.

Developing interventions in a participatory way calls for innovative tools that help to keep up the motivation for action and are interactive, as the intervention must address the specific needs of a particular community. The process of developing a supportive environment for behaviour change in a community will differ from place to place. It will differ in the kind of action developed, because this will depend on the type and root causes of risk-taking behaviour present in the community; the pace will also differ. The use of extra resources needed for the intervention (from district or national level or from donors) should be integrated with the process of community action that is taking place.

Issues in community interventions

Initially, communities may take a passive attitude to interventions. Health workers may feel they could suggest ready solutions, but the majority of the community is not likely to be immediately motivated enough to begin a concerted effort to promote behavioural change and reduce HIV transmission. If a village has felt needs other than the HIV/AIDS problem, they may not develop and implement action. AIDS programmes thus are more apt to succeed if they follow a process approach, such as the one outlined below, in working with communities. Advocacy regarding the need and possibility for action towards behavioural change is first necessary. Planning needs to be done not for but *with* communities: it must follow their priorities, their felt and expressed needs, which may not necessarily be the same as the HIV/AIDS programme priorities or programme-determined needs.

Addressing people's felt needs is apt to be easier when HIV/AIDS and behavioural change initiatives are integrated into primary health care structures. The extent to which this can be done in practice depends on the quality of these structures. The use of existing institutions that provide social services in the village may be difficult because of lack of motivation for action within the village health committee. In many communities, committee members may be passive. The selection of health committee members may be motivated by political or personal interests. If primary health care structures are not functioning and development orientation in the villages is low, the introduction of community interventions will take longer, and will need to find ways to work with and through other village institutions.

A stand-alone, 'vertical' AIDS programme is more apt to change into an integrated programme (see Chapter 22) at community level when a participatory approach is used, since people perceive health problems as linked to their existence as a whole. Communities often point out that AIDS and engaging in high-risk behaviours are related to the unemployment of youth and women, lack of authority, and diminishing social control. Therefore, AIDS programmes need to mobilize resources to attend to these broader needs.

The communities that are chosen as priorities need to be mobilized to participate in designing programmes, but also to support them with local resources. Cash resources for financing any type of self-help activities are apt to be limited; much of community participation will be based on voluntary work. AIDS programmes will therefore need to be innovative, seeking ways to maintain motivation and assist communities in mobilization. A participatory approach is an important part of this effort. The process of beginning behavioural change is important, which takes time and only pays off later.

Working with communities

The aim of a community intervention is to facilitate behavioural change. Such change is a dynamic process, which has to come from within the community. The role of outsiders should be limited to a facilitating and supporting role in problem analysis, and planning and implementing action. That is, the most effective approach is one in which outside facilitators and community residents work and learn together to solve problems that have been identified by the community. This approach has been outlined by Korten, who envisioned a process in which: 'villages and programme personnel would share knowledge and resources, creating programmes in which the needs and capacities of beneficiaries would be linked to those of the outsiders who provide assistance' (1).

The identification of risk behaviours and how to address these is also best done with people living in the community. People are likely to be less interested in being told about risk behaviours which have been identified by outsiders. Moreover, if given the chance, community members can be more critical and more precise about risk behaviours in their own community. The community risk behaviour mapping exercise presented in Chapter 9 is often a very good starting activity as it is very practical, does not need strong outside input in terms of either personnel or financing, and is highly gender sensitive. Community members are also best equipped to propose solutions. Therefore, behavioural change in a community calls for a process in which people analyze their situation, identify risk situations and risk behaviours, select solutions, monitor and evaluate changes and peoples' responses, and develop corrective actions. This whole process of change can be characterized as a learning process for the community.

It is important to follow locally acceptable protocol when entering a community. Following local protocol means first contacting the community/village government, and discussing the purpose of the programme and the approach with them. Local leadership and the available primary health care structures responsible for social services should be involved in all stages of developing an intervention. It is then necessary to quickly begin involving others who represent the many parts of the community, as described below in the discussion of participatory rapid appraisal, so that you – and the community – begin to build up a reliable picture of the situation. Throughout, it remains important to stay in touch with leaders, so they remain interested and committed, and understand what is happening and why.

Training for programme personnel

Trained personnel are an essential part of working with communities. Developing interventions that call for a learning approach, using participatory techniques, has implications for training staff who work in the programmes as well as implications for the management of these programmes. Very often staff use an information-giving approach as opposed to an information-*sharing* approach: educators may tend to use a top–down approach, telling people what to do with an attitude of 'the professional knows best'. Staff need to be trained in participatory principles – particularly in taking the role of 'facilitator' as opposed to 'teacher' – including an attitude of willingness to learn from people and assist them in making their own decisions. This is discussed further in Chapter 12.

To support staff working in this way, programme management will also need to change. Only with the development of a participatory management style, and with delegation of operational responsibilities, can it be expected that programme staff will take a participatory approach in their health education sessions. Supervisors should give feedback that encourages learning, and should treat errors as learning opportunities. Reports on AIDS education and training sessions should indicate what staff have learned from the participants in addition to what participants have learned from the session. In-house staff training can focus on communication styles, gender, participatory discussion techniques, ways to facilitate planning workshops, methods to facilitate participatory monitoring and evaluation workshops, and how to conduct AIDS education and training sessions using learner-centred and participatory approaches. The trainers guide for participatory learning and action (2) may be helpful in organizing an in-house training workshop.

Developing an HIV prevention programme with a community

Making a community profile

Getting to know the community should be seen as the first phase in the development of an intervention. When beginning to make decisions about collecting information and contacting community residents, it is essential to follow local protocol, as mentioned earlier. Preparatory work with community leaders can make the task of programme staff much easier. Box 3 lists the kind of information that is useful to include in a community profile. Using participatory techniques both with village leaders and in collecting the information necessary for making a community profile also builds momentum for later interventions.

If resources, including time and knowledgeable staff, are available, a PRA (participatory rapid appraisal; 3, 4) can be an excellent way of establishing a participatory learning process in a community. This approach helps to assure that all members of the community are taken into consideration, and that both expert and local knowledge are incorporated in the process of building a community profile. PRA is now a well-developed tool, which has been used in rural development programmes across the world. Its characteristics and principles are briefly given in Box 4. Additional information on using this technique can be found in the many handbooks on participatory rapid appraisal for community development (5, 6). Carrying out PRA requires careful planning and broad representation of both 'experts' and local people. Further, it must not be done *too* quickly: otherwise it will be difficult to gain the genuine participation of the target groups.

Box 3. Information for a community profile

Demography: population, sex and age distribution, family sizes, migration patterns, ethnic groups;

Economy: economic activities, employment and unemployment, number of recreational facilities such as bars, local beer shops and guesthouses (mapping facilities might be useful);

History: history of the community, issues of concern, history of community action, history of HIV/AIDS information/campaigns/activities;

Health and social services: number of health facilities available and performance, active traditional healers and their specializations, HIV and STD prevalence, number and geographical distribution of schools. Potential partners within the relevant sectors (and their potential contributions) should be identified; and the relationship between community and service providers should be analysed;

Organizations: religious organizations, women's groups, youth groups, NGOs in the area. Which of these are potential partners?

Power and leadership: existing community organizations (is there an active PHC committee and/or social services committee?). Who are the influential leaders, and what are their relationships with district power structures? What are the differences among political factions, and what influence do they have on leadership and on power struggles;

KAP information for HIV/AIDS programming: gender-specific perceptions, felt and expressed needs with regard to general health, STDs, HIV/AIDS problems; norms and traditions with regard to sexual behaviour; norms concerning the role of women and men and their health-seeking behaviour; differences between past and present risk behaviour; risk perceptions concerning HIV/AIDS; norms/values and practices regarding prevention; specific risk behaviours; and condom distribution and use. What are the most important sources of information for the various groups in the community?

There are numerous other ways to obtain information for a community profile, either as a part of PRA or separately. The historical mapping process outlined in Chapter 9 can assist the community in discussing how a problem has arisen, its extent and its root causes; mapping recreational facilities and so forth can encourage free discussion of where and how problem behaviour occurs. Role playing and other theatre techniques can be used to express risk behaviour in the community and feelings regarding it. Community-directed visual images can be made with a still or videocamera, and can be used to portray risk situations and behaviours.

Much of the information for the community profile can be obtained by talking to district officials. It is a good idea to check, update and fill in the gaps by talking to community leaders and others. Service providers in the area and any NGOs are valuable resources. Information about HIV prevalence may be available at district or regional level. STD prevalence may be available from dispensaries and clinics.

Box 4. Participatory rapid appraisal

- Information is collected, working in small teams of up to six people with different backgrounds, e.g. villagers, health workers and community development workers.
- Participation from representative villagers in the team is essential: village leadership, opinion leaders, women's and youth leaders.
- The composition of the team should be balanced, including a significant number of women. Since sensitive issues have to be discussed it will be necessary to split the team when these issues are handled.
- Flexibility regarding content and method is needed: short guidelines should be used instead of standardized tools for data collection.
- Daily team discussions in the field serve to adjust guidelines, identify areas and/or target groups of specific interest, and so to develop an accurate village profile.
- More than one research method and source of information should be used to cross-check the data collected: information from the district office, discussions with influential villagers and focus group discussions with relevant target groups will help to identify differences of opinion about health matters, previous actions in the community, behavioural problems and possible solutions. The listening survey (see below) is also an effective tool for cross-checking.
- The initial appraisal should be of short duration: data collection and focus group discussions for the community profile might take, for example, one week.
- The results of the rapid appraisal should be discussed with the village leadership.
- A rapid appraisal is action-oriented: it is intended to provide a basis for programme design and implementation.

As suggested by Box 4, it is very important to also include information from those whose needs and views may not be adequately represented by community leaders and official data. Group discussions with relevant target groups will provide relevant information with regard to knowledge, attitude, behaviour (KAP) questions, such as those listed in Box 3. A relevant method to quickly collect information about what people think about HIV/AIDS and related issues is to hold a listening survey. In this technique groups go into the community and try to identify how people talk about AIDS, and what their attitudes and fears are. This listening survey can most effectively be done after group discussions with different target groups. In our experience, formally organized group discussions to which people are specifically invited by community leaders often stimulate lively discussions. Recording or taking notes of what is said in these discussions is one of the tasks of the listening survey. The survey should focus separately on males and females, and can be repeated at subsequent intervals.

Developing an AIDS action committee
To follow up on the information and interest generated by the process of making a community profile, the village government should be consulted about which village

Figure I. From situation analysis to a new vision

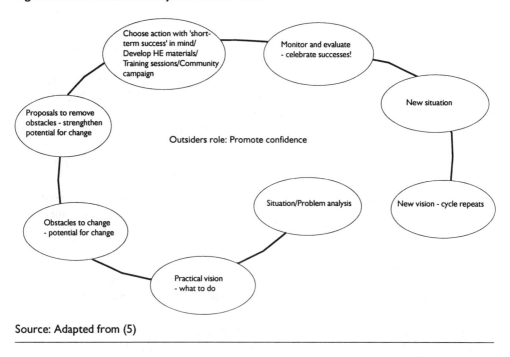

Source: Adapted from (5)

institution will be given a mandate, as an AIDS action committee, to coordinate and supervise AIDS prevention and care activities. If there is an existing village institution with a history of taking action, it is an advantage to set up the AIDS action committee as a part of that institution. This might be a primary health care committee, a social services committee, a health committee or a completely new committee especially created to deal with the AIDS problem. However, in this stage advocacy is often necessary to obtain balanced representation of women and youth on the committee. A search for highly motivated people is also apt to be beneficial. People who themselves have been affected by the disease, or whose family members or friends have been infected, may sometimes be more motivated, and moreover, will have first-hand experience of the impact and consequences of HIV infection and the needs of those affected.

After an AIDS action committee has been formed, it should be assisted by programme staff to plan for action in the community. Figure 1 outlines the participatory planning steps that can be undertaken together with this committee. During the first step, the committee is assisted in analysing the risk behaviour problems in the community. (Techniques for situation analysis described earlier, such as the mapping exercise, can be used.) In step 2, the community develops its own vision of what can be done to create a supportive environment for behaviour change among residents. Step 3 involves a look at the obstacles and potential for creating this environment; then it is time to choose the actions that will be carried out. In this process, it is crucial to help the committee choose actions they can carry out in the community while working on their own. This assures their ownership of the process and builds commitment. Action that requires help from outside should be planned for later – after a self-help period has been completed successfully.

The various actions should be planned carefully with the committee and each action should be monitored and evaluated together. Successes should be celebrated to boost the motivation of the committee. Also, exchanges between the committee and important visitors, or among different committees, can be quite important. After each successful action the situation in the community changes; the committee can start planning for new activities at the same time its vision is developing and becoming increasingly practical, as to what needs to happen in the community to support behaviour change.

Throughout the process, another important role of facilitators is to monitor the confidence of the committee. Local committees can easily lose their confidence if they face obstacles such as problems in working together, motivational difficulties, having difficulty in mobilizing the community, or becoming discouraged by the response of residents. Box 5 summaries the steps involved in this participatory planning process.

Box 5. Participatory planning process for an AIDS action committee

1   Mobilize the committee for action by stimulating awareness of the problem of HIV infection in this specific community. As input to this process, facilitators calculate the number of people infected on the basis of HIV prevalence in the adult population.
2   Involve a broad variety of community residents; analyse behaviour problems based on the villagers' own perceptions (e.g. from a PRA) and vision of what should happen in the village to change the situation.
3   Analyse the potential for and obstacles to change (focus on the potential for change, to motivate action).
4   Select strategies to strengthen potential and remove obstacles.
5   Choose actions that will provide immediate successes. Programme facilitators should be aware that in the beginning, if tasks are too large – so that they fail – people may lose confidence in their ability to succeed.
6   If necessary, include some basic training for committee members who will be working with the community in principles of health education, including a focus on problem-solving instead of simply accumulating knowledge and presenting 'expert' opinions. (See Chapters 5 and 7 and Box 6.)
7   Prepare materials for work in the community, for example by using participatory techniques to develop picture codes or story-telling sessions as discussion starters.
8   Choose peer educators or community educators from vulnerable groups for training.
9   Plan monitoring and evaluation of the initial activities; take time to celebrate successes!
10 Assist the community in planning and carrying out an intensive campaign to create momentum for ongoing activities, using, in so far possible, local resources.

Box 6. Basic steps in AIDS education and training sessions (4)

1   Assess what people already know.
2   Build on what is known.
3   Stop and check people's understanding often.
4   Build sessions around problem solving and decision making, involving the audience in both.
5   Plan in evaluation of education or training activities as part of the process.

Joint planning sessions for communities
An initial planning workshop can involve committees from several communities. The advantage is that this will give committees more access to ideas and they can stimulate each other to act. It also allows committees to realize that others share their problems. Evaluation of activities can also be a joint effort, promoting healthy competition between committees, as well as providing a forum for discussing common problems. A single community working on its own may develop the habit of turning to the programme for answers and assistance (especially financial) for every small problem. Sharing problems with other communities is more likely to encourage them to look for their own solutions. Exchange visits are recommended for this reason as well.

Committees and individuals often develop and express a need for further training, although this may come slowly. As one senior AIDS committee member expressed: 'We will always ask for allowances, but what we really need is more education'. Such an identification of real training needs as the result of peoples' involvement must be stimulated and supported. Training provides a strong motivation. As people's perspectives broaden they will tackle broader issues, and in doing so will reduce the role of the programme. Hence, training those involved is a way of improving sustainability.

Self-help period in the community
After a planning workshop the village should begin to undertake the self-help activities that they have identified. Programme staff should only monitor at this time, from a distance, but should stay informed about what is happening, either through visits or through reports from the committee. The role of the project staff needs to be made clear to the committee early on, so as not to create wrong expectations. Self-help activities might include information meetings for the community; supporting the economic activities of vulnerable groups such as women and youth; developing by-laws to protect youth and women, and to control alcohol and drug abuse; and improving and monitoring the distribution of condoms to guesthouses, bars, shops and dispensaries. A period of three months should be sufficient for committees to create awareness in the village about the need for behavioural changes. After this three-month period facilitators can assist in evaluating initial achievements. Programme facilitators need to help people see that their activities really can make a difference. Again, combining communities for the evaluation is worthwhile. Poor performance by some committees in this stage usually

means the village has priorities other than AIDS-action programming, so that additional support will probably not be worthwhile. Committees that are more active can be supported in organizing a broader campaign to increase the momentum of their ongoing activities. This is discussed further below, under 'Organizing an intensive community campaign'.

Selecting and training peer health educators

Part of the planning process for an AIDS action committee is the identification and selection of vulnerable (high-risk) groups and the selection of peer health educators (PHEs). This can be done after the committee has finalized some of their self-help activities, such as information meetings for the community and the introduction of new by-laws. PHEs are individuals from within a targeted community who are trained and known as HIV/AIDS educators. Peer education is beneficial for groups of people who experience strong peer pressure concerning their behaviour, including out-of-school youth (school youth can be reached through the school intervention programme, outlined elsewhere in this book), fishermen, barworkers and other groups with distinct subcultures.

Selection of PHEs within specific peer groups can follow criteria such as permanent residence in the village, literacy, selection by peers for acceptability, and being interested in training others. The required number of PHEs is difficult to establish, as it will depend on the situation, and on the particular characteristics of the vulnerable groups involved. Resources available for training may also determine numbers, which can easily be up to 15 people. However, it is important that PHEs do not work in isolation and that the group trained is made up of both females and males. Drop-out rates may differ per area and circumstances but a rate of even 50% is possible. Dropping out can be caused by a lack of motivation, inability of a PHE to change his or her own behaviour, migration forced by economic circumstances, marriage, sickness or even death (particularly since PHEs are recruited among high-risk groups). For more information about peer health educators and their training see Chapters 8 and 12.

Training for the PHEs selected by the community should be undertaken by the programme. A training workshop requires about five days and can be organised close to one of the villages. Combining PHEs from different villages has advantages, but separating men and women into different workshops remains a necessity. Groups of up to twenty PHEs can be trained together. An outline of the training sessions used in Magu Tanzania, is shown in Box 7.

Organizing an intensive community campaign

If the committee is satisfied with its initial self-help activities, facilitators can then assist it in organizing and preparing an intensive village campaign to increase the momentum behind community action for behavioural change. Campaigning can be combined with local resource mobilization, and committees can organize fundraising – both in cash and in kind – for such campaigns.

Box 7. Training for community peer health educators

- how adults learn best: an introduction to working as a facilitator;
- basic facts on HIV/AIDS and STDs, reproductive health and the relationship of tuberculosis and HIV infection;
- treatment of STDs;
- family planning methods;
- gender issues in behavioural change;
- care for people with AIDS and the role of stigma; ways to promote positive living.
- basic training in the principles of health education, the use of picture codes and short role plays as discussion starters;
- monitoring and evaluation methods, including the identification of risk behaviours of peers, the role of alcohol and drug abuse, planning activities, choosing evaluation questions and indicators for measuring success, and ways to monitor activities (see also Chapter 6).

Every training session requires follow-up in the field to provide motivation and on-the-job training, and to help solve problems. Those who successfully complete training should be awarded an official certificate and an incentive, such as a T-shirt to be used during PHE activities.

In Mwanza, Tanzania, committees have been able to raise on average one-third to one-half of the total local costs of their campaign (excluding personnel assistance from the AIDS programme). Educational videoshows can also be used during a campaign to raise funds to assist the committee in implementing new or ongoing activities. The clearer the aims of fundraising – for example, to assist a women's or youth group in the village – the better the response.

The organization of the campaign should be left up to the committee as much as possible. Assistance from the AIDS programme focuses on motivation and facilitation, and on training the groups involved in the campaign to deliver their messages more effectively. Local cultural groups should become as involved as possible; this is apt to increase acceptance of activities. In the roadside and fishing settlements of Mwanza Region, organizing committees found a well-trained drama group from Mwanza town unacceptable ('we have our own groups'). Local cultural groups are almost always available to convey messages through popular dramatic forms like songs, poems and theatre or short role plays, depending on what will be culturally most effective in the local situation. Women's groups can be assisted in finding ways to include messages on condom use and to deal with the existing stigma regarding condoms. Appropriate messages have to be thoroughly discussed with the committee and the cultural groups involved in the campaign, since the first tendency is often to use an approach that instills fear. Training on how to deliver messages is often necessary. Committee members can learn to use picture codes as discussion starters and other participatory techniques.

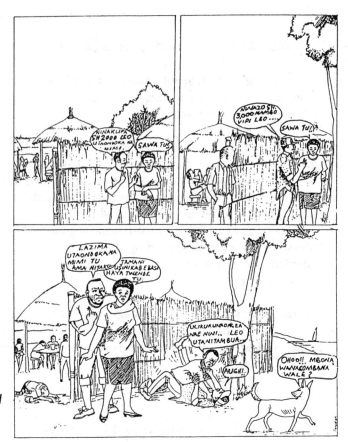

Alcohol, commercial sex and violence: a scene in a local beer shop in a fishing post.

We have found it useful to include these basic components as parts of an intensive campaign in a community, where the goal is to motivate behavioural change:

- A mix of culturally familiar popular drama forms can be used as discussion starters to deliver behaviour-change messages, and to portray locally identified community risk behaviours. Since the main aim of these popular drama forms is discussion rather than simply a show, training in their use should focus on facilitating discussion after the performance. The presentations should also be pre-tested with a few villagers prior to the campaign.
- Exhibition boards for educational activities can be used to portray:
  - risk behaviours;
  - the reasons for risk behaviours;
  - the illnesses that result from risk behaviours, focusing on STDs and HIV;
  - treatment-seeking behaviour and problems related to it, focusing on the familiar, trusted traditional healer, modern medicines and self-treatment;
  - consequences of illnesses, focusing on repeated STDs, infertility problems, and an open door to HIV infection;

- the need for community action to remove the reasons for risk behaviours and achieve behavioural change.
- Videoshows can be presented: a variety of feature films such as *Neria, More time, It's not easy* and the like, which were produced in Zimbabwe, are available in several local languages. Videoshows like these can be used for fundraising in the village as well. A widescreen video might be purchased by the AIDS programme for this purpose. Videoshows usually attract large numbers of people; over a three-day-period the entire population of a village will normally attend at least one show.
- A song or drawing competition may be part of the campaign.
- Picture codes can be used by PHEs or others to start meaningful discussions in small groups.
- Information pamphlets on STDs, HIV/AIDS and family planning can be made available, along with books on these topics. Demand for reading materials is usually very high. National AIDS programmes will be able to suggest sources for there materials.
- Condom demonstrations can be held in a relatively private place, and combined with condom distribution.
- Posters should be posted in relevant places, where they will continue to be seen after the campaign is over.
- T-shirts can be sold or given out to continue to remind people in the village of the basic messages. These messages can be selected by the committee or the PHEs to fit the local situation. (This requires finding a way to produce T-shirts at a low cost – perhaps locally, since the number of T-shirts needed will be very limited).

The discussion starters to be used in community campaigns need to be developed in close cooperation with villagers and trained PHEs. The risk situations and/or risk behaviours identified in the community can be used to develop short role plays, theatre performances, picture codes, stories and the like. They can also be used to develop messages, which might be expressed in songs and poems. Community/village groups may need some help in developing messages. Messages for the community should not aim to instill fear, but rather relate to behavioural change, gender issues and the possibilities of change.

Picture codes need more preparation since they will be used in ongoing activities. When pictures are familiar, people are more likely to understand that the messages are intended for them. Pictures have a great deal of power: it is important that they communicate the intended message in a locally understandable way. Pictures that show one sex or ethnic group in an unfavourable light may cause problems. Furthermore, what is effective for one community may be of little use in another. Picture codes need to be thoroughly pre-tested to see whether the picture is understood, and whether it shows an existing and recognizable problem in the community. Familiarity, simplicity and realism are usually what make a drawing effective. The steps in pre-testing a picture code are shown in Box 8.

Box 8. Pre-testing and using a picture code (4)

The questions below can be used to pre-test picture codes. The aim is to see whether the picture code 'works' – whether people relate to the pictures and understand them, and whether they can identity the problem the code is meant to portray. If these conditions are met (and a good discussion follows), the picture code is apt to be a good one!

1   Who are the people in this picture?
2   Are they from your village?
3   What do you see happening in the picture?
4   Why is this happening?
5   Does this happen in real life?
6   What problems does this lead to?
7   What are the root causes of the problem?
8   What can be done about it?

The last six questions can also be used as 'discussion starters' when using the picture codes in the community.

Ongoing activities after the campaign

After a campaign, committees need and often request further training, and want to revise their initial planning. The original planning cycle (see Figure 1) may be repeated: the committee can begin a new problem analysis and focus on proposed or ongoing activities such as youth programmes, women's economic activities, ongoing education, identifying orphans and initiating community action for them, or community care programmes. New activities may be called for: for example, if the committee identifies women's or youth groups as needing economic support, these groups may need assistance in feasibility studies, locating potential sponsors, training in how to apply for credit and so forth. A community development department, NGOs or other institutions may be mobilized to assist in this role.

After the campaign, exchange visits to other villages and institutions might be organized for committee members to facilitate assistance and assessment, exchange experiences and stimulate interest in community interventions that have been success-ful elsewhere. Visits from prominent visitors to villages with well-organized programmes is usually very much appreciated and can provide strong motivation for ongoing activities; they are also a source of ideas and new methods.

PHEs also require ongoing attention from the programme. They too express the need for further training and follow-up workshops. Furthermore, replacements for drop-outs may be necessary. PHEs who do their work well may be trained as trainers of new PHEs. Allow-ances paid initially can be adjusted to link actual activities to the payment. That is, the amount received can be based on the actual planning and implementation of activities.

Most PHEs are unemployed and seeking employment. It is advantageous to create a career 'ladder' for PHEs. There should be advocacy for their position and status; for example, they could be selected as village health workers. There may be room to enrol those who perform well in training for other jobs in the health sector or other development programmes. Apart from this, special efforts could be made to assist PHEs to organize themselves and help them engage in income-generating activities.

Linking AIDS programmes to community development
Even after a campaign is well underway, the programme should continue to work with other programmes, agencies and NGOs, acting as an advocate for initiatives that come from the community. Ongoing local resource mobilization is needed. If other development programmes are available, community initiatives can be linked up with them. Such action in the community is easier when the programme and AIDS action committee work together to understand and present the impact HIV/AIDS have on all aspects of community life. Containing the AIDS epidemic is vital to community development: when this relationship is clear to the community and to other organizations, their participation and willingness to share resources is more apt to be forthcoming. And when the programme advocates and supports initiatives that give practical help to people who want to change their behaviour, perhaps by helping them develop new sources of income, it helps to build HIV/AIDS activities into the life of the community.

To work with others and support such initiatives, however, AIDS programmes may have to think about a change of direction. This is especially true when they have been organized as vertical programmes. While as noted early in this chapter communities naturally see health as linked to all other aspects of their lives, this is apt to be a new challenge for an AIDS programme. For example, dealing with the HIV/AIDS epidemic by helping communities with development-oriented activities may go beyond the original objective and mandate. However, a shift from vertical project planning to more integrated district development planning can be an excellent way of getting more impact out of the scarce resources that are available. Also, when working together leads to initiation of development-oriented activities by a district social services committee, it may be easier to mobilize districts to fund them.

Monitoring and evaluation of community interventions

In general, monitoring and evaluation of community interventions should be built into programmes during their planning phases. Further, it is important to work with communities in defining what will be evaluated at community level, and how. Those who will collect the information need not only to understand how to collect it, but also why it is important. Planning should also provide for feeding back the information collected to the community. (See Chapter 6 for more information.)

An evaluation of community interventions may focus on the whole process of change in the community, or on the evaluation of specific communication activities such as the organized campaigns. Communication activities can be evaluated by asking such questions as:

- were the communication activities carried out as planned?
- did the message come across to its intended audience?
- did they pay attention to the communication?
- was the message understood?
- did the audience find it realistic and workable?
- did it result in a change in behaviour?

District planning progress indicators. Evaluating the programme of community interventions at district level will require some indicators (Chapter 6) that illustrate the degree of success of the programme. For example, for evaluation related to the high-transmission areas selected as priorities, the following indicators might be used:
- number of high-transmission areas covered by community interventions;
- number of high-transmission areas where an intensive campaign has been organized;
- number of high-transmission areas where activities are planned;
- number of high-transmission areas with proper condom distribution channels.
- number of PHEs active in high-transmission areas.

Community behavioural change indicators. Indicators of community behavioural change to be used at district level include:
- Number of AIDS-action committees that sustain ongoing activities.
- Types of activities identified as ongoing:
  - community care programmes;
  - economic activities for women and youth;
  - identification and enforcement of new by-laws protecting women and youth, especially those dealing with forced sex, rape and alcohol abuse;
  - organized youth programmes such as sports events;
  - successful enforcement of age limits at bars and local beer shops.
- Types of follow-up training identified and implemented:
  - for further ongoing activity planning;
  - for community home-based care and counselling services;
  - for care of orphans;
  - for further training in health education;
  - for feasibility training.

Timing of the activities

For a group of four communities, the timing of activities might follow a schedule such as the one presented in Box 9. An end point for such a programme cannot be stated; this will depend on the ability to hand over activities and support from relevant departments such as community development or other NGOs. Involving the relevant actors from the beginning will help to ensure that this is done properly.

Box 9. Model time schedule for interventions in four communities

Type of activity	Time frame
Rapid appraisals; community profile; report writing	I month
Preparation, meetings with leadership from selected communities, select/form an AIDS-action committee for some four communities	I month
Participatory planning workshop for AIDS-action committees	2 weeks
Self-help activities as a result of the planning workshop in each community	allow for 3 months
Evaluation of self-help activities	2 weeks
Training of PHEs from the selected villages (gender-specific, including preparation)	I month
Initial educational activities by PHEs	2 months
Intensive campaign for behavioural change, including preparations in every village	4 months
Evaluation of the campaign	2 weeks
Follow-up planning for ongoing activities in each village	4 weeks
Support/advocacy to other sectors for ongoing activities	allow for I year
Participatory monitoring and evaluation workshops with PHEs and the AIDS-action committee	4 weeks
Overall evaluation to determine need for further support or handing over to specific sectors	4 weeks

Conclusion

Working with communities as a whole is an essential part of an AIDS programme. Mobilizing individuals and organizations should involve community leaders, and stimulate the active participation of all groups in the community, rather than just concentrating on specific groups or individuals. Community interventions require a participatory approach. This should not be expected to lead to quick results in behavioural change, but instead should focus on getting the process started.

Lessons learned in the context of rural development and primary health care programmes also pertain to AIDS programmes, and can be adapted to fit the context of AIDS and sexual behaviour. A planned, courteous approach should be used, carefully following local protocol. It is also necessary to establish and follow community priorities and felt needs. Participatory rapid appraisals and community profiles are helpful in establishing these priorities and needs.

Staff and management need to be well trained and able to work in a participatory way. Then they can provide good support to the community, for example, to an AIDS action committee and to peer health educators – both of which have been found to be particularly effective in spreading AIDS information among vulnerable groups. Given limited support, communities can organize and carry out their own campaigns. To get the best effects, they must also be involved in the monitoring and evaluation process that needs to be built into this sort of intervention.

Further reading

Chambers R. *Rural development: putting the last first.* London, Longman, 1983.

Bergdall TD. *The MAP facilitators handbook for promoting rural participation.* Lusaka, 1991.

Graeff JA, Elder JP, Booth EM. *Communication for health and behaviour change in a developing country perspective.* San Francisco, Jossey-Bass Publishers, 1993.

Hubley J. *Communicating health. An action guide to health education.* London, Macmillan Press, 1993.

Hubley J. *The AIDS handbook: a guide to the understanding of AIDS and HIV.* Basingstoke, Macmillan Education Limited, 1995.

Laver S. *Let's teach about AIDS series.* London, AHRTAG, (London Bridge Street, London SE1 9SG. UK).

Video

African film and video catalogue
Media for Development International *(D)*
9111 Guilford Road, # 100
Columbia, MD 21046 USA
Tel. 1-310-490-4465. Fax: 1-3-1-490-4146
(There are several DSR affiliate distributors in Africa)

References

1. Korten DC. Community organisation and rural development: a learning process approach. *Public Administration Review* 1980, 40: 480–511.

2. Pretty JN, Guyt I, Thompson J, Scoones I. Participatory learning and action. A trainers guide. *IIED Participatory Methodologies series.* London, International Institute for Environment and Development, 1995.

3. Beebe J. Rapid appraisal: the evaluation of the concept and the definition of issues. In: *Proceedings of the 1985 International Conference on Rapid Appraisal.* Khon Khaen University, Thailand, 1987. pp. 47–68.

4. Grandstaff TB, Lovelace GW. Summary report. In: *Proceedings of the 1985 International Conference on Rapid Appraisal.* Khon Khaen University, Thailand, 1987.

5. Theis J, Grady H. *Participatory rapid appraisal for community development.* Sustainable Agriculture Programme, IIED and Safe the Children, 1991.

6. Guijt I, Manneh L, Martin M, Sarch, T. *From input to impact: participatory rapid appraisal for Action Aid The Gambia.* London, Action Aid, The Gambia and IIED, 1992.

7. Bergdall TD. *The MAP facilitators handbook for promoting rural participation.* Lusaka. 1991.

Part three
Behavioural
interventions

8   Working in high-transmission areas: truck routes

Blastus Mwizarubi, Christoph Hamelmann and Klinton Nyamuryekung'e

---

- Why are truck stops considered high-transmission areas?
- What is social mapping?
- Who can become a peer health educator?
- What kind of health learning materials are needed?
- Why is a community approach more effective than a target group approach?

High-transmission areas play a key role in the spread of HIV in Africa: they are nodal points, feeding the rural epidemic. Work in these areas is therefore a means to achieve an intervention with high levels of impact. This chapter presents implementation experience in establishing project sites: the recruitment of peer health educators, training and motivation, monitoring and evaluation, health learning materials development and distribution, condom promotion, STD services and project sustainability issues. Experiences from similar interventions in other areas of Tanzania and other countries are also incorporated.

The importance of high-transmission areas

HIV is not evenly distributed within populations or geographical areas. The pattern of distribution is related to social, economic and ecological factors. Population movement, population density, border areas, urbanization, poverty, civil disturbances such as war, imbalance of the sexes and the pattern of social networks and life-styles are all important in determining the dynamics of the epidemic and the resulting levels of prevalence.

Certain situations may promote commercial (paid) and transactional sex (in return for favours or goods) as well as occupations or life-styles that can lead to frequent sexual partner change and/or multiple partners. These types of sex are more common when women lack adequate sources of income and, at the same time, many men have a ready source of income and are separated from their wives or cannot form stable partnerships. Obbo (1) has described the pattern of HIV transmission in Rakai, Uganda's hardest hit district, where important factors are distance from fishing villages, rural townships on roads to Kampala, small rural centres and movement of soldiers, traders and migrant labourers. She also described the effects of these factors on migrant labourers' and soldiers' home areas after they return. She was able to identify two 'socio-geographic mating networks': an urban network based on people attending secondary school together and a rural one based on neighourhoods.

Several studies in Tanzania, Kenya, Zambia and Uganda have shown high levels of sexually transmitted disease and HIV among long-distance truck drivers and their assistants, commercial sex workers, bar and guesthouse workers, miners, fishermen, soldiers, migrant labourers and smugglers (2, 3). For example, a study of lorry drivers travelling from Mombasa to Uganda, Zaire, Rwanda or Burundi shows how one mobile group of individuals contributes to the spread of HIV infection across national boundaries, via trading routes, and takes the infection into local communities (4).

When high-transmission areas have been identified, this knowledge can be put to good use: targeting resources specifically to these areas can produce highly cost-effective interventions. For example, an ethnographic study of the truck stop environment in Tanzania found that the growth of the Tanzanian highway system brought outside investment. This created a service sector (hotels, bars, petrol stations and restaurants) which previously did not exist in the small towns. Commercial sex workers (including female bar workers, lodge attendants, women in brothels, local-brew sellers) migrate to truck stops from rural areas, but they also move between stops, to towns and back to their communities of origin (4). Further evidence of other higher transmission areas is provided by studies on the prevalence of STDs and HIV in gold mining areas, and in fishing posts in Tanzania (5).

With knowledge of the existence of these high-transmission areas, a national intervention project was developed in Tanzania in 1993. Five organizations, funded by various donors, are now working in different regions of Tanzania; coordination is provided by AMREF. The project aims at long-distance truck drivers, bar/guesthouse workers, travellers, mining and fishing populations, businessmen and workers at major construction sites; it provides information on HIV/AIDS risk awareness and the adoption of safer sexual practices, including condom use. Peer education is the main strategy employed in project implementation. In this chapter the experience is used to show how work in high-transmission areas can be organized.

Establishing project sites in high-transmission areas

The approach used in Tanzania to establish a high-transmission area project site involved community sensitization and social mobilization for support of the activities.

Step I: Community entry and sensitization
Before starting intervention activities, the community must be aware of the project's objectives, strategies, implementation issues and the role the community is expected to play. Project staff should hold meetings and make personal contact with local leaders or authorities in the community, including religious, traditional, health and educational leaders, and business owners.

Possible target groups include bar and guesthouse workers, and women working in brothels; men and women involved in petty trade; youth, both in and out-of-school; local groups such as choirs, football teams and dancing groups. They should be contacted to solicit their views and perceptions of HIV/AIDS/STD, and to gauge their interest in participation in intervention activities. Care should be taken that they are not made to feel targeted and stigmatized. Contacts should be informal, and take place through such methods as observation, focus group discussions or meetings, and interviews with key informants (see Box 1). The objective is to sensitize and mobilize the community – to increase awareness, knowledge and interest so that people become interested in working with the project.

Box 1. Commercial sex workers as informants

Information on commercial sex workers, brothels and guesthouse activities is probably most accurately acquired through peer health educators. In a project in Tanzania a 'snowball' technique was used: one commercial sex worker identified colleagues who identified still others. These 'informants' made it possible to get information on the number, origin and background, and organization of sex workers.

The project recruited commercial sex workers from different establishments. These women were trained as peer educators and were then able to elicit information on sensitive questions such as:

- Who are the clients and where do they come from?
- What negotiation and/or payment takes place?
- Is there any harassment by police, local leaders or others?
- What are the common sexual practices (vaginal, oral, anal, traditional practices)?
- Which places are used for sexual intercourse (brothels, guesthouses, commercial sex workers' residences)?
- Who are the gatekeepers (key persons influencing decision making)? What is the role of bar owners?

The data collected made it possible to construct a picture of the social interaction network involved, showing the important transmission sites on a village map as well as any services available (e.g. dispensary, clinic or private practitioners).

Step 2: Physical and social mapping
The process of mapping enables the project staff to understand the high-transmission area community – its location and the sexual and other social dynamics related to HIV/AIDS/STD infection – and to gather baseline data upon which intervention strategies, messages, and training sessions will be built. The baseline survey should reveal gaps related to knowledge, attitudes and practice. At the same time, it can help to increase

community awareness. Specific, detailed methods should be prepared by project staff or the implementing organization, with help from the community.

Data can be collected using both qualitative and quantitative instruments, including observation, focus group discussions, open-ended and structured interviews, face-to-face information collection and a review of records, depending on the nature of the target group. Information is needed on:

- location: it is important to accurately enter the name of the locality for future record-keeping purposes;
- geography: region, district, division, ward, village (list name plus distance from a town);
- type of settlement: trading centre, truck stop, fishing camp;
- historical background: how it came into being and how it is developing or declining;
- population: an estimate of numbers of people, age, sex, migration characteristics;
- social structures: ethnic groups, religious denominations, women's and youth groups, cultural groups;
- economic activities: trading, shops, wholesale businesses, alcohol brewing and selling; age and sex divisions in occupations; types of farming; markets;
- commercial sex: sex workers, guesthouses, brothels (see Box 1).
- HIV/AIDS/STD prevalence rates, if any data are available; STD types and local names; groups infected and their treatment-seeking behaviour; drugs and local herbs used.
- Orphans/homeless children: estimated numbers and any available services for them.
- Initial target groups: e.g. truck drivers, sex workers.
- Knowledge, attitudes, behaviour, practices (KABP) studies. Areas of information include knowledge of HIV transmission, misconceptions, condom use, risk perception, preventive measures taken (see Box 2).
- Condoms: availability, accessibility, cost, acceptability, community perceptions.

Box 2. Addressing misconceptions about HIV/AIDS/STDs

Misconceptions or lay health beliefs concerning HIV/AIDS/STDs will continuously be uncovered and need to be addressed in educational sessions. These misconceptions undermine prevention activities and contradict information, education and communication (IEC) messages (7). Persistent misconceptions include:

- Mosquitoes or bed bugs can transmit HIV virus.
- Men cannot get AIDS from fat women, women from rural areas or schoolgirls.
- Men cannot be infected if they ejaculate outside their partner and then drink a lot of water.
- Condoms are deliberately impregnated with HIV during manufacture.
- A healthy looking person cannot be infected or transmit HIV.
- Anal sex is a safer practice. (Studies conducted in 1990 and 1991 showed that the proportion of commercial sex workers and truck drivers reporting anal sex increased from 37% to 57% and 37% to 55%, respectively.)

Step 3: Community motivation and support for the intervention
Data collected during community sensitization meetings and physical and social mapping can be analysed and used in planning the intervention. Motivator meetings can be held, making use of these data to solicit community support and participation. The data (e.g. STD prevalence) will facilitate presentation, problem analysis and planning preventive measures. The strategy used is usually participatory problem-solving.

Motivator meetings should be attended by local leaders, influential persons and religious leaders. Their potential role is highlighted and discussed. The goal is to obtain the agreement of all or most to play their part in the intervention. For example, they might be asked to provide sites for educational sessions or video/film show halls, to give permission for their employees to attend sessions, or to allow posting of educational materials and condom distribution in their buildings. Securing this support is not always easy (see Box 3).

Box 3. Convincing bar owners

In one truck stop a bar annex guesthouse owner would not allow his employees to attend educational sessions, especially those on condom use, even though the sessions were being conducted on his premises. It was only after long consultations that his religious convictions against condoms were overcome and he allowed his bar workers to attend the sessions without the risk of losing their jobs.

Motivator meetings should also be used as training opportunities for local leaders and business owners. Training content might include:
- basic information on HIV/AIDS/STDs;
- HIV/STD preventive measures;
- social and economic impact of HIV/AIDS;
- basic counselling skills and care;
- condom use, disposal, storage;
- project goal, objectives and strategies;
- project monitoring and evaluation;
- motivator roles and responsibilities.

Motivator meetings can also be used to request that business owners extend invitations to their employees to attend a target group meeting. The date, time, venue and duration of the meeting should be given.

Step 4: The target group meeting and selection of peer health educators
The main objective of target group meetings is to identify peer health educators (PHEs). PHEs are members of the target group who share similar concerns, life experiences,

expectations, values and norms. Peer educators are agents for behaviour change, and can serve as models among their peers who provide credible dissemination of information, using the same language (see Box 4) and sharing the same situation as the target group: information regarding HIV/STD prevention is more likely to be seen as relevant and acceptable when it is given by someone with similar life experiences rather than by an outsider. Also, because peer educators live and work at project sites, they can provide consistency and continuity in AIDS education and social support among peer group members.

Box 4. Expressions used by commercial sex workers at truck stops

Mimi siwezi kumpa kwa jirani: 'I cannot give him to the neighbour', said by a woman, meaning she cannot indulge in anal sex.
Zungumza na huyo dereva, hatari sana kupima oil: 'Talk with that driver, he is very smart/he likes measuring oil', meaning the driver was a sex maniac.
Leo wamekula stafu: 'Today they have eaten staff service', said by a woman, meaning they have had sexual intercourse with her without payment.

Peer educators can be found by using various techniques. They may be identified in target group meetings or in motivator meetings. In either case people may volunteer to become peer educators, and the group may vote on candidates. Another method is to identify potential peer educators ahead of time and ask for them to be approved at the meeting. In our experience, motivator meetings tend to suggest bar/guesthouse owners, managers, relatives, or children of local leaders as peer educators. Occasionally, professionals such as health workers and teachers are identified as peer educators at motivator meetings. Target group meetings, attended by target group members, are more likely to produce real peer educators, for example, bar and guesthouse attendants, women working in brothels or involved in petty trading, including selling local brew. Criteria for identifying PHEs include:
- being a member of one of the target groups;
- being acceptable to peers and the high-transmission area community;
- having a basic primary school education or literacy skills;
- being willing to work on a voluntary basis.

Peer educators are a vital link to the community. Health staff should consider PHEs as their field counterparts: relate to them in a friendly manner, work with them harmoniously (and not in a military style), address their problems and exercise patience. However, one constraint experienced in peer education is attrition. For example, in our project at least 15% of PHEs dropped out of the project during 1993–1994. Reasons for dropping out include: being outside the peer group, marriage, finding better opportunities elsewhere or other mobility, employment termination or illness. On the other hand, an attrition rate of 15% is quite low for doing such work on a voluntary basis. This suggests that peer educators find rewards in the programme, including the feelings of self-worth, friendship and community they may gain from it.

Step 5: Peer health educator training

Once our PHEs are identified and selected they undergo a one or two day training session as a brief orientation to peer education. Orientation has been more successful when given immediately after selection rather than delayed. Enthusiasm is maintained and high morale is apparent during training activities.

Initial orientation can be conducted when work in a high-transmission area is established or when two or three neighbouring high-transmission areas can be grouped together. The main components of PHE orientation include:
- basic information on HIV/AIDS;
- preventive measures;
- condom use;
- communication skills, including the use of educational materials.

After six months or a year PHEs should attend a zonal or regional training session. In our case, this training session is a one-week residential programme, enabling PHEs to share implementation experiences, problems encountered and solutions attempted.

The session covers the items of the orientation programme in more detail, and provides an introduction to project monitoring and evaluation, and familiarization with tools and techniques. Participants share information in the course of drawing maps of high-transmission areas and in the process come to understand their area better. Gender sensitization can also be included. The methodology employed in zonal/regional training sessions includes demonstrations, role plays, drama, practical sessions (for this reason training should be held in one of the high-transmission areas) and case studies. The improved lecture method (as described in Chapter 12) is also used, but as little as possible.

Ideally all PHEs who work within one organization also receive a one-week, third-level central training session. We draw the content from zonal/regional training sessions and cover national or international issues pertaining to HIV/AIDS/STD control, such as women and AIDS, AIDS-day themes and Ministry of Health policy issues. However, due to financial limitations and the geographical locations of high-transmission areas, central training sessions have not been conducted by all organizations involved in our project.

Health learning materials

PHEs' communication with their peers is verbal. Due to the sensitivity of the content (HIV/AIDS/STD) and issues pertaining to sexuality, PHEs prefer person-to-person encounters and small group discussions using interactive techniques such role plays, drama, songs and poems.

To enhance PHE verbal communication, educational materials have been used such

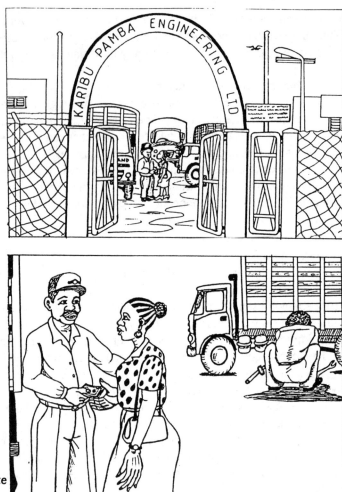

A commercial sex worker and a truck driver negotiate sex at a truck stop.

as posters, stickers, booklets, ashtrays, key-holders, recorded cassettes with AIDS songs/ messages, leaflets, brochures, wearable items including T-shirts, *khanga* (a women's traditional printed cloth) and caps, and PHE carrier bags. Even though lack of funding places constraints on the development of health learning materials, care should be taken to be sure that the educational materials used by and given to PHEs and target groups is appropriate. Materials not considered relevant by target groups have ended up being used for wrapping up things like buns or salt!

Experience has shown that truck drivers and commercial sex workers do not like bulky materials such as books. They prefer comic illustrations, posters, leaflets, wearable items, lorry stickers and key-holders. A mid-term evaluation revealed that truckers and commercial sex workers found one series of posters, depicting a family scene with changing messages, monotonous and recommended that it be changed.

Health learning materials should also be culturally sensitive. For example, miners at Mererani-Arusha thought the booklet *Majuto ya Sande* ('Worries of Sande') targeted truck drivers, not them. A poster was also developed showing two Mererani miners drinking beer. During pre-testing miners did not identify themselves with the illustration because the men didn't have torches on their heads, which they saw as the sign of a Mererani miner. Their feedback was incorporated.

Round stickers have been used in the project aimed at increasing risk awareness among truck drivers and commercial sex workers. However, feedback questioned the use of Islamic names such as Abdallah in materials for HIV/AIDS/STD control. Due to patent restrictions no modifications could be made on one sticker and production was stopped. Health learning materials should also address knowledge, attitudes and behavioural gaps identified among target group members.

Condom promotion

Preventive measures include abstinence, fidelity, and safer sexual practices including condom use. Among truckers and commercial sex workers abstinence and fidelity are difficult to achieve through peer education strategies. However, PHEs have been effective in motivating condom use. During the pilot truck driver project, condom distribution increased steadily from less than 20,000 in June/July 1990 to 120,000 by December 1990. By August 1991, over 2 million condoms had been distributed along the Dar es Salaam–Tunduma highway and to two trucking companies in Dar es Salaam. At truck stops, guesthouse owners reported drivers requesting condom availability before booking rooms.

Condom promotion is carried out through PHE demonstrations of correct condom use, utilizing wooden penis models, role plays, small group discussions and ensuring condom availability in high-transmission areas. Distribution takes place at bar counters and guesthouse reception desks. In addition, a strip of four condoms is placed on a small table in rooms, along with a condom leaflet and reading materials on HIV/AIDS. Guestrooms have become small HIV/AIDS/STD libraries. Dispensers and individual contacts also serve as channels for condom distribution. PHEs are easily identified as 'mama or baba condom'. At first PHEs were shocked by this name but they have since become used to it. The main issue now in condom promotion is consistency in use, including use with regular partners (see Box 5). PHEs continue to work to change misconceptions about condoms among truckers and commercial sex workers, with emphasis on the risk of HIV/STDs from unprotected sex with regular or permanent partners. To this effect, T-shirts have been produced with an anti-AIDS message emphasizing condom use with regular partners: *Umdhaniaye siye ....Ndiye* (The one you think cannot be HIV positive might be the very one who infects you. Use a condom).

Box 5. Promoting consistent use of condoms

To be a highly effective HIV/STD preventive measure, condoms must be used consistently in all sexual encounters and throughout each act. Several problems affecting the
use of condoms were identified in the truck stop programme. Truckers and
commercial sex workers reported:
- less condom use with regular or permanent partners;
- removing the condom before ejaculation;
- using a condom during the first round only;
- truckers cutting off the tip of the condom because they claim they cannot throw
  away their children or that their sexual partners need the semen.

Promotion of STD treatment-seeking behaviour

When we considered ways to deliver STD services along transport routes in Tanzania,
the main question was which strategy would be most acceptable to commercial sex
workers. A study conducted along the Dar es Salaam–Makambako–Njombe highway
showed that commercial sex workers prefer to seek STD services outside conventional
health facilities. Thus, in our project PHEs discuss common signs, symptoms and
complications of STDs and, after making a risk assessment, they refer potential patients
to health units or treatment centres. Women are advised to seek STD examination and
treatment even when no symptoms are present, since many STDs are assymptomatic. In
the coming years, financial and technical donor assistance via the coordinated NGO
network will make it possible to extend STD treatment to women in all high-transmission
areas throughout the country.

Monitoring and evaluation

Monitoring and evaluation in the project are aimed at following up the implementation
progress of project operations and identifying ways to improve implementation. Monitoring covers the distribution of project materials such as condoms, the implementation of
specific activities such as project site establishment, identifying PHEs (and their support
and training), the performance of those in charge of implemention and the participation
of group members. Project implementation has three levels: PHEs and their communities
(community level), implementing organizations (field staff level), and the coordinating
unit (central level). A coordination unit has been established and a computer-aided data
collection, processing and evaluation project monitoring instrument developed. Monthly
data collection and analysis starts at the community level and flows to the central level
using pre-coded forms. Codes for these forms were developed in collaboration with
project staff.

During implementation of the monitoring system some problems occurred. Working with codes was not feasible at the community level, and PHEs now collect data by recording in ordinary language the distribution of educational materials and condoms, activities accomplished and the like, using register books. This information is transferred to project monitoring forms with the support of project staff, who can analyse the information and act on the information during supervisory visits.

At the level of implementing organizations, constraints included a lack of accessible computer equipment, lack of computer competence (program installation problems and operational problems), delay or non-submission of diskettes to umbrella unit, no feedback to PHEs or no relevant use made of data. Computer training has solved some of these problems.

We therefore recommend using simple monitoring instruments, developed in a participatory process that includes local leaders. These may be administrative tools enabling PHEs to report on the use of educational materials, condom distribution and activities carried out during the reporting period. Findings should be fed back to those who collected the data and used to strengthen peer education; monitoring is best used to assure that resources go where they are needed, not to identify faults (see also Chapter 1).

Sustainability of peer education

A sustainable project is one in which the core project activities are continued by the community after donor funding support ceases. Core activities include:
- information, education and communication on HIV/AIDS/STDs within the community using the peer model;
- promotion, availability and use of condoms (both free and those promoted by 'social marketing');
- procurement and distribution of health learning materials.

A mid-term evaluation showed that the truck stop project was heavily dependent on external funding and input, and was thus not likely to be sustained after external funding was reduced. Therefore, project staff have started establishing structures and mechanisms for project sustainability at truck stops. These include the establishment of AIDS advisory committees, women's health groups and income-generating activities using social marketing of condoms, and attempts to integrate these into existing health structures such as village health committees. That is, to support and sustain core activities it is advisable to establish groups such as the following:

- AIDS advisory committee: formed by community members themselves; has overall responsibility for project implementation at community level. This should be a small group consisting of activists in HIV/AIDS control in the high-transmission area, who are ready to contribute and offer voluntary services. The committee provides an informal forum for meeting and exchanging ideas. Local leadership and health workers are represented on it.
- Women's health group: formed by women in high-transmission areas, starting with

commercial sex workers and later expanding to include other women in the high-transmission area. These groups will be channels for AIDS education, STD services, family planning services, recreational activities and later will be incorporated into income-generating activities.

- Income-generating activities: the economic empowerment of women can be expected to enhance their capacities for safer sex negotiation. If women's groups were to participate in the social marketing of condoms, it might generate additional funds for AIDS programme activities.

It may be too early to assess the feasibility of these structures and mechanisms for achieving project sustainability in high-transmission areas in Tanzania. It is increasingly being felt that the task of establishing structures for sustaining HIV/AIDS control activities will require more time. Success in achieving project sustainability will finally depend not only on community response but also on the impact of government structures, such as health services for STD control.

Conclusion

The Tanzania HIV high-transmission area intervention project in truck stops is a good example of collaboration among various donors and a network of implementing organizations being used to successfully tackle a large and complicated problem. It also shows the multiple constraints that need to be anticipated when working in high-transmission areas. Such areas have certain features which make community-based and sustainable project planning and implementation more difficult than in other communities.

The first major lesson learned was that in high-transmission areas there are often many mobile young people. They are used to taking risks and are not likely to change their behaviour rapidly. These communities have many members who have come from somewhere else, as well as many temporary or transient members; this makes traditional or governmental organizational structures less effective. Each high-transmission area has its own specific characteristics. Because truck stops are situated along highways, mobility is even greater there than in other high-transmission areas. Truck drivers and their assistants only stay for a short while. Female commercial sex workers are highly mobile as well. Fishermen are used to risking their lives, making nightly boat trips on an unpredictable lake or ocean. Taking risks is part of their daily life and messages aimed at changing their sexual behaviour or alcohol use may not come across easily.

A second lesson is that it is important to consider the whole population of a high-transmission area and not just target groups like men in high-risk professions and commercial sex workers. Experience in the truck stop project and other areas such as fishing villages has shown that virtually the whole adolescent and adult populations of such villages are at increased risk of HIV and STD infection. Focusing on the population as a whole may also be more successful, as it avoids the problem of stigmatization of high-risk subgroups. Finally, addressing the whole community increases the prospect of sustainability. However, it is difficult for interventions in high-transmission areas to be sustained by the community alone: additional funding and support are required. Such support is justified, if only because high-transmission areas continue to play a key role in the spread of HIV in Africa. High-transmission areas feed the rural epidemic, and without strong interventions in these areas HIV transmission cannot be reduced significantly.

Further reading and resources

AIDSTECH. *STD/AIDS peer educator training manual*, 1992. Can be ordered from: Family Health International, P.O. Box 13950, Research Triangle Park, NC 27709, USA; National AIDS Control Programme, Ministry of Health, P.O. Box 9083, Dar es Salaam, Tanzania; AMREF, P.O. Box 2773, Dar es Salaam, Tanzania.

Obbo C. HIV Transmission through social and geographical networks in Uganda. *Social Science and Medicine* 1993, 36: 949–955, 1993.

References

1. Obbo C. HIV Transmission through social and geographical networks in Uganda. *Social Science and Medicine* 1993, 36: 949–955, 1993.

2. Mbugua GG, Muthami LN, Mutura GW et al. Epidemiology of HIV infection among long distance truck drivers in Kenya. *East African Medical Journal* 1995, 72: 515–518.

3. Carswell JW, Lloyd G, Howells J. Prevalence of HIV-1 in East African lorry drivers. *AIDS* 1989, 3: 759–761.

4. O'Connor P, Leshabari MT, Lwihula G. *Ethnographic study of the truck stop environment in Tanzania.* Durham USA, Family Health International, AIDSTECH, *1992.*

5. Barongo L, Senkoro K, Boerma JT. *HIV infection and sexual behaviour in four fishing villages on Lake Victoria, Tanzania. Report of a cross-sectional survey.* Mwanza, 1995.

6. Nicoll A, Laukamm-Josten U, Mizarubi B et al. Lay health beliefs concerning HIV/AIDS – a barrier for control programmes. *AIDS Care* 1993, 5.

9 Addressing gender and gender-related issues

Dorica Balyagati and Dick Schapink

- Why do women require special attention in AIDS programmes?
- Are men and women equally well-informed about AIDS?
- Are women's groups an important resource?
- How can gender awareness be promoted in a district?
- Is it worthwhile to try to strengthen the socioeconomic position of women?

Gender issues are an essential element in planning behavioural interventions aimed at preventing HIV transmission. As shown in Chapter 5, a gender perspective is necessary to understand sexual behaviour and to develop appropriate interventions.

Gender-based programmes that strengthen or improve the position of women by working with both men and women can increase the effectiveness of interventions. For example, messages to promote reduction in the number of sexual partners (be faithful) or condom use need to be directed at men as well as women. AIDS programmes using this approach can be much more gender-sensitive than family planning programmes, which for the past three decades have predominately focused on women.

Yet, the important differences between women and men necessitate special work with women in district AIDS programmes. This chapter therefore describes not only approaches that can be used to promote gender awareness in district AIDS programmes, but also interventions aimed at advocacy and mobilization to enhance the socio-economic status of women, improving reproductive health services, and information and communication to involve women.

Important gender-related differences

A survey is the most common methodology used to assess differences in male-female knowledge, attitudes and risk perception concerning AIDS and sexual behaviour. WHO has developed a standard set of questions (1) which has been used in many countries. The results of such surveys often show a similar picture when it comes to gender differences:

- *Knowledge*: both men and women know about AIDS and that HIV can be transmitted by sexual intercourse. Not everyone knows that a person who looks healthy may have AIDS, however, and women are often less likely than men to have more detailed knowledge. For example, in surveys in Togo and Burundi men reported higher levels of exposure to information than women, both through the media and through more frequent discussions among friends (1).
- *Risk perception*: more men than women feel personally at risk of AIDS. In addition, their reasons for feeling at risk differ. Among men, having multiple partners is the most common reason, while among women multiple partners are not frequently mentioned. They more often feel at risk when they consider their partners unfaithful.
- Sexual behaviour: a much larger proportion of men indulge in high-risk sexual behaviour (multiple partners) than women. Although under-reporting of multiple partners by women is thought to be common (due to different norms regarding promiscuous behaviour, see Chapter 5), it is generally accepted that promiscuous behaviour is more common among men.

Because women have poorer access to information and risk HIV infection through their partners, special interventions (see Box 1) may be necessary for them.

Box 1. Women's knowledge and risk perception

Campaigns to change behaviour in Mwanza, Tanzania, have had difficulty reaching women because women are not supposed to talk in front of men. This implies that in mixed audiences men's views prevail. In addition, basic prevention messages such as: 'be faithful, reduce the number of partners and/or use condoms in relationships of risk' were not really relevant for a large proportion of women because of their subordinate position to men, who controlled these issues in relationships.

Because basic behaviour change messages did not coincide with most women's decision-making power in relationships, they either developed wrong risk perceptions or ignored safer sex practices. Questionnaires distributed among women in urban and rural areas, and workshops with women leaders revealed that many married women who were at risk due to the promiscuous behaviour of their partners did not perceive themselves to be at risk. They thought only women who are promiscuous, single and/or prostitutes are at risk. Unmarried women and those who engaged in sex work realized they were at risk but found it difficult to change behaviour because of their strong dependence on economic support from multiple partners for survival. Women also found it extremely difficult to negotiate for safer sex through condom use because they may be branded as prostitutes and stigmatized if they demand that condoms be used.

Interventions

Several interventions can be used to address gender issues and the specific needs of women in the context of the AIDS epidemic. Activities should:

- Promote gender awareness, especially by advocating that women have the right to discuss sexual issues with their partners, such as the practices of having multiple partners and extra-marital relationships; they should also support a norm allowing women to protect themselves and their families, and to be protected through responsible behaviour by their partners.
- Advocate and mobilize resources to enhance women's socioeconomic status in the community, including income-generating activities for the most vulnerable groups, decision-making power in matters related to development and ways for men and women to share the workload, especially the responsibility to care for the sick.
- Mobilize resources to improve women's access to good quality, accessible and affordable reproductive health services and to meet their needs for information on health issues.
- Improve women's access to information and communication on health issues to narrow gender differences in acquiring knowledge.

Promoting gender awareness

The process of gender analysis
To provide a context for promoting gender awareness, data should be gathered on gender inequalities from a health perspective, a cultural perspective and a socio-economic perspective as described in Chapter 5. Here we will focus on the process of carrying out a gender analysis. Making such an analysis can be seen as an intervention in itself. Gender sensitivity is often low among project staff as well as in communities and among the target groups for HIV prevention programmes. A gender analysis therefore is the start of an ongoing learning process involving both project staff and target audiences. The most important point is to get people to start thinking about gender and its role in HIV prevention.

Several methods can be used for gender analysis. Questionnaires to get at issues like those outlined in Chapter 5 can help provide an impression about what women and men think and know about HIV/AIDS, the differences in their access to information, and how they perceive their personal risks and possibilities for prevention. After analysing questionnaires, workshops can be organized with both women and men representatives to verify the findings. It may also be useful to hold separate workshops for men and women, especially when women find it difficult to talk in the presence of men.

Another method is to use various types of group interviews in meetings or work-shops. Box 2 lists six possibilities. The dynamics of group interaction among members are important aspects of all these methods. In practice, a combination should be used to overcome the limitations of each method.

Box 2. Types of group interviews[a]

Natural group	A group which already exists: perhaps project staff who know each other well. Meetings are usually informal and notes are taken rather than using audiotapes.
Community interview	Most widely used in projects, with discussion open to all or large segments of a community. The interviewer uses a structured question guide. There is little interaction among the public. Usually notes are taken, rather than making audiotapes.
Brainstorming	Can be used to generate examples of ideas and norms concerning female and male characteristics, abilities and (proper/improper) behaviour.
Drama performances	An example of action research. The audience may be mixed or of a single sex. A gender-sensitive problem is presented in a short role play. Afterwards, a facilitator discusses with the audience whether they recognize the problem, what the possible consequences may be and what can be done about it in the community.
Consensus panel	Key informants from health committees, including opinion leaders and experts can be invited to act as panel members. Seeks responses to the question of how AIDS affects men and women differently within the cultural context.
Nominal group	Encourages individual reflection followed by group consensus, which may be differentiated according to gender. A good way to stimulate participation.
Focus group	Participants are selected from the target groups of a project and preferably do not know each other well. The discussion identifies facts, feelings, meanings and solutions in a controlled order, and can be audiotaped and transcribed for analysis. Discussion is open-ended and seeks to identify differences more than to achieve consensus.

Source: adapted from (2)

[a] More information about these techniques can be found in the 'Further reading' at the end of the chapter (see IIED and KIT).

An action research and intervention method that was particularly useful in Mwanza, Tanzania, used drama performances followed by focus group discussions with the audience (either single sex or mixed). For research purposes the audiences' reactions should be closely monitored by making a record (written or taped) of all questions, including the different reactions of men and women after the performance. Since it is often difficult to make an accurate record, someone with social science training should be appointed, if possible, to take notes and/or to audiotape and analyze the interviews. It is also helpful if an anthropologist or other social scientist can be involved in the analysis of transcriptions.

Community risk behaviour mapping exercise. Constructing a map of risky places in the community is a good way to involve the community in discussion, as well as to provide information. Mapping can be done by men and women separately, followed by discussions on the different problems the two groups face in avoiding risk behaviour. In Mwanza, Tanzania, such mapping led to an effective analysis and action being taken after men's and women's groups exchanged their maps and held discussions with each other. Mapping was arranged as a low-cost intervention for the whole district. From this process it became clear that women and girls are much more sensitive to the dangers of HIV infection than men and boys, and they are also more actively seeking solutions. A mapping intervention gives women a way to explain themselves better and translate this directly into action. The steps we used in the process of mapping and discussing risky places in the community are given in Box 3.

Training for gender sensitization
Gender sensitization has two phases: community workers are likely to need gender sensitization as a preliminary step before beginning their work in helping community members to become more aware of gender issues. The results of the gender analysis should be used in deciding what sort of gender sensitization is needed and what training will be required. Health workers, peer health educators and/or community educators may need training to enable them to start the second phase: to organize health education sessions in which gender issues are integrated. Both phases of gender sensitization training can focus on:
- attitudes towards promiscuity of men and women;
- age differences in transmission;
- inequality in relationships between men and women, especially with regard to decision making;
- obstacles to behavioural change for men and women, such as economic insecurity and its effects on sexual behaviour;
- negotiating safer sexual practices and condom use
- empowerment of women.

The methods listed in Box 2 can also be used for gender sensitization. Picture codes (which show gender-related problems about which people have strong emotions) and drama are very useful in discussing gender differences and related problems.
To sensitize the community about gender issues a drama group can be trained to act out gender-related behaviour problems. In Mwanza these groups first held performances for women's groups before giving general community performances. Training and development of gender-specific drama forms such as theatre plays and role playing, as well as the questions for discussion, require gender specialist support. In societies heavily dominated by men, it may be advisable to make women responsible for this task since it is more difficult for men to personalize and practise gender-sensitive behaviour.

Box 3. Steps used in a mapping exercise in Mwanza, Tanzania

1   Participants for a mapping exercise can be selected in various ways. One possibility is to divide an existing group into males and females. Then females decide on females in the community who can assist them in the mapping exercise. Males decide on males in the community and work with them in completing the exercise. The women's team and the men's team should each include at least eight people, of different ages. They should be knowledgeable about the community in general and about risk behaviours in particular; this makes it important to select the participants with care.
Steps 2–8 are to be carried out by each team, working separately.

2   For each team: draw a map of your community/subvillage; use black pencil or ink to show boundaries, roads, churches, markets and other important sites.

3   Group work – questions to discuss:
    – what risk behaviours take place in our community/subvillage?
    – where do we feel at risk?
    – where do risk behaviours take place/where are they negotiated?
       (include places you know of outside the community but nearby)

4   Indicate on the map where risk behaviours take place and/or are negotiated, and where participants feel unsafe or at risk of contracting HIV/AIDS:
    – girls and women show these places using a *blue* pencil;
    – boys and men show these places on the map using a *red* pencil.

5   Identify places where people can get HIV/AIDS and STD information/services/assistance/condoms.
    – show these places on the map using a *green* pencil.

6   Each team discusses the problems they face in avoiding risk behaviours. List these problems beside the map.

7   Discuss possible actions: what could be done in the community to start changing risk conditions? Write these possibilities below the list of problems.

8   Each team presents its map and the results of its discussions to the other team, for discussion by the group as a whole.

There is no need to reach consensus, but it is important to try and understand the differences (or apparent differences) in the conclusions of the two teams. What is essential is for the group as a whole to try and reach conclusions on action that will address the needs of the community as a whole, including women and girls, boys and men.

Women are used to anticipating men's wishes and demands, thus they are likely to have a good idea of male expectations and behaviour, and may therefore be more powerful educators on gender issues. Gender-specialist teams, consisting of a woman and a man, may also be useful.

Gender education using gender-sensitive drama

In most African cultures, drama is a popular means of getting messages across. In Tanzania *ngonjera* (poems) are very popular. Theatre plays are normally accompanied by songs and poems. Before a show starts drums are used to alert people. Culturally well-known drama forms are especially powerful. Often there are many people with expertise in developing role plays, poems, ngonjera and songs; however, special efforts are needed to develop their gender sensitivity and to update artists on HIV/AIDS issues. Many artists may prefer to create powerful theatre by instilling fear in the community, but positive and open-ended messages that present the audience with a choice are more apt to promote changes in behaviour. Special training is necessary to develop skills to shorten role plays, which tend to be too long, and to facilitate discussions afterwards.

To develop gender-sensitive drama forms it is necessary to identify problems in the community that are related to gender inequality. Groups of women and men may be asked to identify obstacles to behaviour change. These obstacles can then be analysed to determine which have their roots in gender differences. A person trained in gender analysis should assist the drama group in analysing and developing messages. Experience has shown that performances for selected audiences (in most cases women, in closed surroundings) can be instrumental in analysing the cultural gender specifics of behaviour problems. This approach can also be used as a pre-test before plays are performed for a wider and/or mixed sex audience.

Advocacy and mobilization to enhance the socioeconomic status of women

In addition to increasing overall gender awareness, other areas of specific importance to women need to be addressed. Since community leaders are the guardians of cultural norms and values it is important to specifically involve them. These leaders can subsequently assist in addressing the community on gender-related obstacles to behaviour change. It is important to ensure representation of women on committees that deal with village development issues in general or with AIDS issues in particular. An example of involving local leaders is presented in Box 4.

HIV infection is often directly linked to poverty, unemployment, and the dependence of women on sex work and multiple partners for their economic survival. Therefore, another important objective for community AIDS programmes is to assist youth and women with income-generating activities. It is important that communities try to mobilize local resources before district and outside help is negotiated. One role of HIV/AIDS programmes can be to assist committees with feasibility studies to establish what kind of economic activities are viable and can be recommended for support.

Box 4. Involving local leaders

As a first step in self-help activities, the village AIDS action committees in Magu District, Tanzania, visited their subvillages to inform community leaders and all those interested at a community meeting about the need for behaviour change. Originally they used a very formal approach in which the community was invited to attend a meeting on the problems of AIDS. After realizing the power of drama they changed this approach. They now show short role plays presenting behaviour problems which they have identified as problematic and discuss with the audience what should be done. In the process of analysing behaviour problems, the community has proved itself quite able to identify practical gender-related problems such as wife inheritance, alcohol abuse by males, sexual violence against women and girls, pressures for men to have multiple partners, and the economic insecurity of women and youth. The committees have found this to be an effective and enjoyable way of working with the community.

When the obstacles to and potential for such income-generating activities have been identified, communities can be assisted in mobilizing district resources. Advocacy can be directed to government departments, NGOs and district councils. District councils, for example, can be asked to include support for women's economic activities in their yearly planning and budgets (see Box 5).

Income-generating activities require support such as training in business skills and/or establishing a revolving fund for a mini-credit system. Activities should further be supported by participatory monitoring and evaluation systems (see Chapter 6) with the specific aim of promoting ownership of the support programme by the women involved.

Improving reproductive health services

Another issue specific to women is the need in many communities to improve reproductive health services. Reproductive health is a broad concept which includes responsible reproductive and sexual behaviour, widely available family planning services, effective maternal care and safe delivery, as well as effective control of sexually transmitted diseases including HIV/AIDS (3). As in any vertical programme, AIDS programmes may tend to focus too narrowly on one subject – in this case HIV and its sexual transmission. Although HIV/AIDS may be perceived as a problem by communities, it is often not seen as a priority. Thus programmes that include other elements of reproductive health may be more effective.

Box 5. Enhancing women's economic status

In Magu District, Tanzania, the community development department was asked to do a feasibility study on options for women's economic activities in fishing posts along Lake Victoria. Information was collected through individual interviews, reading available literature or documents, observation and focus group discussions with economically active women's groups.

The study showed that women were involved in a multitude of economic activities, including selling fried fish, ground nuts, local brew, firewood and food. Other sources of income were fishing, fish smoking, running retail shops and commercial sex. The activities were characterized as small hand-to-mouth businesses. Obstacles for women engaging in these activities were lack of technical and business skills, lack of investment capital and not being sufficiently perceived as having the potential to run a business ('because they are women'). However, after comparing women's activities in different fishing posts, the study concluded that there was considerable potential for the development of smoking, drying and selling fish, and for forestry activities. Advocacy for the idea of a programme to support these types of activities mobilized support from the Fisheries Department for licenses, from the Forestry Department for advice and support for tree growing, and from financial donors to establish a revolving fund for a mini-credit scheme. Feasibility workshops organized by the Community Development Department assisted women in assessing the choice of product or service to sell, finding the right market, how to operate the business, calculation of business expenses, estimates of sales income and assessment of business viability. Women calculated their own credit needs and in practice proved to be very reliable in paying back their loans.

HIV/AIDS prevention and control measures need to be integrated into MCH (maternal and child health) and family planning programmes. There they will reach many women who would otherwise not be exposed to AIDS education campaigns: the only health care-related advice some women receive is from MCH/FP (family planning) programmes, when they take their children there or seek health services for themselves during their reproductive lives. On the other hand, HIV/AIDS control programmes are much more successful in reaching men: this could benefit family planning programmes, which have mostly failed to involve fathers and potential fathers.
The gender dimension pervades all elements of reproductive health. It is obvious that women bear the brunt of the reproductive health burden. The consequences of STDs, which are often asymptomatic, are more profound among women than men. The consequences of childbearing and pregnancy for health are largely borne by women. Women are also more often victims of sexual abuse and sexual violence than men (see Chapter 5).

Antenatal and delivery care services are available in many places but tend to focus on female hormonal birth control methods that do not protect women against STDs. STD services are much more commonly used by men than women, even though STD prevalence (symptomatic or asymptomatic) is thought to be higher among women. Unwanted pregnancies may result in illicit abortions, which may be carried out in unhygienic circumstances with adverse consequences for women. Women who are victims of sexual violence often have no place to seek protection.

In summary, it is obvious that special efforts need to be made to increase the availability, accessibility and quality of reproductive health services. This includes providing health education to both women and men, training health staff on reproductive health issues, and integrating services. In some instances, it may be warranted to establish a special facility for certain groups of women or for all women. Experience with such centres in districts is limited and costs may be prohibitive. If such a centre is well integrated with local health services, however, costs need not be excessive. Such centres are probably more effective where fairly large groups of women are not reached by the regular system. Box 6 presents the experience of a women's centre in Tanzania.

Box 6. A women's centre

In Mwanza town, Tanzania, there are an estimated 1,000–1,500 female bar workers. Since these women were thought to play an important role in the spread of HIV/STDs and were not adequately covered by existing services, two organizations (AMREF and TANESA) supported the municipal health services in setting up a mobile STD service. After a few years it was decided to replace the mobile service with women's centres for female bar workers. Not only had women requested this; it was also a way to reduce costs. The centres offer medical care as well as a base for training peer educators and the community, counselling and testing services, social activities, and so forth. On women's requests and to further reduce costs, the centres are now expanding their services to include family planning, MCH and other services. The target population is also expanding to include other groups of women (such as female traders).

Information and communication for involving women in gender issues

Exchange of information on HIV/AIDS and STDs, and communication about gender issues can be facilitated by working with and/or establishing women's groups, which are an important entry point for addressing these issues.

Women's groups

Many districts have women's groups that can be involved in AIDS programmes. There are several reasons for doing this. First, educating women's groups is one way of disseminating AIDS information and reaching women. Second, the members of women's groups can be mobilized and trained to become community educators. Third, women's groups also can play a role in organizing home-based care programmes.

Mobilization of women's groups may be difficult because groups have different goals. Most organized women's groups in Mwanza, for example, consist of married women who have organized themselves with the aim of economic advancement. In addition, their risk perceptions do not generally provide enough motivation to mobilize them into action. However, sensitization on gender issues can change their risk perceptions and mobilize them to discuss these issues among themselves.

Some groups have more socio-cultural functions and have specialized in forms of drama aimed at delivering messages to the community. An example of this type of drama is given in Box 7. These cultural groups can be trained to sensitize the community on gender issues. Powerful groups include the formal or informal support groups that exist in most African cultures and aim to assist women in times of social or economic difficulty. These groups have good mobilization potential in the community. They can be trained on gender issues and given assistance to develop community-based home care programmes for people living with AIDS.

Mobilization of women's groups on gender issues and for home care initiatives can best be done using a specially trained gender drama group that is also trained to help women's groups develop action plans. Showing videos on gender issues, HIV/AIDS topics, counselling and home-based care can be instrumental in starting discussions and raising awareness. Workshops are another means to mobilize women's groups for action.

Box 7. Example of a gender-sensitive role play

One role play developed in Mwanza shows a husband (Baba Shida) who is always drunk and refuses to take responsibility for caring for his family. Instead he beats his wife (Mama Shida) when she asks for money for family expenses. She starts to make snacks to earn money to support her family, but her husband takes all the money she earns to buy drink. This situation leaves the wife helpless and she decides to return to her family home, but her parents send her back to her husband.

Use of picture codes
The development of picture codes follows the same process as the role plays. A behaviour problem about which strong emotions exist in the community is identified and a professional artist is asked to draw a picture of it, showing the problem without using words. Many of the illustrations in this book were developed in this way. It is essential to find an artist who is close to the target audiences culturally to ensure that they will recognize and relate to the pictures. Picture codes can be used by health workers and peer educators as discussion starters during health education sessions and community meetings. The basic questions for picture codes should be the focus of the discussion: What do you see happening in the picture? Is this happening in this community? Why is it happening? To what problems can it lead? What should be done about it?

Print media and newsletters

Although women seem to prefer receiving information by radio, and perhaps even more through discussions with friends, the demand for information on HIV/AIDS-related issues in the form of booklets and leaflets is substantial in many African societies. Newspapers primarily reach men. In rural areas women often do not have access to radios or newspapers. Due to economic hardships many are unable to buy books; even second-hand books are not affordable for many families.

Most projects fail to meet the demand for written materials. However, developing a newsletter for specific target groups such as women, youth or factory workers is a cost-effective way of informing people. It is essential to include the target group in the preparation and distribution of the newsletter. Topics for newsletters can be based on research findings concerning obstacles to prevention, and a target group's specific needs. (Work in discussion groups often suggests what these needs are.) For instance, a newsletter for women can include information on family planning, infertility, the effects of STDs on HIV transmission, vertical transmission of HIV, gender topics, cultural obstacles for prevention, how to raise sons and daughters in a way that provides them with equal opportunities and the obstacles to such upbringing.

Where most workers are male, topics for a newsletter for factory workers might focus more on obstacles to prevention among men. Alcohol, the price of promiscuity, family planning, HIV/AIDS policy in a factory, relationships between bosses and secretaries and forced sex may be topics of interest to them.

A newsletter for youth can address issues relevant for teenage boys and girls, such as adolescent dating issues, alcohol and drug abuse, unemployment problems and reproductive health issues. Other topics may be communication with parents, problems with teachers and sexual abuse.

Leaflets to address topics relevant for specific target groups should be developed. Topics can be identified from experience with interventions and research findings. Examples of topics are negotiating condom use, consequences of unprotected sex, legal issues such as inheritance, and other culturally determined practices.

Conclusion

Women require special attention in district HIV prevention and AIDS care programmes, because they have specific, different needs. This chapter has focused on the need to promote gender awareness, as well as the need for advocacy directed toward mobilizing more resources to enhance women's socioeconomic status. It also emphasizes the need to improve reproductive health services (in part by integrating services) and to pay special attention to gender in designing and carrying out specifically focused information, education and communication activities.

Ways to increase awareness of gender issues can include discussion groups, group interviews and mapping exercises. Drama, poems and pictures can be useful tools in identifying gender issues and starting discussions on these issues. In developing printed information, just as with drawings and other media, it is extremely important that the material is acceptable, recognizable and of interest to potential readers.

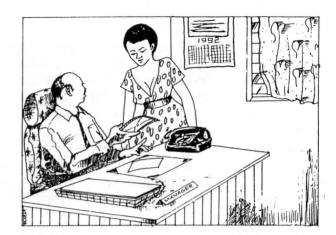

Sexual relationships in the workplace: boss proposing an affair to a secretary.

Further reading

Berer M, Ray S. *Women and AIDS: an international resource book.* London, AHRTAG, 1993.

Coreil J. Group interview methods in Community Health Research. *Medical Anthropology* 1995, 16: 193–210.

Cleland J and Ferry B (eds.). *Sexual behaviour and AIDS in the developing world.* Published on behalf of the WHO. London, Taylor & Francis, 1995.

References

1. Ingham R. AIDS: knowledge, awareness and attitudes. In: Cleland JC, Ferry B (eds.). *Sexual behaviour and AIDS in the developing world.* Published on behalf of the WHO. London, Taylor & Francis, 1995. pp. 75–123.

2. Coreil J. Group interview methods in community health research. *Medical Anthropology* 1995, 16: 193–210.

3. Khanna J, Van Look PFA, Griffin PD (eds.). *Challenges in reproductive health research. Biennial report 1992–1993.* Geneva, UNDP/UNFPA/WHO/World Bank.

10 Youth and HIV/AIDS programmes

Dick Schapink, Jumanne Hema and Bartimayo Mujaya

- Can youth be mobilized for behavioural change?
- What are the facts about sexual behaviour among youth?
- How can a schoolgirl be protected from the advances of older men?
- What is a student guardian?
- How can the majority of youth in a district be reached?

A significant proportion of new HIV infections occur in young people, especially young women. Thus, the AIDS epidemic has highlighted the need to reach district youth with effective sexual health and HIV prevention programmes. More importantly, educating youth, who may comprise up to 16% of the total population in developing countries, is an investment in the future. During the period of sexual and social maturation, special programmes make it possible to reach large numbers, and many countries have succeeded in using this 'window of opportunity' to build young people's knowledge about HIV transmission and prevention. The main challenge, however, is to achieve success in changing the behaviour which puts young people at risk of HIV infection.

This chapter outlines some of the specific features associated with the period of adolescence and what this implies for sex education and AIDS programmes. A district programme for primary schools is described, involving students, teachers, parents and the community, using the peer education approach. Including out-of-school youth in this approach is also discussed.

The period of adolescence

Adolescence has been defined as a period of transition from childhood to adulthood, marked by physical, psychological and social maturation. In this chapter people between 12 and 20 years are considered adolescents, but may also be referred to as youth or young people.

In most traditional societies the period of transition from childhood to adulthood was short. Very young people often took on the same responsibilities as adults. The change was often abrupt, marked by ceremonies of initiation which included practical instruction on adult behaviour and sex education. However, these young people were not provided with relevant sexual facts enabling them to make their own decisions, but rather were taught what was considered to be morally right (1).

The traditional pattern of sex education has been disrupted by social and economic changes: rapid urbanization, increased mobility, rapid population growth, education and the introduction of religions which are new to the community. Traditional systems are disappearing so quickly that new institutions to guide young people through the period of adolescence have not yet had enough time to develop. In this situation, parents may also feel left behind by the development of their children in adolescence.

To understand young people's behaviour it is necessary to understand the period of adolescence, the challenges it brings and the changes that come with it. Physical, mental and emotional development occur at different and uneven rates in adolescents. They become physically mature before they have fully developed the mental, emotional or social skills necessary to understand or practise safer sex behaviour. Social skills increase during adolescence; youth learn by interaction with others in society to show empathy, and to become more certain of their own beliefs and values. As part of the maturing process, young people often question established social norms and attitudes. Maturing also means developing one's own adult identity, as part of a gender-specific process. The process of changing from child to adult often takes the form of testing alternative views, behaviour and norms. As part of this process adolescents tend to increasingly identify themselves with peer group values or behaviour.

Risk taking may also be linked to 'rebellion' against adults, which is a normal part of teenagers' acquiring their own identity. The risks may differ among young people in different cultures, but often include experimentation with sexual activities, alcohol and drug abuse. Risk-taking behaviour among adolescents is strongly linked to the fact that the pleasure or importance of the moment may outweigh their ability to foresee or care about the long-term consequences of their actions. Because adolescence is a period in which an identity is being acquired, it is also a period of uncertainty. When young people have a sense of self-efficacy and self-esteem (rather than powerlessness and a sense of worthlessness), they are better able to make their own decisions: they have less need to 'prove themselves' to their peers by taking risks.

Adolescents and sexual activity

Survey data indicate that adolescents are sexually active: in most countries the median age at first intercourse is about 15–16 years, indicating that half of these youth have experienced sexual intercourse prior to that age. This means that a significant proportion of youth may be sexually active by ages 13–14. Therefore, postponing sex education to later in the adolescent period is not an effective strategy for coping with the problem of HIV/AIDS.

The common belief that sex and AIDS education can encourage sexual activity in young people can hamper the introduction of HIV/STD prevention programmes for them. However, a WHO review of 19 studies has shown that sex education increased neither the onset of intercourse nor its frequency, and in several studies it actually delayed the onset or frequency of sex (2). These factors, together with the high percentage of young people in developing country populations, make it extremely important for HIV programmes to consider targeting this age group for interventions.

Prerequisites for behavioural change

Projects using peer approaches have been identified by WHO as some of the most success-ful in promoting and assisting behaviour change to reduce the risk of HIV transmission. Much of the information youth receive on sexuality comes from peers. In view of this and other aspects of development during adolescence, a peer approach using peer educators can play an important role. Explicit HIV/AIDS education for young people and the promotion of condoms for sexually active adolescents is a controversial issue in many countries, and adults often find it difficult to address these issues with youth. In Tanzania, teachers were reluctant to give practical condom demonstrations to students, fearing loss of respect. Parents, however, easily agreed to the idea that youth would obey their teachers. Many projects have found that when youth are motivated for AIDS prevention and given the right support, they become eager to disperse information among themselves and capable of discussing the need for behaviour change. Experience in Tanzania, Zambia and Benin indicates that peer educators can play a vital role in educat-ing their own families and communities. Four prerequisites can be identified as key to health behaviour changes (3), as well as showing the importance of the peer approach:

Building knowledge. Basic knowledge is necessary, although this alone is not sufficient for behavioural change. Information should include HIV/STD transmission and preven-tion, the consequences of unprotected sex, sexuality and maturation of the two sexes. Particular behaviours which put youth at risk of HIV infection, and factors that make these more likely, need special attention, e.g. the apparent preference of some girls for sexual relations with older men. Since young people receive most of their knowledge related to sex from peers, these channels should be utilized to disseminate important information. When youth understand more about the role of peer pressure, they are more likely to be able to resist it and adopt a point of view which supports HIV prevention.

Perception of risk. Even though risk taking is a normal part of adolescent behaviour, a major component in motivating behavioural change is to have youth develop the perception that certain behaviours put them at risk. It is important to strengthen such perceptions as: unprotected sex leads to unwanted pregnancies, and also puts one at risk of HIV and STDs; however, this can be avoided by postponing sexual relations or by using condoms. It is advantageous to link the risk of HIV and STDs to the often more immediate risk and fear of becoming pregnant. It is also useful to educate youth about the fact that teenage pregnancies often involve more medical complications. Accepting material gifts in exchange for sexual favours may also be discussed as a risk behaviour. Selecting more mature peers to act as peer educators may help promote adequate perceptions of risk.

Perception of norms. During adolescence social maturity and skills are developing. Respecting group norms and gaining social acceptance are key issues in adolescent development. It is necessary that young people see the desired behaviour as acceptable and are convinced that others like them have adopted or are planning to adopt a particular behaviour (like postponing sex or using a condom). Safer sex practices have to be legitimized, by presenting them as the social norm accepted by those who are especially respected by the group ('everybody is changing behaviour, so you had better join the crowd'). It is important to link messages to what is actually happening among youth. The advantage of peer approaches to achieving behavioural change is that the norms of the group are automatically included.

Feeling of self-efficacy/self-esteem. Emotional and social maturity develop at uneven rates during adolescence, and are often poorly established in early adolescence. To be able to change behaviour young people need to have confidence, self-esteem and the belief that they can determine or change their behaviour. The ability to negotiate safer sex practices with one's partner is a key factor. This ability will be strengthened if the right to say 'no' is accepted by the community, including men and boys. This ability is negatively influenced by the exchange of material gifts between boys and girls, and even more so between adult men and girls. Gender differences with regard to decision making on safer sex practice, and age differences between partners hamper the power of girls to negotiate for safer sex (including such intimidating problems as how to approach discussing the use of a condom with a man who is 10 to 15 years older, or – worse yet – with one's teacher?). For adolescents, the peer group is a key reference and support group in the development of social skills. Skills to use in negotiating safer sex practices can be introduced and promoted by trained peer educators.

Targeting youth at district level

Developing behaviour interventions for youth in the adolescent age group at district level should focus on both in- and and out-of-school youth. The target group of youth attending school (12-19 years) is found in both primary and secondary schools. As shown in Box 1, it is not sufficient to focus on secondary schools alone: in fact programmes in secondary schools will reach only a minority of adolescents. Neither is it sufficient to focus exclusively on youth who attend school. A significant proportion of youth do not attend school at all, or drop out before reaching the higher levels of primary education.

Education systems differ from country to country, and large variations among primary schools with respect to age at enrolment may lead to large age differences among pupils in the higher classes of primary schools. Therefore an age at which primary school is typically completed cannot be given. Yet, the majority of children do attend primary schools; focusing on these youth offers a way of reaching large numbers. Ages 6–12 present a 'window of opportunity' in which it is easier to reach children. Intervention at this time is also apt to be successful in influencing later behaviour, and can create a cohort which will remain uninfected throughout their lives.

In sum, in most countries a two-pronged approach is needed to reach youth: a pro-
-amme directed at adolescents in the higher classes of primary and secondary schools,
a programme for out-of-school youth. Because countries vary with respect to children's
particular classes, programmes should target specific ages rather than classes.

Box 1. Schooling patterns among adolescents

- In Zimbabwe in 1994, 85% of rural girls aged 11–15 were enrolled in school; at ages 16–20 this dropped to 28% (4).
- In Malawi in 1992, 20% of boys aged 15–19 had never attended school, and only 4% were attending secondary school (5).
- In urban Nigeria in 1990, 66% of boys and 70% of girls aged 15–19 were not in school.
- In Zambia, in 1992, only 27% of boys and 24% of girls aged 15–19 had at least some secondary education (6).
- In a rural ward in Tanzania in 1994, 78% of girls aged 12–14 were in school, but only 45% of those aged 15–17 and 13% of those aged 18–20 (Kisesa, unpublished data).

School programmes

Peer education and counselling using peer health educators (PHEs) are at the core of interventions. The peer health educator programme we have developed for schools in Mwanza, Tanzania, came to have several components in addition to peer educators:

- Information and advocacy to parents and school authorities about adolescent development and the need for sex and AIDS education.
- Mobilization of partners for the AIDS programme (see below) including mobilization of schools to establish AIDS committees involving teachers, parents and community leaders. This should take place at the lower level of the education system, before a national curriculum is introduced.
- Peer education: formal and informal education activities.
- Scope for expanding out-of-school activities such as clubs and sports events to support AIDS education (this depends on existing capacity).

In the initial phase of starting a school intervention programme a set of basic questions should be asked (see Box 2). The answer to some questions may vary by district. This information is needed to understand which approaches are most apt to succeed in a particular community. There may be strong opposition to a school sex and AIDS education programme, but some people may just be poorly informed. Advocacy for interventions in schools is intended to help overcome resistance, to help mobilize resources and relevant partners for the school programme (teachers, parents, students, government and NGOs) and to aid subsequent programme implementation targeted at youth.

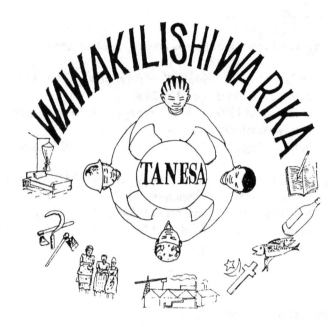

TANESA Peer health educator logo.

Box 2. Basic questions for starting a school programme

- When do boys and girls become sexually active?
- What is known about HIV and STD prevalence in the community by health workers or by parents?
- How do youth perceive their risk of HIV/STD infection?
- What are their main health concerns?
- What is their attitude to sex?
- What is known about the most common sexual practices in adolescence?
- What do parents think about sex education?
- What does the community of which the school is part think about sex education?
- What do teachers think about sex education, and are existing teaching methods appropriate?
- Is there any room for expanding out-of-school activities to support the school sex education programme?
- What kind of organizational structure is available to support the programme?
- What is the approach of the official curriculum? Is it necessary to supplement the deficiencies in the top–down approach of a national curriculum?
- How could a peer health educator programme be set up to supplement the official curriculum?
- Do teachers have sexual relations with students?
- Is there a need for school counsellors or guardians to help in protecting students' sexual health (with priority given to girls)?

Answers to the basic questions will come over time: during workshops with parents, and discussions with and seminars for teachers. In starting up a PHE programme, information that completes the picture will continually be collected. In addition, special efforts can be made to gather relevant information on these issues through small-scale research projects. This may be done through in-depth interviews, structured question-naires (7), self-administered questionnaires, focus group discussions (8) or using the narrative research method (9).

Use of narrative research method
In Magu District, Tanzania, the narrative research method gave very good results. Working with a selected group of about ten students, the aim was to develop story lines about sexual relationships. Depending on the local culture, this may be done with a same-sex group or a mixed group of boys and girls. Head teachers may be asked to select pupils from various classes representing different age groups. Another method is to ask the pupils to select representatives among themselves. In both cases, brighter and more mature pupils are likely to be chosen.

A workshop may last one week. The first days are spent developing an atmosphere where sensitive issues can be openly discussed, the participants understand the importance of the exercise and know that they themselves are taken as serious and knowledgeable. Some transfer of knowledge on reproductive health and AIDS may occur, although the facilitators should be careful not to influence the students: it is important for students to understand that the aim of the workshop is to identify current sexual practices, not to define 'good' or 'bad' behaviour. Facilitators for the research should have some experience in the use and interpretation of role plays. Other programme planners or health educators may participate as well. During the course of this research, a common experience is that adults and pupils come to see each other as equals. This experience is very valuable on both sides for future cooperation and planning activities.

After the foundation is laid the participants are divided into subgroups and asked to develop a story showing how sexual relationships start and develop. It is important to stress that the research focuses on the most typical patterns rather than on atypical events. The stories are used to identify the relevant events in logical order. Then the groups are asked to role-play these events. In Magu District, the role plays were video-taped and analysed at length, focusing on the real and sometimes hidden motivations of the players, and challenging the content to come up with realistic life events.

Box 3 presents the main conclusions drawn from a series of three workshops using the narrative research method: one for girls, one for boys and one for a mixed group (see also Chapter 4, on narrative research, and reference 10, on these workshops).

Box 3. Conclusions from narrative research in Tanzania

- Most boys and girls at primary school may become sexually active by the age of 13–14. By the time they enter the higher classes of primary school, most youth have experienced a number of sexual relationships.
- Girls often have sex with schoolboys and later on develop sexual relationships with adult men from the village. Boys usually have sexual relationships with schoolgirls and with younger girls in the village. Teacher-student relations are not uncommon.
- Exchange of gifts and/or money is always part of sexual negotiations. Accepting gifts and/or money is a signal that a girl agrees to have sex.
- Because of sexual relationships with older men, girls are more at risk than boys at this period in life.
- Neither girls nor boys are afraid of getting STDs or HIV: pregnancy is the main fear.
- The norm for youth is to have unprotected, penetrative sex.
- Although girls have strong negotiation power for money or gifts in exchange for sex, they do not negotiate for protected sex.
- Negotiations by girls for postponement of sexual encounters are dominated by the fear of getting pregnant. Boys often use a wide range of deceptions (lies) to confuse girls such as: 'You cannot get pregnant by a schoolboy, or from one-time sex'. 'I'll take good care of you/marry you if you get pregnant'.
- Experience has taught girls not to expect a good outcome if they become pregnant. They are likely to be sent away from school and from home. Parents may divorce if the mother is held responsible.
- Although abortion represents a strong taboo for girls, they accept certain misconceptions about how to deal with unwanted pregnancies. A common belief is that drinking strong tea without sugar after sex helps prevent/abort the pregnancy. Traditional herbs are frequently used, and chloroquine tablets taken, even though this is known to be dangerous. Illegal abortions are practised as well.
- During role plays it was always girls from poor families who became pregnant. This points up the role of poverty as a contributing factor to these problems. The exchange of money in negotiations for sex is apt to be a greater incentive for girls from poorer families. In later discussions with parents, this problem was acknowledged.
- The values, norms and attitudes of adults regarding the sexuality of primary school youth are not realistic. It is therefore necessary for youth themselves to take active responsibility for a programme to prevent the further spread of HIV among their peer group, and to educate teachers, parents and the community.
- Young people find it easy to express themselves in role plays and stories. Story lines developed as described in the text help to identify culture specifics in the development of sexual relationships. These culture-specific events, dialogues, beliefs, expectations, misconceptions and peer pressures can be used for direct interventions in forms such as picture codes, drama performances, songs and poems.

Advocacy and mobilization of resources

During the process of advocacy and mobilizing resources and relevant partners for a school intervention programme, several issues have to be addressed. In this section the basic questions are discussed, illustrated by the experiences gained in Magu District, Tanzania.

What do parents think about sex education? Parents find it very difficult to talk openly with their children about sexual matters. In the culture of the Sukuma in Magu the role of the old aunt who guided girls through the maturation process, and traditional rites for boys have disappeared without being replaced. Sex is not discussed at home – usually children are only told what not to do – and it is generally understood that upbringing, including sexuality, is the mother's job. She is supposed to know all that happens to her children and to prevent any problems. In fact she bears all responsibility for her children's behaviour. The father does not interfere; he limits his role to reinforcing the 'do-not's' and to acting at those moments when things have gone wrong.

What does the community think about sex education? The community expects schools to support the cultural norms; the messages communicated at home should in large part also be communicated at school. Schools play a restrictive role and preferably avoid sex education topics. Rules are very restrictive and reproachful. A pupil may be punished for carrying a love letter because it is believed that this is the first step towards a forbidden sexual relationship.

Although the Ministry of Education in Tanzania has proposed changes, the common practice is to dismiss a girl from school as soon as it becomes clear that she is pregnant. Usually the boy responsible remains unknown, but if he is known, he may face the same fate and even be charged.

What do teachers think about sex education? Both male and female schoolteachers are conservative in their approach to sex education. Teachers fear they will lose authority over their pupils if they have to teach about sex. Teachers are often embarrassed and feel uncomfortable talking about sex. Sex is often called the weakness of the flesh, and teachers are unprepared to teach sex education, especially when the content is ill-defined.

Teaching methodologies are typically top–down, an approach which is unsuitable for sex education – a much more interactive approach is needed. Teachers' understanding of adolescent development is low. They tend to ignore that sexuality is one of the most important concerns of pupils during adolescent development. The norm is to act as if that which should not happen (according to the communities' norms and values) does not happen. The acceptable attitude is to be very strict and instill fear into youth about sexual experimentation.

Experience shows that it is extremely difficult to convince teachers that their pupils are indeed engaging in sex. Introducing condom use is most controversial.

Organization for out-of-school activities. In Tanzania, as in many countries, schools face difficult conditions. There are few facilities or opportunities for extracurricular activities. No money is available, even for the most basic activity needs: programmes involving hobbies and other meaningful out-of-school activities like clubs and sporting events are typically not available. Further, teachers cannot afford to spend their time on such things, because they are usually too busy supplementing their inadequate salaries. This makes it essential to involve school committies in children's activities, including sex education. In Magu District, prior to the intervention described, primary school committees were not active in the field of sex education. When approached properly, in our experience committees can become very interested and are usually supportive of interventions.

The introduction of an official AIDS curriculum for primary schools
An official AIDS curriculum was introduced in Tanzania in 1993. Development of a curriculum for the primary schools took a long time; at ministerial level it was difficult to reach consensus about the content and approach to be used, and which messages should be communicated.

The controversial issues seemed to be related to concerns such as 'Sex education will lead to more sex' and 'Condom promotion in primary schools will lead to promiscuity'. These controversies were expressed at national level, but are present at all levels. There is a concern that a more liberal approach to teaching matters of sexuality will lead to an increase in unwanted sexual behaviour. Therefore, the curriculum that was finally accepted is basically knowledge-based with the prominent message being: postpone sex until marriage. Condom use is only taught in theory. Practical demonstrations on condom use, and skills training in condom negotiation have been left out. The curriculum is teacher-based and does not include the use of peer educators. Although diverse teaching methods have been introduced, the training programme still remains very much adult-controlled. The self-confidence required to use more interactive and/or participatory teaching methods (and the belief that these are appropriate) varies greatly among teachers.

In Magu District the teacher training programme ran short of finances, with the result that training was reduced to information meetings about the new curriculum. Only two-thirds of primary schools in Magu could be reached. Lack of finances also resulted in insufficient distribution of teaching aids such as teaching guides and books for students. Delays at national level were repeated at the district level where the curriculum was not introduced, even after two teachers at every school had been trained.

What is taught should also be practised by teachers. However, during development of the intervention it became known that some teachers had sexual relations with pupils in the upper classes. The programme recognized this as a behaviour problem requiring specific attention.

Conclusions
The cultural norm expected by parents, the community and schools is that pupils will not have sex while still in school. The community expects this norm to be supported by the school. People believe that a restrictive atmosphere will help to reach the objective of no sex at a young age. If there are signs that the norm is not being reached, the solution, it is believed, is to become more restrictive: no deliberate efforts are made to

determine if the cultural norm matches the reality. This restrictive reaction seems to come from adults who themselves have not experienced an extended adolescent period. The resulting attitude may work in traditional cultures, but is likely to have little effect on adolescent behaviour today.

In this setting, providing information and acting as an advocate with parents and school authorities regarding current adolescent development is a necessary component of a school intervention programme. Difficulties in introducing the official curriculum reflect this basic issue: before a curriculum is introduced, partners at the lower levels of the educational system need to be mobilized and consensus reached on the content and method of teaching behaviour change.

Advocacy and mobilization also help in establishing opportunities for out-of-school activities that, among other things, can provide HIV/AIDS education. Starting such activities in the context of a project may have sustainability problems but is greatly needed. Here too, working with students, parents and other partners is vital. Another intervention that is needed for programme success is to address the problem of sexual relations between teachers and pupils. This problem may indicate a need to develop interventions such as the guardian programme described below, to help youth assume more control for themselves.

Starting a PHE programme for school youth

Our experience shows that a PHE programme can be vital. It may grow to include components such as the organization of school AIDS committees, anti-AIDS clubs, informal and formal PHE educational activities aimed at behaviour change, and an out-of-school activities programme; it may also be linked to a guardian or counselling programme aiming to assist girls and boys in matters of sexual health. New issues should regularly be discussed by those concerned.

A programme for school youth should involve all parties concerned: education authorities, school authorities, parents, teachers and the community – but above all, the youth themselves. Prior to developing an intervention programme for youth at the schools in a district, the entry process must be decided upon. An analysis of the basic questions presented in Box 2 will aid decisions on the advocacy needed to build support for the programme at district/community and school levels. Advocacy for sex education is needed with parents and community leaders. There will be an ongoing need for advocacy for the needs identified by youth (e.g. the introduction and distribution of condoms as a means of protection and the need to address the issue of teachers having sexual relations with pupils) and for pupils' wishes to join the school AIDS action committee, to be able to advise on actions to be taken.

A good method of doing this was found in Mwanza Region, Tanzania, where AIDS committees were mobilized in the schools to discuss the need for AIDS and sex educa-tion. These AIDS committees, which included teachers, parents and community leaders, were trained for their role of supervising the AIDS programme in the school, including the PHE programme. Open discussion about the advantages and disadvantages of sex education in school helped to create a positive response from parents and school authorities. Parents were actually more in favour of the programme than teachers, who did not feel confident about teaching sex education. Presentation of the results from the narrative research convinced parents and communities that action was needed; then they insisted on the speedy introduction of the official curriculum as well as the PHE programme. The committees spontaneously decided to enter the community and provide AIDS education for the general public, as well as to inform them of the need for AIDS education for their children, and of the special risks for girls who are enticed into sexual relations with adult men.

Student guardians

Parents also identified the problem of some teachers having sexual relationships with school girls The programme then assisted in advocacy with the education authorities, who took the matter very seriously, since it was presented by parents. In all schools in Mwanza Region guardians are now selected from among the women teachers whose task it is to assist girls in particular, and boys if needed on issues related to sexual health. Apart from maturation issues, girls may also report unwanted sexual harassment by teachers, other adult men or boys. The guardian reports directly to the district and regional authorities who can take action. Guardians also have formed a support committee of representatives at district level, which negotiates with district authorities concerning necessary action and support for guardians, who may face threats from males engaging in sexual relations with schoolgirls.

Information from a narrative workshop for girls and boys about the obstacles to and potential for postponing sex was used to train guardians, especially in counselling skills. Girls indicated during the workshop that they are approached by boys and adult men for sex and that they do not really feel empowered with the right to say 'no'. Boys, indicated that their biggest problem in trying to postpone sex is peer pressure. When approached for sex, girls use strategies such as running away or taking another route to avoid contact, or making promises such as 'let's do it tomorrow'. Their strategies, however, are only temporarily effective, and bring them more problems if males are not prepared to give up. Boys indicated that the price for escaping peer pressure is isolation and loss of friendship.

During the training workshops, guardians realized that they recognized many of the same problems girls face in trying to postpone sexual activity: these problems very much resemble those of adult women. As teachers and out of solidarity, the guardians initially tried to solve the girls' problems, basically by taking disciplinary action. Training for guardians aimed at developing skills to enable them to assist girls in solving their own problems – in that way the girls would become empowered to deal with future situations. Girls are encouraged to solve their own problems by discussing and sharing problems among themselves.

Exchanges between girls and boys are organized with the aim of exchanging views about the obstacles that both groups experience when trying to postpone sex or to negotiate protected sex. A radio programme and newsletter have been developed to give guardians ongoing support and information about how to develop gender-based responses to the sexual health problems faced by pupils of both sexes.

School by-laws

AIDS committees in Mwanza also discussed and put into effect new village by-laws intended to protect children, especially girls; this alerted the community to the situation. The new community awareness of the need for action immediately resulted in the conviction of several adult men. However, due to the lack of out-of-school activities these new by-laws also acted as 'do-not's' for youth (e.g. do not go to video shows, do not attend festivities in the evening, do not go to bars). Therefore, in several schools the PHE programme initiated out-of-school activities like sports events and school discos, as well as exchange programmes with other schools. The PHE programme also raised small amounts of funding for these sorts of activities, for example by asking for a small contribution when an educational video film was shown in school.

The process of advocacy

The process of advocacy leads naturally to the process of mobilizing resources and selecting the best partners for collaboration at district and community level, as well as to identification of what partners can potentially contribute. When the process of advocacy and mobilization of teachers, parents and communities prepares them for action, it is then a good time to start the official curriculum and link it to the PHE programme as a supplement. Without the advocacy and mobilization phase the programme may be seen as alien and ill-suited to the cultural values of the community, resulting in delay of the curriculum's introduction.

After advocacy and the mobilization of resources have gained momentum, a PHE programme can be started, with the general aim of assisting young people to protect themselves by encouraging them to develop safe sex behaviour patterns early and helping them to change behaviour which puts them at risk of HIV infection. To cover a whole district it is wise to limit the number of PHEs to one male and one female per class, selected by their own peers. A good selection process starts by explaining the role of PHEs and discussing the criteria for choosing them. After these issues are decided, the class may be asked to select two PHEs from among themselves to be trained by the programme. Following this, the PHEs will train their peers, using both formal educational activities and informal discussions. The selection process should if possible be facilitated by trained trainers, who also train the PHEs for their educative tasks. Selection of PHEs by their classmate peers is an essential element of their acceptance; it is also advisable to select both male and female PHEs. PHEs' training should be very practical and the tasks of the PHEs should be made very clear.

Training

Peer education focuses on assisting groups of young people to build their knowledge, attitudes and safer sex skills through educational activities undertaken by trained PHEs. The PHEs act as educators, role models, organizers and discussion leaders. Their educational activities should preferably combine formal and informal activities because it is easy to lose contact if only informal activities are used. A base of formal activities also stimulates informal discussion. Moreover, formal activities also have the advantage that experienced PHEs can easily use these circumstances to train new PHEs, who will be needed each year as new classes enter the programme. Training should focus on teaching skills related to risk assessment, negotiation, safer sex practices, violence and the use of reproductive health services. PHEs also require training in facilitating group discussions.

Teachers and others on AIDS committees also need training. Teachers' training for the implementation of the national curriculum needs to focus on interactive and participatory skills. Workshops for those on AIDS committees, which include teachers responsible for AIDS education, parents and community leaders, can focus on problem analysis and setting an agenda for action. It is helpful to combine different schools in AIDS committee training, since this will increase the feeling that similar problems are experienced at all schools. It can also help motivate people into action.

PHEs and the national curriculum
To mobilize cooperation and acceptance, peer approaches should be used as a part of school programmes or as a complement to AIDS prevention education in the school curriculum. In so far possible, the PHE programme should complement the official curriculum. That is, teachers can focus on more formal instruction about HIV/STD transmission and prevention, while peer educator activities focus primarily on the necessary changes in attitudes and behaviour. Although some teacher supervision over PHE activities may be advantageous, teachers and other adults should be careful to maintain some distance and avoid taking charge of activities.

The cost of a PHE programme. The cost of the programme per school or per student can be kept quite low; much depends on the type of educational materials produced and the expenditures for training. However, the cost of a school programme that covers an entire district is always high, because of the number of schools. If funds are limited it will be necessary to look for ways to reduce costs and to develop the programme over a few years in stages. Costs can be reduced by:
a. cost sharing;
b. implementation by the education department, without recruiting new personnel;
c. use of experienced PHEs to train new peer health educators in the schools (TOTs);
d. use of appropriate, low-cost teaching materials.

In Magu District, Tanzania, it was extremely important to reduce costs as much as possible – funds were very limited. Once the programme had been developed in one division and personnel had gained experience, the district education department decided to offer the programme to the entire district on a cost-sharing basis. An advocacy campaign informed schools about the programme and the conditions under which it could be offered (Box 4).

Cost sharing reduced the costs to the education department by at least 60%. This was possible because training costs for the AIDS committee members and peer health educators was now covered by the schools. While the programme had once paid participants an allowance per training day, cost sharing meant that this allowance was no longer paid, and the school organized food for participants.

Box 4. Cost sharing conditions for the PHE programme in Magu District

Contribution by the education department
- Two-day training for AIDS action committee from the inspectorate department.
- Five-day training for two PHEs for standards five, six and seven done by well-trained TOTs.
- Activity manual for all PHE activities on: HIV/AIDS/STDs/childrens' rights, changing behaviour and reproductive health.
- Exchange visits among active committees.
- T-shirt for all PHEs trained.
- Follow-up for the PHE programme by their trainers, and by ward education coordinators for AIDS action committees.

Contribution from the school
- Organize selection of responsible members for an AIDS sub-committee (representing teachers, parents, community opinion leaders, and preferably PHEs in the school).
- Organize food/refreshments during AIDS action committee and PHE training sessions.

Out-of-school youth

Out-of-school youth include the following groups, each with their own distinct needs:
- schoolchildren in their spare time;
- children who have left school early because of their families' labour needs, or because the family cannot afford school fees;
- other school drop-outs;
- children who have never attended school at all;
- street or homeless children in urban centres.

When children leave school their period of adolescence may end abruptly; they often seem to assume adult status and become more sexually active. Becoming pregnant is then no longer linked to such disastrous events as when it happens while they are still in school. For many girls getting married is the next obvious step, especially when employment opportunities are limited. Multiple sexual partners may become an economic survival strategy for many young girls without a steady income. Boys and girls may begin to migrate to towns in search of job opportunities. Box 5 outlines problems reported by out-of-school youth in Zimbabwe.

It is difficult to reach out-of-school youth. They are not easily attracted by any type of organization, with the possible exception of church and sports clubs. They often tend to migrate in search of employment, moving to nearby towns and entering into the urban youth culture.

Box 5. Problems of out-of-school youth

In Zimbabwe in 1993, 42 focus group discussions were held with out-of-school youth between the ages of 12 and 20 years. These discussions showed that young people who are not in school and are unemployed gain very little satisfaction from their daily activities. They feel the community looks down upon them, and are bored and frustrated with life because they cannot get jobs and earn an income. Even though their knowledge of AIDS is satisfactory, they consider AIDS a minor problem compared to their unemployment and lack of money (11).

Messages adapted to music, posters and T-shirts are good ways of addressing this distinctive youth culture. It is, however, difficult to identify the cultural specifics involved. Interventions should therefore be developed together with the youth them-selves. A narrative research method (see above) may provide a good way to understand the challenges they face after leaving school. This should identify most of their typical problems, including unemployment and alcohol and drug abuse. Some promising approaches for reaching out-of-school youth are:

- Inform primary school leavers about out-of-school programmes that may be of interest to them.
- Use people that young people admire, such as singers or football players, to speak on health issues.
- Ask popular music groups to perform songs about health issues.
- Use young people as fieldworkers, so that youth will listen and respond.
- Involve the young people themselves in performing drama shows about their lives.
- Train a group of young volunteers (PHEs) to carry out informal health education in bars and discos where young people go.
- Produce magazines and comics on health topics.
- Include health issues in any initiation ceremonies carried out for boys or girls, and which serve as traditional sex education.
- If a radio station is available, projects may negotiate to broadcast special programmes for and with out-of-school youth, addressing issues of interest to them.
- If a school programme is introduced, it can be linked with out-of-school youth, since there are many informal contacts between school-going and out-of-school youth, especially those who do not attend school because of family labour needs.

A PHE programme for out-of-school youth
Some countries have gained experience with an interesting approach, making use of the pool of PHEs created in primary schools. PHEs who have finished primary school are sup-ported to enable them to continue their peer education task among the peer groups they enter after leaving school. Support is not financial, but might include new health educa-tion material, adjusted to their new situation – perhaps as unemployed out-of-school

youth, secondary school youth or working youth. For example, in Ghana, the organization Action-Aid offers PHEs who have finished school new health education materials suitable to their new situation and gives training on how to approach their new peers.

In a ward in Mwanza town, Tanzania, a group of 20 PHEs who left primary school have organized themselves in an interest group for out-of-school youth. They have started with health education to their peers, distribution and sale of social marketing condoms and also provide information on available reproductive health services. The group realized the need to raise their own funds for the programme and do so through the sale of second-hand clothing.

Development of health education materials for PHE activities

Whether in school programmes or outside, working with PHEs means involving youth in research (narrative research and pre-testing health education materials), in planning and in the implementation of interventions. In Magu, Tanzania, it seemed logical to recruit young people involved in the initial narrative research to train as trainers for PHEs in the schools. The same group was instrumental in pre-testing and developing appropriate health education materials. A similar approach can be used for out-of-school PHEs.

In working with PHEs it is essential to design the programme so that PHEs clearly understand what is expected from them. WHO has developed a guide for AIDS educational activities based on a set of exercises (12) which may be used as a resource for developing exercises that are more culture-specific. Narrative research is likely to produce many ideas to culturally adapt the exercises. Box 6 lists a few examples.

Box 6. Peer pressures and common beliefs

Sexual pressures
- 'Do not be a *shamba* (bush) girl, let us agree to have sex'.
- 'You accepted my gifts already, so let us have sex now'.
- If a girl is afraid to refuse (saying 'no' too strongly may be culturally difficult, as it may be received as an insult, leading to violence), she will promise to agree to sex tomorrow. The boy or man then will force her to agree to sex if they meet tomorrow, because of her promise.

Common beliefs about ways to prevent/abort pregnancy
- Drink strong tea without sugar, drink ashes, use chloroquine tablets.

Common beliefs and promises about becoming pregnant
- A school boy cannot make you pregnant.
- You cannot become pregnant from one-time sex.
- 'If things go wrong I will marry you'.

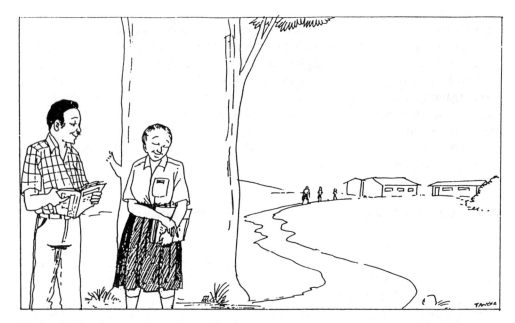

A school girl on her way home from school is approached by an older man. During the pre-test many pupils identified the man as a teacher – the first report of this problem.

The story lines developed and the peer pressures identified during narrative research can be directly used in interventions. Story lines present many situations where an individual has to make choices about what to do. These choices are related to risk perceptions and perceptions of norms and values. Such choices and perceptions are good topics for discussion. For example, while peer pressure may normally dominate decisions, discussion may lead to change: e.g. a young girl who is approached by an older man may be offered a present. The discussion may focus on questions like: 'is it wise to accept this present; what may this lead to?' Discussion starters may be used, in the form of picture codes, short dramas or role plays, and then discussed. Such discussion starters can be found throughout this book.

Young people are action-oriented; they like innovative and entertaining educational activities. Picture codes, as well as short drama or role play performances, are usually well received as discussion starters. Pupils like telling or reading stories very much: this was the preferred method of expression during the narrative research. Youth also enjoy participating in campaigns in the community, as long as they can make their own contributions to songs, drama performance, poems and the like.

Monitoring progress

To estimate the success of advocacy, mobilization, and behavioural change, a few indicators (see Chapter 6) can be selected to monitor the progress of a school AIDS programme.

Indicators to measure success in advocacy
- number of schools with an appointed/selected guardian
- number and type of school AIDS committee activities in the community:
  - information meetings for the community
  - parents' meetings to discuss sex education
  - organized youth events
  - support to the PHE programme at regional and district levels
- number of schools that allow teaching about protected sex
- number of schools that allow condom distribution by PHES
- change in treatment of girls who get pregnant (allowed to stay in or to return to school)
- are both boys and girls permitted to carry condoms while on the school compound?
- is the school AIDS committee satisfied with the programme?

Indicators to measure success in mobilization
- number of schools that have started teaching about AIDS as a topic
- number of schools with an active AIDS committee
- number of schools with a PHE programme
- involvement of other sectors and NGOs in the programme
- number of parental requests for training in how to talk about sex with their children

Indicators to monitor behaviour change
Schools where the programme has and has not implemented can be compared with respect to some of the following factors.

Building knowledge
- an increase in knowledge on how to prevent HIV/AIDS, using condoms and using contraceptives
- knowledge of where to purchase condoms and find family planning advice
- knowledge about gender differences in maturation and sexual issues

Perception of risk
- improved attitude towards delaying sex, having protected sex and the use of contraceptives
- able to state general risks for boys and girls as well as personal risks

Perception of norms
- responsible behaviour in delaying sex or having protected sex has become the norm among peers
- pupils are able to give a logical argument regarding their stated choices of ways to protect themselves
- condom use is a generally accepted means of protection

Feelings of self-efficacy and self-esteem

- pupils who say they had never engaged in sex when the intervention started are/were able to delay their first sexual experience
- pupils are able to negotiate safer sex practices with their partners
- girls are able to reduce the number of older partners
- girls are able to negotiate condom use with boys and older partners
- boys respect girls' rights to negotiate protection
- boys are able to reduce the number of partners
- sexual harassment of girls by teachers is reported
- adults in the community who sexually harass girls are reported

Timing of the activities

There is generally strong pressure to develop health education materials and PHE activities quickly, to show that the programme is a success. However, as already stated, the distribution of health education materials to schools without proper advocacy and mobilization of the relevant partners may lead to disappointment. Development of materials *with* students always takes more time than developing materials *for* them. However, time spent on initial baseline research, advocacy and mobilization is time well spent: it is apt to accelerate the programme in a later stage. Research, advocacy of the findings and mobilization of relevant partners always takes more time than expected. In addition, the programme has to develop peer educator activities, pre-test them and train the trainers for their role, training PHEs in the schools. It is therefore wise to allow a full year for these preparations. Implementation could then start in the second year.

Development of materials and activities can also proceed in stages: first, activities can be developed to inform students on the basic facts of HIV/AIDS, STDs and reproductive health; then materials related to postponing sex can be developed, and finally, materials for protective sex produced. This phased development provides more opportunity for students to participate. When materials and staff are ready, it is wise to start small, covering a ward or division (depending on the administrative system) to develop staff capacity and experience. It must be realized that the educational system will typically not be able to fully cooperate with pilot projects: they may expect that one such project is apt to lead to more, coming from different NGOs, each with their own objectives and approaches. This may confuse district authorities and in the end hamper district coverage. We were fortunate in Magu District, Tanzania, in that the education department was strongly in favour of the approach developed by our programme, and asked other donors to participate in its implementation.

It is extremely important to work with educational authorities at district level and, if possible, to focus on district coverage from the beginning. As noted above, this may not always be possible with pilot projects. When the programme is ready to expand to district coverage, however, this is responsibility of the education department.

Coverage should be planned in accord with the administrative set-up of the education system in the district. In Tanzania this meant developing the programme by division, some 20–25 schools at a time. When the programme has been established in the first division (or other admistrative area), and has been evaluated, the education department should plan for expansion to other divisions as allowed by the available personnel.

Conclusion

In developing countries adolescents in the age group 12–19 years make up 16–20% of the population. A considerable proportion are sexually active and at risk of both HIV infection and other sexually transmitted diseases. Sex education should start with younger age groups: the age group 6–12 – the 'window of opportunity' – needs education and prevention information to produce a cohort which has a better chance of going through their lives without becoming infected. Cultural beliefs and attitudes, denials and secrecy have always surrounded children's sexuality; nevertheless, if they are to be successful, AIDS programmes must be based on interventions agreed upon by the community, following discussion. This requires a culturally empathetic approach. A careful understanding of parents' desire to protect their children from dangerous behaviour and its consequences must form the basis for AIDS programmes for youth.

This chapter demonstrates not only the need but also the possibility of an approach which builds knowledge, perception of risk and understanding of norms, and raises children's feelings of self-efficacy and self-esteem. In schools, this must be done with all three major partners – the children, the teachers and the community. Including programmes for out-of-school youth is also essential. These processes do demand time, but promoting safe sex for youth is a priority: it deserves to receive resources in accord with its importance.

Further reading

Adolescent Health Programme. Counselling skills training in adolescent sexuality and reproductive health: a facilitator's guide. Guide to running a 5-day workshop. Geneva, WHO.

Grazyna B, Hanes H. *Child to child resource book.* TALC, (P.O. Box 49, St Albans, Hertfordshire AL1 4 AX, UK) 1992.

Hubley, John. *Communicating health. An action guide to health education and health promotion.* London, Macmillan, 1993.

International Federation of Red Cross and Red Crescent Societies. *Action for youth – AIDS training manual.* (P.O. Box 372, 1211 Geneva 19, Switzerland.)

UNICEF. *Methods in AIDS education: a training manual for teachers.* Information on methods and implementation/evaluation of school-based programmes. Order from: P.O. Box 1250, Harare, Zimbabwe.

World Health Organization. School health education to prevent AIDS and sexually transmitted diseases. *WHO AIDS Series,* no. 10. Geneva, 1992.

World Health Organization. *Counselling skills training in adolescent sexuality and reproductive health*. Geneva, 1993.

World Health Organization. *School health education to prevent AIDS and STD*. Resource package for curriculum planners; comes with student activities and teacher's guide. Geneva, 1994.

World Health Organization. *The health of young people: a challenge and a promise*. Geneva, 1993.

World Health Organization. *The narrative research method: studying behaviour patterns of young people by young people. A guide to its use*. World Health Organization/ADH/93.4. Geneva, 1993.

References

1. Ford N, Fort d'Auriol A, Ankomah A. *Review of the literature on the health and behavioural outcomes of population and family planning education programmes in school settings in developing countries*. Exeter, University of Exeter, Institute of Population Studies, October 1992.

2. Kirby DB. Sex and HIV/AIDS education in schools. *British Medical Journal* 1995, 311: 403.

3. Fee N, Youssef M. *Experiences of peer approaches in developing countries*. Geneva, World Health Organization/Global Programme on AIDS (GPA), 1993.

4. Central Statistical Office and Macro International Inc. *Zimbabwe Demographic and Health Survey 1994*. Calverton, Maryland, 1995.

5. National Statistical Office and Macro International Inc. *Malawi Demographic and Health Survey 1992*. Calverton, Maryland, 1994.

6. Gaisie K, Cross AR, Nsemukila G. *Zambia Demographic and Health Survey 1992*. Calverton, Maryland, 1993.

7. Seha AM, Klepp KI, Mdeki SS. Scale reliability and construct validity: a pilot study among primary school children in Northern Tanzania. *AIDS Education and Prevention* 1994, 6: 524–534.

8. Barker GK, Rich S. Influences on adolescent sexuality in Nigeria and Kenya: findings from recent focus group discussions. *Studies in Family Planning* 1992, 23: 199–210.

9. World Health Organization. *The narrative research method: studying behaviour patterns of young people – by young people. A guide to its use*. Geneva, World Health Organization/ADH/93.4, 1993.

10. Nnko S, Pool R. School pupils and the discourse of sex in Magu district. *TANESA Working Paper,* no. 3. Mwanza, 1994.

11. Gadidze M, McGrath N, Peters A. *A report on focus group discussions with out-of-school youth on perceptions and strategies for communicating about AIDS*. Harare, Ministry of Education and Culture/UNICEF, 1993.

12. World Health Organization. *School health education to prevent AIDS and STD. WHO AIDS Series,* no. 10. 1994.

11 Condom promotion and distribution

Venance Nyonyo and Dick Schapink

- How reliable is the male condom?
- Why do many people dislike condoms?
- What is social marketing of condoms?
- Can peer educators distribute condoms?
- How many condoms are needed in a district?

Sexual transmission accounts for 75% of HIV infection worldwide, according to recent epidemiological figures (1). The most effective ways to prevent sexual transmission are abstinence or mutually faithful sexual relationships with uninfected persons. However, these approaches are not feasible for most of the sexually active population, and promoting abstinence and faithfulness alone will therefore affect too few people to contain the epidemic. Promoting safe or safer sex practices among the sexually active population can also be an effective way to prevent sexual transmission. Consistent condom use reduces the risk of HIV infection up to 90% or more. Even without a 100% guarantee of safety, any delay in HIV transmission is of benefit to an individual, and can also change the dynamics of the epidemic. Furthermore, condom use protects against the transmission of other STDs, which is one of the strongest contributing factors to the spread of HIV (see Chapter 13).

This chapter looks not only at the technical effectiveness of the condom and the obstacles to its use, but also at issues related to condom promotion, distribution and health education at district level. We refer to the male condom throughout this chapter; the female condom is not included, as we have no experience with implementing its use in districts. The female condom is a welcome addition to barrier methods for women, but in Africa its cost and lack of availability has hampered use.

Do condoms prevent HIV infection?

Results from laboratory studies show in general that high-quality latex condoms are impermeable to the passage of HIV and other organisms (2). Hence, sexually transmitted diseases can effectively be prevented by the use of a condom. Nevertheless, product failure related to manufacturing, distribution and storage, as well as user failure, diminish the effectiveness of condoms to varying degrees.

Quality control measures are required at all levels to avoid manufacturing mistakes, damage due to accidents during distribution or poor storage of condoms. Project managers, distributors and storekeepers have to be trained to ensure proper storage and care of condoms. A regular supply of well-disseminated information on quality control measures is essential.

Throughout the world quality standards are set for condoms, and in most countries a bureau of standards electronically tests condoms for reliability and safety. Leakage, strength and size is tested, as well as holding qualities in storage for a period of up to five years after manufacture. Every batch of condoms then is delivered with its quality control results. Every condom package indicates the manufacturing date, the size of the condom and the batch number. Typically only the date of manufacture is indicated on the condom package; this is confusing for many consumers. The date of expiry is usually set at a maximum of five years after manufacture. Under tropical conditions three years may be more appropriate.

User failure is a big problem in promoting condoms. Estimates of failures rates caused by incorrect or inconsistent use have ranged from 0.1% to 13%. Proper training in the use of condoms may reduce the rate of failure due to breakage. Inconsistent use should be targeted by health promoters as the biggest problem related to condom use. Studies among discordant couples (where one partner is HIV-infected) have shown that inconsistent use carries considerable risk of infection, while consistent use confers substantial protection for the uninfected partner. In several studies no seroconversion was observed among discordant couples who correctly used a condom for every coital act, while the seroconversion rate with inconsistent use was estimated at 4.8% (3).

Obstacles to condom use

A range of obstacles to promoting condom use has been encountered. These include personal dislike of condoms by men and women, the association of condoms with promiscuity, the lack of the negotiation power of women, religious opposition, misconceptions on the effectiveness of condoms, the link between risk-taking behaviour and alcohol abuse, and low availability of condoms. Box 1 lists all the obstacles.

Who should be protected?

Not everybody is at equal risk of HIV infection. It is thus important to select priority target groups for the promotion of condom use. Commercial sex workers and their clients are the most important target group. Adolescent youth are a second target group. People with AIDS and their partners are another priority group.

In addition, it is important to identify relationships that put people at risk of HIV infection. There is increasing evidence that men are more commonly infected outside marital relations, but women usually become infected by their spouses. This situation would argue for condom promotion to the entire population and for all relationships. However, condom use is rarely accepted in marital and/or regular relationships (except for family planning reasons). Hence interventions are targeted at other risky relationships and the importance of recognizing where and when such risky relationships take place.

Box 1. Obstacles to condom use

Low motivation:
- Condom use is new to many people and the cultural norm may discourage use: popular opinion is that 'flesh to flesh is the real thing'.
- Condom use may be associated with disease, leading people to reject it ('I'm healthy; I'm not infected').
- Starting to use condoms is very difficult for many people. Problems with condoms are most common for beginners, thus demotivating people from continuing.
- Many communities have had a strong stigma against condom use, linking condom use to undesirable social behaviour and sexual practices.

Alcohol abuse:
- Alcohol abuse makes negotiation for protection more difficult.
- Alcohol or drug abuse hinders the motivation to use condoms and enhances irresponsible behaviour.
- The use of alcohol makes proper condom use more difficult.

Condoms prohibit conception:
- In cultures which highly value fertility the argument that condoms prohibit conception is used often by men and women to resist condom use: 'How can one get pregnant when using a condom?'
- There is often resistance to using a condom in addition to another family planning method.

Women often lack the power to negotiate condom use:
- Many men become infected in extramarital relations and then infect their wives. Cultural norms and values related to sexual relations make it difficult for husbands and wives to discuss sexual matters, extra-marital relationships and condom use.
- Men usually hold the decision-making power in sexual relations, and thus men make decisions about condom use.

Men and women are uncomfortable about condom use:
- Both men and women may feel uncomfortable about using condoms. Women often say: 'I do not want to see the face of a condom entering my body'. Men assert they won't enjoy sex with a condom: 'You do not eat a sweet with the wrapper on'.

Beliefs, misconceptions and mistakes:
- Many common beliefs keep people from using ~~ impregnated with the HIV virus'. 'Condoms lea~ into a women's body and cause sterility'.
- AIDS is linked to the practice of witchcraft and m for undesirable sexual behaviours: 'A condom can~
- Use of the wrong lubicant may damage the cond~ no petroleum-based lubricants are used with con~
- Sex workers in Tanzania were convinced that a co~ oral or anal sex.

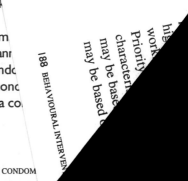

Negative impact of anti-condom factions in a community:
- A campaign against condom use can strengthen misconceptions and common beliefs about health, and stress the ineffectiveness of the condom. Such an 'anti-condom lobby' is mostly fuelled by religious opposition. Religious opposition to condom use does not come from a lack of proof of the effectiveness of condoms, but because condom use is linked to promiscuity and to 'technological' family planning.

Erratic supplies of condoms:
- A sustained supply of condoms is often unavailable because of distribution problems in rural areas. In some countries condoms are supplied free of charge, but money for distribution is often lacking.
- Condom promotion campaigns lack proper follow-up with distribution.
- As more condoms appear on the market, poor quality condoms that burst may become a problem.

Promoting condoms in a district

A WHO protocol is available for rapid assessment to be used in planning condom services (5). This protocol outlines the components of a comprehensive and coherent condom service: planning to meet demand; procurement of condoms; development of appropriate distribution channels and outlets; and strengthening health promotion. The protocol provides guidelines for the methods needed for this rapid appraisal, including review of existing information, focus group discussions with different target groups, informal surveys and direct observation of distribution outlets.

The dynamics involved in HIV and STD transmission and high-risk behaviour patterns are particularly important in planning condom promotion in a district. For example:

- Assessing levels of new HIV and STD infections among various target populations can allow targeting interventions at vulnerable groups such as commercial sex workers, youth, fishermen or truck drivers.
- Identifying areas, places, and practices of high-risk behaviour so that interventions can be targeted at places where sex takes place or is negotiated, including guest-houses, bars and local beer shops.

Priority target groups and intervention points

Condom promotion campaigns help to reduce the stigma of condom use in a community, and may be the obvious choice in countries with high HIV prevalence. However, as noted above, not everybody is at equal risk of HIV infection. It is those who are at higher risk who should first be targeted for condom promotion. Condom promotion works best if it is customized to fit the behaviours and beliefs of specific target groups. Target groups for condom promotion are people who share common characteristics that make them more vulnerable to HIV infection. These characteristics are based on demographic indicators such as age, sex, occupation or location; or on sexual orientation or practice. Priority target groups may include refugees, migrants, fishermen, travelling businessmen, military personnel, and people who practise specific risk behaviour, such as having multiple partners. Box 2 presents examples of efforts to find good starting points for condom promotion among target groups.

Box 2. Choosing a starting point for condom promotion

Research among adolescents in Magu District, Tanzania, showed that some girls have regular unprotected sexual contacts with adult men, making them vulnerable to HIV infection. These girls, however, did not fear HIV or STD infection; instead they worried about becoming pregnant, which would have immediate implications (such as abortion and/or expulsion from school). It was therefore decided that promoting protected sex to prevent HIV infection had to start from the girls' needs for protection against unwanted pregnancies.

Fishermen on Lake Victoria indicated during focus group discussions that they were not at all impressed by the danger of HIV infection and were strongly opposed to condom use. They are used to accepting risking their lives because of the type of work they do. They felt little fear of death from HIV in ten years when they cannot even be sure of returning safely from fishing every day (most cannot swim). However, they did indicate that their main health problem was STD infection. They also indicated that their partners suffered a great deal from infertility (caused by frequent STDs). Condom promotion therefore focused on the need to protect against STDs and/or to avoid infertility.

The promotion of condoms for casual sex should be done at drinking places, in guesthouses, discos and other places known as meeting places for casual sex. One effective approach to promoting condom use among peers and clients is to train commercial sex workers and bar and guesthouse attendants as peer health educators (see Chapter 12).

Knowledge, attitudes and practices of target groups

Understanding of the knowledge, attitudes and practices (KAP) of target groups is essential to designing a suitable promotion campaign. Epidemiological data and STD rates may give an indication of the magnitude of the problem among the target group. Knowledge about the sexual behaviour and beliefs of specific target groups in a district may be available from market surveys or other existing data. KAP studies can be conducted using questionnaires and in-depth interviews, focus group discussions and listening surveys in bars and markets. Research can include knowledge and attitudes concerning AIDS and STD in general, and attempt to identify obstacles to increasing condom use.

It is also important to listen to peer educators and use the information they collect. From experience with bar workers in Mwanza, Tanzania, it was learned that bar and guesthouse workers remained at risk of HIV infection even though they responded positively to early STD treatment and condom use with casual partners. When the bar workers tried to identify reasons why some were still becoming infected with new STDs and remained at risk of HIV infection, they found alcohol abuse and not using condoms properly were related problems. Alcohol abuse by clients also often led to forced sex without a condom. However, most bar workers indicated that they relied on several regular partners, mostly married men. For workers who became reinfected with new STDs, these infections often came from their regular partners with whom condom use was not possible.

Marketing and distribution

A number of factors are involved in assuring that condoms will be as appealing as possible and available where they are needed. Thinking in terms of 'marketing' to increase the appeal of condoms is a worthwhile approach. However, attention to the many details of distribution is also essential – questions such as how many condoms are needed, how they must be stored and how to ensure they reach their required destinations must be included.

Marketing

A concept called 'social marketing' builds upon the successes that have been achieved in commercial marketing, and is now being used to promote more desirable practices regarding drug and alcohol abuse, heart disease, malnutrition and overpopulation. Social marketing is defined as the design, implementation and control of programmes calculated to influence the acceptability of social ideas, involving considerations of product, planning, pricing, communications and market research (6).

To promote condoms, social marketing involves trying in a very systematic, strategic and research-driven way to find out for whom and how a condom can be made attractive, easily available and affordable. In a fully developed social marketing campaign, a researcher may use quantitative, cross-sectional and longitudinal surveys, interviews, mail and telephone surveys, and/or qualitative methods such as ethnographic fieldwork, focus group discussions, unstructured interviews and direct observation (see Chapters 4 and 9). A full range of monitoring and evaluative methods may be used to guide and assess the promotion programme.

The funding required for this kind of extensive research effort will typically be beyond the capacity of a district. Nevertheless, we can learn from it: attention to the attractiveness of the product and price setting, distribution and promotion are issues that need attention at district level. The basic idea of discovering what makes a product more or less acceptable to people is what is important. Paying careful attention to feedback from peer educators, for example, can be helpful in obtaining information in all of these areas.

For example, what preferences do different target groups have with respect to condoms? What colour should they be, how should they be packed, what name appeals to the target audiences, what names should be avoided? Condoms in social marketing programmes have names like Salama, used in Tanzania, which means safe and reliable. In Zaire and other francophone countries a brand name for condoms is Prudence. Commercial companies also use specific names to appeal to target groups, such as Topsafe (against pregnancy and HIV/STDs) and Rough Rider (emphasizing masculinity).

Another important consideration is price: condoms must be affordable. Often people prefer to pay something for a condom, and tend to mistrust free condoms. Hence, it may be advisable to begin selling condoms at a small price. This may even be recommended in countries where condoms are supplied free of charge: the charge could help to cover distribution costs.

Other elements that can be adjusted to target groups include the media used for promotion and the places where condoms are available. Among the possibilities for spreading information are the use of mass media (public campaigns, posters, billboards, banners), traditional media (songs, poems, theatre plays) and interpersonal channels (health workers, counsellors, peer health educators, village health workers). Research (which might include simple interviews and discussion; it need not be expensive) about the obstacles to condom use will be needed to develop messages for condom promotion that are appropriate to the target group. If people change their thinking about condom use, the message has to change accordingly.

Condoms may be supplied through health facilities, hotels, bars, guesthouses, market stands and shops. What distribution outlets do people prefer? Can condoms be promoted as part of a kit for STD treatment or family planning? How can condoms best be made available to the target group? Box 3 gives an example of using feedback from target groups.

Box 3. Choosing the best place to sell condoms

To better understand their preferences, target groups should be encouraged to give advice on possible distribution outlets for condoms. An AIDS action committee decided to make free condoms available at all small market stands to improve availability of condoms, but this failed because people did not trust condoms from market stands. Distribution through dispensaries, guesthouses and peer educators was more successful, even though it required more effort from people to obtain condoms.

Distribution
As a rule condom promotion should be combined with distribution: organizations engaged in the promotion of condoms have a role to play in distribution as well. Wherever and whenever condom use begins to be promoted, people should have access to a supply of condoms. Promotion creates interest in condoms, and condoms should be made available at that time.

In these cases, condom promotion is normally part of a set of interventions geared at behaviour change; it is seldom introduced as a single intervention strategy. For instance, promoting condoms in a factory could be part of an intervention package that includes peer health education on behaviour change, STD early treatment services, home-based care services, and HIV voluntary testing and counselling services. Often it is not difficult to ensure condom distribution during IEC activities, but to sustain a regular supply afterwards is more problematic. Hence, it is important that distribution points are identified and maintained. WHO training modules can be used in training programme managers, storekeepers and supply officers to ensure sound management and distribution of condom supplies (7).

In a district it is also essential to ensure the cooperation of hotel and guesthouse management as well as bars and local beer shops for the distribution of condoms, since these are the places where risky sexual behaviour is initiated and/or practised. It is also important to have a place where condoms can be stored and distributed to other outlets, such as a health facility. Wherever condoms are kept, care should be taken to ensure they are stored under proper conditions to preserve quality (see following section), and that their location is acceptable to users (see Box 4).

Box 4. Condom distribution in hotels and guesthouses

In Mwanza, Tanzania, condoms are supplied free of charge. The question, however, was how to make condoms available to clients in bars and guesthouses? Should they be distributed by barworkers or more anonymously through condom dispensers?

It was decided to locally produce condom boxes where condoms would be available free of charge. The boxes were placed in the toilets of all bars and guesthouses. One-half year later, when the system was evaluated, it was learned that most boxes had disappeared from toilets because these were not clean enough and people had ruined the condoms. The boxes had been moved to dark corners, and in some cases people had to ask the receptionist for a condom. After discussions with bar and guest-house owners it was agreed that condoms would be provided to all guesthouse rooms every day. Condom dispensers were also placed in more secluded corners in bars. Female bar workers trained as peer health educators became responsible for distribution.

The role of peer educators. Peer educators can play an important role in the promotion and distribution of condoms, as illustrated by the examples from Mwanza, Tanzania, shown in Box 5.

Box 5. Peer educators and condom distribution

Fishermen. Peer educators among fishermen on Lake Victoria were asked to distribute condoms to their peers directly, as they are isolated from other distribution outlets. Since fishermen are extremely mobile and often go to places where no condom distribution system is available, peer educators decided to use flexible condom distribution. Although they normally give out four condoms per individual, they decided to distribute 100 condoms per boat crew (about five men) when they go out on the lake for several days. Peer educators are pressed by their peers to make sure that a stock of condoms is always available – excuses that condoms are 'out of stock' are unacceptable.

High-transmission areas. Condom promotion is organized through a network of peer health educators in bars, local *pombe* shops and guesthouses. This ensures that customers find condoms in their rooms in all guesthouses. The number of condoms provided per room may differ from place to place: peer educators know best how many are needed per day. Condom stocks are kept by the peer educators, who also procure more condoms from the dispensary or central store when necessary.

Community educators. To develop a sustained condom distribution system, community educators in Tanzania were given the freedom to sell condoms to their peers and to the community. Although discussed at length with all parties involved to ensure acceptability, this system failed because the educators found it very difficult to negotiate a price with their peers for a condom that they receive free of charge. Another problem was that the system depended on a few individuals being motivated enough to spend time and arrange transport to procure condoms from the central store.

In working with peer or community educators it is important to discuss condom storage to ensure that it is done properly. Even in the short term, problems occur with condom storage: in guesthouses condoms may be kept in a window where the sun dries them out; fishermen have no proper storage places for condoms in their temporary shelters on the beach.

Another concern that can be addressed by peer educators is condom disposal. People need education about how to properly dispose of used condoms. Hygenic disposal of used condoms in guesthouses is also necessary.

The system of distribution.
Condoms are valuable commodities. This, plus the fact that they have an expiry date make shipping and distribution important concerns. Making sure supplies of condoms are well distributed, even in rural areas, is apt to require the mobilization of collaborators. At district level the Ministry of Health is often able to distribute condoms to its network of hospitals, clinics and dispensaries throughout the district. Private hospitals

and dispensaries can also assist in distribution. However, sometimes there is no budget for transporting condoms from central stores to peripheral areas. In this case, other government departments with an outreach service might be mobilized to assist, as may NGOs, clubs and associations. The management of workplaces should be asked to assist in the distribution of condoms to their workers.

How many condoms are needed in a district per year?
There are three ways of estimating yearly demand for condoms in a district (7): from past issuance (past consumption); from population-based data (based on assumptions of the number of risky acts); or from programme targets (in accord with national AIDS programmes).

- Past issuance: in most cases district officers in charge of condom supplies can estimate demand according to past consumption. For example, 100,000 condoms were distributed in a district in 1991, 130,000 in 1992, 155,000 in 1993 and 190,000 in 1994. Annual increase over the years was on average 30,000. Based on these figures it seems fair to estimate that the demand for 1995 would equal the demand for 1994 plus the average annual increase, yielding an estimated demand of 220,000 condoms. This calculation will do in most districts, especially when stock is monitored closely and additional condoms can be ordered during the year.

- Population-based estimate: a population-based estimate can be used if past issuance data are unavailable or inaccurate. The advantage of this method is that it estimates the maximum number of condoms needed, since it is based on all who are at risk. However, this method may easily overestimate demand since not everyone who is at risk will use condoms. Furthermore, it does not incorporate the capacity of the distribution system. The method also requires assumptions about the number of risky acts. For example:

1. identify sexually active men in the population	50,000
2. estimate the percentage of these who engage in risky sex	30%
3. estimate the percentage of condom users	33%
4. estimate the number of condoms needed per user, per unit of time (month or year)	250
5. estimate of total condoms needed (5 = 1x2x3x4)	1,250,000

- Making an estimate based on programme targets means working with the targets set for IEC activities. For instance, in a school programme where condom use is targeted to increase from 5% to 50%, condom needs may be estimated based on this increase. The condom usage rate per individual is very hard to estimate and hence, the quality of calculations will depend on the quality of KAP data. Also, if targets are unrealistic, the estimated demand based on these targets will also be inaccurate.

Health education

Health education materials and presentations to promote condom use should be chosen or designed based on information about target groups; and should aim at removing the identified obstacles to condom use.

Dealing with the stigma of condom use

If condoms are to become more widely used, it is necessary to develop basic messages to deal with the stigma related to their use. It is important to link condom use to responsible behaviour, conveying a message like: 'It is good to protect yourself, your partner and your future children from HIV infection by using a condom.'

It is also important to try to negotiate cooperation with religious groups opposing condom use. For example, they can be asked to campaign for their values, but not to campaign against condom use as this is confusing and may work against both campaigns. During community interventions local women's groups may be asked to campaign for responsible behaviour by promoting condom use as a positive way to protect one's family from HIV infection. When developing or choosing posters to promote condom use, it is important to present positive images and stress that both women and men are protected by condom use.

Married women are often the silent victims of the HIV epidemic, becoming HIV infected when their husbands engage in extra-marital sex (see Chapter 9). The practice of extra-marital relationships is usually not discussed, and in many societies cultural norms support men engaging in this practice. Picture codes (a picture which illustrates a familiar problem about which strong feelings exist) are an ideal means of breaking this taboo. The picture code shown below has stimulated worthwhile discussions among both men and women about various subjects such as the cultural norm of not discussing the (accepted) practice of extra-marital sex within a relationship, the need to reduce the number of sexual partners, and taking responsibility for protection by using a condom in relationships of risk.

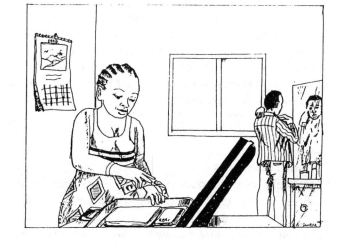

Faithfulness and condom promotion: a wife putting condoms in her husband's suitcase before he goes on safari.

Targeting consistent use

Linked to the issue of stigma is the problem of inconsistent condom use. Using a condom in a relationship signals that it is regarded a relationship of risk, creating mistrust. People usually stop using condoms when a relationship gains emotional value or changes into a loving or prolonged relationship. Condom use within marriage or regular relationships is virtually impossible: trust is regarded as more important than protection. Hence, messages to promote condom use can link trust to protection, for example: 'Love is to trust and to protect'; 'To use a condom is to care'; 'The answer to AIDS is to protect'.

Positive messages like these are thought to be more effective than negative messages, such as: 'don't die of ignorance' or 'AIDS kills, use a condom before it is too late'. Negative messages instill fear in the community, and may have an adverse effect on the stigma attached to AIDS.

The basic messages selected can be pretested and presented via mass media such as posters, advertisements and radio messages. They can also be used in face-to-face communications such as role plays, themes for poems or any other cultural drama performance. Short role plays performed by peer health educators have a strong impact. Following the role play basic questions can be posed to the audience (see Box 6), and the message further strengthened by printing it on a T-shirt. The players can wear such T-shirts and/or someone who participates in the discussion could be given a T-shirt. Both married and unmarried women in Tanzania were very enthusiastic about a T-shirt with the message: '*Jilinde unilinde*' meaning 'If you protect yourself, you will protect me' in English.

Box 6. A role play – Love is to trust and to protect

Situation: A man and a woman who have known each other for three months have used a condom every time they had sex. The man feels they can stop using condoms because they now trust each other and 'in a trusting relationship one does not use a condom'. The woman refuses, arguing that trust is as important as protection and an HIV test is needed for both before they stop using condoms.

Dialogue: Dialogues can be developed by peer health educators.

Discussion: The audience is asked: How will this end? Will they continue to use condoms? Will they go for an HIV test? Who decides about using condoms in a relationship? Is it easier for a man or for a woman to go for an HIV test?

Popular beliefs

Terms like 'misconception' should be avoided in discussions. Using the term misconception implies that the person asking the question is wrong and that an expert can help resolve the issue. Health educators and peer educators should always remember that some people in their audience may be more experienced than they are in sexual matters and condom use. For example, in one situation, when people remarked that condoms break easily, health educators were quick to explain that condoms only break when not properly used. But these health educators were married and had never used a condom themselves. It would have been better for them to accept the audience's remarks and look for reasons why condoms may break. This is an example of how questions can lead into a discussion of important issues, such as the quality and reliability of condoms. Another point that often comes up is the fact that condoms protect both males and females.

There are many popular beliefs regarding condoms (see Box 7). Since questions and answers may have different meanings in different cultures, all beliefs need to be thoroughly discussed among teams of health educators and peer educators to find and share proper answers. Answers may be found in many kinds of publications, but these should not be adopted without discussion.

Box 7. Popular beliefs about condoms

- Condoms are implanted with the HIV virus.
- Condoms may come off and remain inside women.
- Condoms break easily, and HIV virus will leak out.
- If you want to become pregnant you cannot use condoms.
- If I ask to use a condom, it may imply that I am HIV-positive.
- If I provide a women with enough financial support, I can trust her.
- A condom causes irritation and rashes.
- You can have sex only one time using a condom.
- Condoms are either too big or too small.
- Condoms reduce sensation.
- Condom use prolongs sex for too long and can lead to irritation in women.

The media may strengthen certain beliefs about the origins of the HIV virus or about the possibilities of a cure or vaccine. When an irresponsible doctor argues that the HIV virus does not exist, or that it is engineered to wipe out Africans from the earth, the story always receives attention from the press. It is necessary to address these media errors, especially since these inaccurate messages easily find fertile soil. Regularly providing interesting yet factual material to journalists is one possibility.

The level of motivation for condom use
User failure is reduced when people are motivated to use condoms. Alcohol or drug abuse strongly influences the motivation to use condoms. Targeting alcohol or drug abuse is difficult, but condom promotion should be done where the abuse takes place: in bars, local beer shops and guesthouses, and should preferably be supported by bar-workers who understand the behaviour of customers. Role plays used as discussion

starters are an effective tool for reaching customers in bars and other drinking places. Community action can also be mobilized to reduce alcohol and drug abuse by setting regulations for opening hours, increasing security for women, improving assistance (reporting procedures) in cases of coercive sex, preventing young people from entering bars and so on.

Focus on specific groups

Targeting specific groups means working to move potential users through the process of behaviour change from knowledge to awareness, trial and continued use. Important target groups for condom promotion are:

People who have tested HIV-positive: ongoing counselling of HIV-positives is needed to promote their consistent use of condoms. However, often they do not wish their partners to know their status, or if they feel healthy, they tend to ignore their HIV status.

STD clinic attenders: risk assessment counselling and voluntary HIV testing could be offered to those attending STD clinics and other people at special risk. Condom demonstration and distribution should always be part of health education for those attending STD clinics.

Commercial sex workers: a 100% condom use policy is essential but one problem is that sex workers may also have regular relationships in which condom use is regarded as unacceptable. Many unemployed women depend on selling sex as a source of income but do not regard themselves as commercial sex workers. Such women are difficult to reach, as they are unorganized and mobile.

Youth: may experiment with sexual relationships; responsible behaviour should be promoted – responsible in the sense of delaying sex or having protected sex, using condoms. Skills training to promote responsible behaviour is necessary: it is especially important for girls to receive training on condom negotiation and how to say 'no'. Promoting condom use among youth requires messages that fit into their specific culture, and the messages needed to fit urban and/or rural cultures may vary. The appropriateness of a poster or a message needs to be pre-tested; revisions may be needed. The messages should preferably be developed with the involvement of the youth themselves. Youth often fear pregnancy more than AIDS. Condom promotion should therefore link protection against STDs and HIV infection with protection against pregnancy.

Training for condom use

Health workers and peer educators need training to be able to provide appropriate health education on the use of condoms. Educators should be aware of the reasons for user failure and should address these in their educational sessions with audiences. User failures are known to be influenced by level of education, experience with condom use, motivation, sexual practices, and ability of partners to discuss sex, condom use and the implications of inconsistent condom use.

User failure is highest when people first start using condoms, and the less educated they are, the more training they require in condom use. Providing basic training in condom use to people who have never used them before is an important first step.

Special wooden dildos or rubber models are available for condom demonstrations. With the help of these models, each step in using condoms can be explained. Health workers may prefer to use their own models. When one peer educator in Magu District, Tanzania, lost her model she decided to use a soda bottle, and found it even more suitable because a bit of leftover soda made it easier to explain how semen remains in the condom after ejaculation. A humorous demonstration may help ease people's shyness and strengthen the idea that condom use can be made pleasurable. There should always be an element of fun in such demonstrations.

The condom demonstration should always be followed by a discussion on condom negotiation for both men and women. When a group of young girls were asked after a condom demonstration whether they would be able to start using condoms, they answered: 'No, because we would not know how to bring up the topic of condom use in our relationships'. A short role play can be very effective in starting a discussion on the ways to negotiate condom use.

It is also useful to distribute flyers about condoms after demonstrations. Most national programmes and many NGOs have developed satisfactory and tested flyers on how to use a condom. Before distributing these within a district, however, they should be retested among the prospective target group. The local language should also be used. Box 8 lists some tips for health educators and peer educators to use in condom promotion.

Box 8. Tips on condom promotion for health and peer educators

- Condom promotion should be fun: Ask some people from the audience to do a condom demonstration as a kind of game. Ask the audience who did it well and why. Humor can also be used to show that condoms are large enough or strong enough (by blowing them up like balloons or filling them with water).
- A wooden or rubber model may be used for condom demonstration; if unavailable, a soda-pop bottle can be a good alternative.
- Give people a few samples to play with after a health education session, before they actually start using condoms.
- Do not reply to every misconception or question by giving expert advice or an opinion. A question may also be posed to test you. It may sometimes be better to ask the questioner for his/her opinion or to ask other people in the audience to assist in finding an answer.
- After a condom promotion session, supply condoms to men and women who want them.
- Explain to people that it will take some time to get used to condoms.
- Explain that user failure is highest in the beginning and that people should not immediately become discouraged.
- Always give correct information, such as 'condoms reduce HIV transmission.'
- Try to reach people in bars and drinking places before they have had too much to drink.
- Always carry condoms during IEC activities.

Monitoring and evaluation

Monitoring is an ongoing survey of accomplishments, helping managers to evaluate whether projects are on target. Failure to reach objectives may indicate that targets were unrealistic or that management and distribution problems have occurred.

Indicators are a way of indirectly measuring the extent to which objectives have been reached (see Chapter 1). For condom promotion these may include:

- The extent to which distribution or sales targets have been reached. If a programme has a separate distribution component, such targets should be established for each month (or year), geographical area or specific programme.
- Changes in consumers' opinions or behaviour regarding condoms, collected through ongoing research, and feedback from training sessions (see below).
- Accessibility of condoms in the community.

Evaluation can be used to assess the programme performance of integrated intervention packages such as community or school intervention programmes, or may assess a condom promotion component separately. Since in most cases the limited funds available for evaluation will not be spent on condom promotion evaluation alone, condom promotion indicators can be included in the evaluation of an integrated intervention programme.

A survey of self-reported condom use may be too expensive. Moreover, there is a tendency by the target population to overreport condom use when it is understood that it is being promoted, or to underestimate use when people link condoms to culturally unwanted sexual behaviour. Evaluation of trends in condom use also need to be considered in the light of other changes in sexual behaviour, such as a reduction in the number of sexual partners. However, changes (before and after condom promotion activities) can be estimated based on changes in demand; and knowledge of how to use a condom, brand name recognition and negative attitudes can be investigated.

Conclusion

Condom promotion is an important and potentially highly effective intervention. However, in Mwanza increases in condom use are proceeding slowly, and there are still too few consistent users in vulnerable groups. Promotion of consistent use must remain a priority.

Condom promotion should preferably be integrated into other interventions, and it should be realized that people may prefer changes in their personal relationships over a technological response to the epidemic. An approach combining interventions aimed at reducing the number of partners with those aimed at increasing condom use can help people to make more responsible choices.

Condom promotion messages should stress the relational aspects of protection instead of presenting it merely as a technological solution to unwanted behaviour.

The obstacles to condom use for various target groups need to be understood and addressed in ways that make sense to each of these groups. Youth, for example, require a far different strategy than workers in bars and guesthouses. Role plays can be effective in getting people to begin thinking about condom use. Condom demonstrations should include an element of fun. Peer educators can play a vital role in condom promotion in all target groups.

Moreover, it is essential that condoms are made available when interventions are started. Condom promotion interventions create an interest in condom use, and it is important that condoms become and remain available at the same time. Distribution is thus an integral part of condom promotion, and districts need to learn how to ensure that adequate numbers of condoms are available within their areas.

Further reading

PATH. *A response to recent questions about latex condom effectiveness in preventing sexual transmission of the AIDS virus.* Arlington, VA, John Snow Inc., 1994.

World Health Organization. *Condom promotion for AIDS prevention.* Geneva, 1995.

World Health Organization. *Rapid assessment protocol for planning condom services.* Geneva, 1991.

World Health Organization. *Managing condom supply. Training manual.* Geneva, 1995.

World Health Organization. *Report of a WHO consultation on condom quality.* GPA/TCO/PRV/95.4. Geneva, 1995.

World Health Organization. *Guide to adapting instructions on condom use.* WHO/GPA/CNP/92.1. Geneva, 1992.

AIDS Health Promotion Exchange, issue no. 4 on 'Condoms...if you care'. Amsterdam, Royal Tropical Institute, 1992.

References

1. World Health Organization. *Condom promotion for AIDS prevention.* Geneva, 1995.

2. Pool R, Nnko S, Boerma JT et al. The price of promiscuity. Why urban males in Tanzania are changing their sexual behaviour. *TANESA Working Paper,* no. 8. January, 1996.

3. Morris M, Pramualratana A, Podhisita C et al. The relational determinants of condom use with commercial sex partners in Thailand. *AIDS* 1995, 9: 507–515.

4. Feldblum PJ, Morrison CS, Roddy RE et al. The effectiveness of barrier methods of contraception in the preventing the spread of HIV. *AIDS* 1995, 9 (suppl A): S85–S93.

5. World Health Organization. *Rapid assessment protocol for planning condom services.* Geneva, 1991.

6. McKee N. *Social mobilization and social marketing in developing communities. Lessons for communicators.* Southbound, Penang, Malaysia, 1992.

7. World Health Organization. *Managing condom supply. Training manual.* Geneva, 1995.

Part four
Health Interventions

12 Training health workers

Martin Mkuye, Dick Schapink, Christoph Hamelmann and Eva Masesa

- In a district, who requires training?
- What are the advantages of health unit-based training?
- Which qualities should a facilitator have?
- Is there still room for workshops and seminars?
- How can appropriate teaching aids be developed?

There is an enormous need to train health workers in Africa on HIV/AIDS/STDs. In the last ten years HIV/AIDS has exploded into a serious problem, a problem for which new knowledge is the most promising weapon. Knowledge about STDs and their role in the epidemic has changed rapidly in the last five years. But many health workers received their basic training before the impact of HIV/AIDS and its association with STDs was known. Furthermore, workers in remote units have always been less likely than their counterparts in towns to receive continuing education or to be able to attend workshops. The more peripheral, the lower the grade and the older the workers, the more likely they are to have fallen behind in their skills and to have missed advances made in health care.

Inadequate knowledge, attitudes and practices are caused by a number of factors, ranging from insufficient educational background to lack of HIV/AIDS training and re-training opportunities. Another reason training health workers is important has to do with the difficult emotional issues which surround AIDS. Training needs to address the beliefs, attitudes and prejudices of the workers themselves, their fears of infection, how to deal with sensitive topics such as sex and death, and the workers' own personal problems (for example, unfaithful partners).

In Tanzania, training needs assessments showed that health workers who had attended training of some kind had significantly more knowledge and more positive attitudes about HIV/AIDS compared to those who had not. This fact emphasizes the urgent need for and importance of training and re-training health workers in HIV/AIDS.

Another important argument for training is that the role of health workers is in flux – they are now often required to take part in social mobilization activities in villages, to become good communicators, to facilitate meetings or discussion groups and to take part in other training. Training for health workers should prepare them to use participatory, problem-solving approaches. Traditional health education must evolve to keep up with the changing role of health workers.

Who needs training?

Since most Ministries of Health now have a specific and comprehensive HIV/AIDS curriculum for pre-service basic training institutions, the emphasis in health workers' training should be placed on continuing education programmes for in-service health personnel. Highest priority should be placed on middle and lower health cadres, particularly trained nurses and nurse midwives, medical assistants, assistant health officers, village health workers, orderlies, laboratory and dental assistants and any other middle or lower health cadres.

A needs assessment (see below) is a good way to determine course content, method (see 'Training strategy and approach' below) and media. Course content may need to be tailored to a specific clinical setting (e.g. a maternity ward) or to specific types of workers (e.g. medical assistants treating STD cases) and may require self-learning materials, discussion and clinical experience under supervision. One subject to be discussed in all courses is STDs, since they are a factor which facilitates the transmission of HIV.

Examples of health personnel who can benefit from training include:
- staff of small health centres and clinics who provide outpatient care; maternal, children's and women's health services; community outreach services; tuberculosis and STD treatment.
- senior staff members of health units and the district health management team. This will aid them to estimate the size/extent of the impact of AIDS on their respective catchment areas and to learn more specific clinical skills (diagnosis, treatment, uses of tests) as well as community organization and peer education skills.
- hospital staff, enabling them to learn about prevention of occupational transmission, care of opportunistic infections and counselling.
- community leaders; women's, youth and development groups and teachers, enabling them to learn about peer education and community-based prevention and care.
- youth, both in and out-of-school, helping them to learn peer education skills.

In a district, it may be necessary to bring together the top ranks of health workers, such as hospital doctors and private practitioners, senior professional nurses and other sector heads; a workshop may be the best way to do this. However, it may be difficult to combine staff who see themselves as having very different status. For example, senior hospital staff may react negatively to being combined with dispensary staff.

Needs assessment

A needs assessment will indicate in which areas training is needed. Taking this first step helps in making decisions about more specific content. A needs assesment is likely to show a need for training in the following subjects:
- HIV and AIDS: basic knowledge of the disease and its epidemiology;
- HIV infection control in health settings;

- STDs and HIV/AIDS;
- tuberculosis and HIV/AIDS;
- simple morbidity care for HIV/AIDS in clinics;
- community-based HIV/AIDS/STD activities;
- condom information and distribution;
- information, education and communication (IEC) aimed at promotion of safer sexual behaviour in communities;
- examination of personal beliefs, attitudes, prejudices and fears.

A needs assessment should also indicate:
- what types of training were given in the past;
- the number of trained tutors or those with some experience as facilitators;
- availability of health education materials in the district, and whether they have been evaluated;
- the availability of condoms and STD drugs in the district;
- what problems exist and whether training is the right solution; problems such as lack of resources, supervision and motivation are often translated into the need for training.

A needs assessment should not only reveal specific needs for knowledge, attitude changes and skills but also pinpoint which categories of workers need training and whether particular health units' needs are more urgent. It can also help to ensure that a comprehensive HIV/AIDS programme is integrated into the district health system. A needs assessment should also collect information on numbers of people needing training. One way to do this is to administer a knowledge-attitude-practices (KAP) questionnaire to a sample group of workers. The sample should contain government health facilities staff as well as adequate numbers of:
- workers from the private sector or commercial clinics;
- health workers from other sectors (prison, army, police, secondary schools or college clinics);
- NGOs working in health and community development.

It is best to have a group of people prepare the questionnaire. Resources – mostly in the form of people who can help – can be drawn from training schools, NGOs, AIDS committees, doctors and nurses from the District Health Management Team and the regional health office. Existing questionnaires supplied by the National AIDS Programme or by NGOs working in the field of AIDS/STDs may also be useful.

Methods to assess skills such as calculating correct dosages, giving injections and taking blood can be obtained from any nursing college. Other behaviours and skills, e.g. communication skills (taking a history, establishing rapport, listening with empathy and without social distance) can best be assessed by observation. Usually only a few workers within a district have been taught counselling skills; it is best to have their capability assessed by trained counsellors if possible.

To conclude, one possibility for needs assessment is to set up a workshop involving different cadres and supervisors. Based on the needs assessment, this group can analyse job descriptions, responsibilities and new roles to be filled, in relation to the skills and gaps therein.

The range of training

It is obvious that the spectrum of new knowledge, skills and changed attitudes needed for a HIV prevention and AIDS care programme is very wide, even before a needs analysis indicates the areas in which training is needed to ensure a comprehensive programme integrated into the district health system. Many staff members are active in small health centres and clinics, providing outpatient care, maternal, children's and women's health and community outreach services. Health centres and clinics deal with tuberculosis and sexually transmitted diseases. Staff members face occupational risks, dealing with injections and coming into contact with blood and other body fluids. These circumstances call for training:

- Senior members of health unit staff and the district health management team need to understand the impact of AIDS and how to estimate the scope of the problem in their respective catchment areas, as well as to gain specific clinical skills – diagnosis, treatment and use of tests. They also need knowledge about community organization and peer education.
- Hospitals employ a range of workers who may require specific training on preventing occupational transmission, the care of opportunistic infections and pre- and post-test counselling.
- Communities need training as the programme is certain to include community mobilization and peer education in schools and high-transmission areas. Community leaders, community-based organizations, women's groups and youth groups will benefit from training provided by community-based activities for HIV prevention and AIDS home care.
- Youth, both in and out-of-schools, are of special importance for peer education and teacher training as this offers a great opportunity to influence behaviour.

Thinking through the objectives of training as part of a comprehensive programme is a useful first step, and can be of help in deciding which specific content and methods which will be most effective in each district situation.

Selection of training techniques

The selection of training techniques is influenced by several criteria: the learning objectives, the size of the group, the composition of the group of learners, and the resources available (see Box 1). Matching the training techniques to the learning objectives is very important. For example, if the goal is to change attitudes, a series of lectures is not appropriate; discussion groups may be a better strategy.

Box 1. Criteria for selection of training techniques

Learning objectives
- Knowledge, retention of knowledge, understanding: training techniques could include lectures, reading, case studies, discussions.
- Awareness of attitudes and feelings: training techniques could include role plays, case studies, group discussions, participatory work in communities.
- Ability to use different techniques: training techniques could include demonstrations, practice, role plays, videos.
- Improved ability to transfer ideas and interact with others: training could include micro-training exercises, role plays, group discussions.
- Improved capacity to continue learning: training methods to include self-discovery and learning experiences, brainstorming in groups, immediate feedback with distance learning modules.

The learners
- The extent to which learners are familiar with self-learning, reading materials, audiovisual materials, role plays, etc. influences their ability to use these tools.
- The age of the learners is important: adults learn best with learner-centred, problem-solving, self discovery and action-oriented participatory methods.

The size of the groups
- Individuals or groups of two: training via reading, writing, programmed learning modules.
- Small groups (3–15): training by group discussion, role plays, exercises.
- Large groups (16–24): workshops and division into smaller groups, each given different tasks to discuss and 'feed back' to the whole group. (In larger groups personal interaction and knowing individuals by name become difficult and the personal touch may be lost).
- Large assemblies (25 and over): film shows, lectures, panel discussions, classroom talks, buzz groups (talk to 2–3 neighbours and report).

Resources
- Availability of teaching materials: self-learning materials, audiovisuals, libraries, newsletters.
- Availability of resources person(s) (strengths and weaknesses).

Content, method and media

It is very important to make learning interesting and active, and to use a variety of methods and media. For example, the three modes of HIV transmission should be included in training and can be illustrated by short case stories. Mother-to-child transmission is often not understood and is a topic for both women and men because children are so important in families. An example of a story is given in Box 4 (see below), illustrating how transmission from mother to child takes place. Other stories could be used to illustrate transmission via sex and via blood.

Condom promotion should be included in all training, including discussion, demonstrations using, for example, a wooden dildo, written material and flyers (to hand out) about the value and correct use of condoms (see also Chapter 11).

Training strategy and method

A variety of training methods can be employed to train health workers and others about HIV/AIDS:

1 Study group
2 Independent learning
3 Distance learning
4 Classroom teaching
5 Workshop

The first three methods are health unit-based. The independent and distance learning methods can be made more effective by integrating group learning with a face-to-face component into the training programme.

Since facilitators and supervisors require group learning techniques, a section on group discussion is included in the study group method. However, these skills are used in all training methods.

Classroom teaching normally takes longer and may cover more in-depth topics, while workshops are short and concentrated. The workshop is held in a larger venue and employs a variety of methods, including practical work, field visits, group discussions and speaker presentations.

In all teaching methods, case studies are used to support the learning process. These help to engage learners in problem-solving situations and enable participants to reflect on their own experiences. Case studies make learning more lively, as participants discuss problem-related cases providing different views and opinions during discussions.

Health unit-based training

Every country has vast numbers of health workers. This makes it difficult to reach the majority within a short period using conventional training methods. Thus, innovative and pragmatic methods should be used. Health unit-based training is a training approach which focuses on the health worker at the health unit, dispensary, health centre or hospital. The method employs either a 'facilitator' health education system (using group learning approaches) or self-learning devices (mainly printed materials). The latter method may include occasional tutorial support in some form of face-to-face sessions.

Health unit-based training has several advantages, especially concerning cost-effectiveness. Other advantages include wider coverage of the target audience within a short time, learning while continuing to work (on-the-job training), immediate application of what has been learned and retaining learning materials after completion of the course, especially in the case of self-learning methods. Health workers in remote places can be reached easily.

Learning is participatory, and working experiences are used as part of the method. This makes learning effective in terms of knowledge gained. Interactive group exchange of experiences in the health unit is central to health unit-based learning. Therefore the main thrust of the approach is participatory learning by all health workers in the health unit, using their own working activities as a basis. This also facilitates training directed at attitude changes and skills development. Group teaching improves team work and motivation. This method has been used successfully in Mwanza Region and one course is now used there for all workers.

The main limitation of the health unit-based approach is a lack of active learning exchanges among health workers in different health units (denying them the opportunity to draw on each other's experiences). The in-charge staff of different health units, however, can be trained together, providing some exchange. Furthermore, unless some face-to-face tutorial support is included in self-learning approaches, learning gained through demonstrations will be limited.

Method 1: the study group

In the study group method, health workers learn about AIDS individually in their health units, with the support of a trained facilitator. In smaller health units such as clinics or dispensaries and some health centres with fewer staff, all members of the health unit participate in the same study group.

Selection and training of facilitators

The method entails selecting and training facilitators from a whole district. Those in charge of health units – dispensaries, health centres and hospital departments/units – should be selected to attend this training. In addition, one additional staff member from a health centre can be trained, along with perhaps six hospital staff members, representing different departments/units. The number of health unit staff involved can vary depending on the number of staff in a health unit.

The facilitators can be centrally taught at a district level HIV/AIDS workshop lasting four to five days and utilizing the group learning method and group leadership skills. Facilitators are also provided with basic study materials in the form of books or booklets. After completion of the course, the facilitators return to their health units to plan the training programme together with their colleagues. A model training programme developed during the facilitators' training can be adapted by the various health units for their own use.

The role of facilitators

Facilitators (sometimes called motivators) are responsible for motivating their colleagues to learn, organizing learning experiences and assisting their colleagues in learning. They also carry out administrative responsibilities such as keeping progress and attendance records. The facilitator helps the group work out their objectives, plan the programme, structure the learning experience and determine how much time is needed to cover the material. The facilitator should further stimulate all group members to learn, and create a climate which respects each individual and encourages the willingness and capacity to share.

The facilitator's ability to fulfil this role is linked to facilitation style. Facilitators can exercise different degrees of control. In the past, educators were often seen as acting in a 'top–down' way, directing the entire process completely. There may be situations in which this is appropriate. However, facilitators are more often seen as working cooperatively with the group to decide the objectives and the process, or allowing the group the freedom to find their own way but to use the facilitator as a resource. The way the facilitator fulfils his/her role usually depends on individual management style – there is a place for many different styles in different circumstances.

Group discussion is a technique involving purposeful conversation and deliberation about a topic of mutual interest to group members. In using this technique participants should be involved in choosing topics of interest which meet their needs and desires.

The main advantage of the group discussion technique is that participants share experiences based on their own work. The main limitation of the technique is that some members may keep silent while others – sometimes even the facilitator – dominate the discussion. It is also easy for members to drift away from the main topic of discussion. To overcome these difficulties, facilitators, supervisors and motivators should be helped in learning how to deal with such problematic situations. Role playing group sessions can be very helpful.

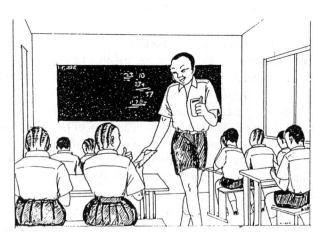

Sexual relationship developing between a schoolgirl and schoolboy by the exchange of gifts.

Evaluation

Evaluation of the study group discussion training method has shown it to be effective in terms of knowledge gained. It is also cost-effective. However, unless the facilitator is specially prepared to do so, the study group method may change attitudes but not improve skills.

In organizing to use this method, hospitals should make special arrangements, such as short, 4-day seminars alternating between hospital units or departments within the hospital. The major organizational limitation of this method is that it takes time: a district may not be able to effectively supervise all health units involved in the training. Therefore, if technical problems arise, feedback to learners is often delayed, which may cause frustration.

Method 2: independent learning

The independent learning method is closely related to the distance learning method (see below). Written texts are most often used, which can be supplemented by brief face-to-face sessions, preferably lasting about two days.

Method

Health workers learn at their own health units using self-learning materials: 'Independent Learning Modules'. They can complete the modules on their own but working in small groups, such as groups of health unit workers, is preferable. Modules can be prepared in a workshop or commissioned from an expert on the subject. In either approach the course writer(s) should be briefed on the techniques of developing self-learning educational materials, and on the language, writing style, examples, etc. suitable for the target group. Pictures and other visual elements should be included in the materials. Such devices make learning active, provide motivation to the learner and help to break monotony. Illustrations should be tested in conjunction with the designer to be certain they communicate their intended messages. Independent learning materials can also be adapted from other sources to minimize production costs. Modules must be tested for relevance, readability, usability, comprehension and effectiveness before being produced in large numbers.

For effective learning, the course should be divided into sections covering broad themes. In Tanzania, for example, the material for the health unit staff was divided into five modules (see Box 2). Modules then may be divided into lessons, ideally taking about one hour to complete, either individually or as a group. Lessons should not normally involve much memorizing but instead should focus on thinking and talking about ideas and application to the group members' working situation. Also included are problem-solving exercises in three forms: in-text questions, questions at the end of each section and questions requiring integration of knowledge from several modules. Activities are aimed at activating learners, making learning more effective.

Box 2. Modules for an independent learning programme in Tanzania

MODULE 1 Basic facts and feelings about HIV/AIDS
     Lesson 1: What are our thoughts and worries about AIDS?
     Lesson 2: What do we know and what do we need to know
           about AIDS?
     Lesson 3: How can we use what we have learned about AIDS?
MODULE 2 How to find out about AIDS in your community (divided over three
     lessons)
MODULE 3 HIV infection and AIDS counselling (divided over two lessons)
MODULE 4 Review of infection control in health units (six lessons)
MODULE 5 AIDS home-based care (seven lessons).

Organization

In a district, a decision to initiate this method requires a discussion between the heads
of the units and the district AIDS programme. Availability of the modules and arrangements for support can then be announced to unit staff.

At a preliminary district level meeting, representatives (facilitators/motivators) from
each unit should then review the modules for relevance and any problems. They are
given an outline of a study plan to relate to their units' actual routines. When they
return to their clinic or health unit they discuss this plan with workers, including the
days when face-to-face sessions at the health centre are planned and when demonstrations relating to the modules will take place. Health workers are encouraged to read
each module independently and attempt the activities for every lesson before it is
discussed in the study group.

Integration with other media

The course can be followed effectively without any other media support. However, for
optimal results, self-study should be integrated with brief (about two-day) face-to-face
sessions. These can be organized at centrally located satellite dispensaries. Face-to-face
sessions provide learners with opportunities to reinforce the lessons in written texts.
Furthermore, difficult concepts are clarified and questions are answered, while health
workers from different health units share their experiences, enriching learning.
Demonstrations and practicals are carried out during these sessions. In hospitals it may
be possible to supplement learning with tapes or videos, if equipment is available or
can be borrowed from NGOs. Using the independent learning method takes six to eight
weeks.

Support services

The support services required by this programme include course announcements to
health workers with a brief statement about how to approach the course. Motivators
also act as student counsellors and report to the district AIDS programme coordinator if

difficulties arise. Two record-keeping forms are used: enrolment and progress record-keeping forms. The district AIDS programme coordinator and the continuing education officer are provided with a comprehensive supervision form. Motivators should be charged with record-keeping.

Advantages and disadvantages

The advantage of this method lies in its coverage: more health workers are reached with minimum travel and accommodation costs. Health workers continue to work while they learn, and knowledge and skills gained can be applied immediately.

A disadvantage of this method is that if the district must prepare its own modules, and no one with these skills is available, the modules may be of poor quality, insufficient or inadequately tested. Furthermore, if individual work is not supported by face-to-face sessions most practical elements will be missing.

Evaluation

The method includes pre- and post-training tests, which permit an assessment of the changes in knowledge levels as a result of the independent learning programme. A more detailed evaluation of a programme was carried out in Tanzania: results are shown in Box 3.

Box 3. Results of an independent learning programme in Tanzania

An independent learning programme was implemented in Magu District, Tanzania. It covered 557 workers in health facilities. The bulk of the training was health facility based, as described above.

The knowledge score among health workers increased from 59% to 68% during pre- and post-testing respectively. A further improvement of the knowledge score was observed at a second post-training test six months later. This increase in knowledge was only observed in health centres and dispensaries, not in the hospitals. The long-term increase in knowledge was ascribed to team work and continued exchange of knowledge in smaller health units. Also, attitudes towards HIV/AIDS patients were positive.

The costs of the programme were about US$ 30 per health worker. Ways to reduce costs are now being explored (for example, correspondence courses).

Source: Masesa Eva, Schapink, D, Mayunga Deograties, Hugo Aloyce. Evaluation of health-unit based learning for health workers in Magu District. TANESA Internal Series Paper no. 9. November 1996.

Method 3: distance learning

Distance learning methods are necessary when the learner is physically separated from the tutor. Learners study on their own, using mostly written self-learning materials. Other media might include audiocassettes, videos and radio programmes (although these may be less available in rural areas, rural people often request them).

The development of distance learning materials is similar to that of independent learning material, except that each module ends with questions which require marking and commentary from a tutor. This provides two-way communication between learner and tutor. A field tutor should return marked assignments promptly, providing feedback which enhances learner motivation. The role of their tutor is demanding (marking, commenting, writing, returning assignments) and requires a field or teaching allowance, which makes this method costly. It is helpful for the tutor to have clear guidelines on how to perform her or his duties.

Improving the distance learning and other self-learning methods
Sharing experiences and ideas enhances learning. Therefore, the addition of short (about two-day) face-to-face sessions towards the end of the self-learning course is useful. Such sessions can be organized at the health centre, also giving learners the chance to gain practical experience. Perhaps several clinics can complete their courses simultaneously and meet together at the end. Record-keeping is important and helps motivators or tutors to ensure the programme is progressing.

Advantages and disadvantages
Distance learning is a way to make training more widely available. In Tanzania, as in several other countries, the Open University of Tanzania and the Institute of Adult Education run professional courses, but to administer a single HIV/AIDS course exclusively for districts would not be cost-effective. Moreover, it is difficult to learn skills if no face-to-face component is built into the programme to provide practical and demonstration opportunities. Furthermore, supportive supervision may be limited if, for example, the tutor and district AIDS programme coordinator only work part-time on the programme, so that neither is able to visit and observe learners due to other commitments.

Evaluation
Evaluation of distance learning has shown that the method is effective in terms of knowledge gained.

Method 4: classroom teaching

Classroom teaching is perhaps the oldest and most conventional educational method; we are all familiar with it. It has mainly been used in formal training institutions. Classroom teaching traditionally employs mostly lecture methods; learners are often passive listeners with teachers playing a dominant role in the teaching-learning transaction. Communication is largely one-way.

This method can also be adapted to suit non-formal training situations. It is now increasingly being used in these situations to train facilitators, peer health educators and health promoters. In non-formal training situations the method can be adapted to incorporate participatory learning processes and improve lecture method presentations.

The improved classroom method

The improved classroom lecture method is most often used in a non-formal training situation. In this method, an adaptation of the conventional method, the facilitator and learners actively participate during the session. Communication takes place in more than one direction: the teacher/facilitator gives messages to learners and asks them questions, while learners ask questions which the facilitator answers. There is also communication among the learners, who ask each other questions and make comments. Such opportunities are limited, however, because the facilitator must complete the curriculum within a specified time period. An example of a case which can be used to involve learners in a classroom situation is given in Box 4. Learners can read the case and then discuss it, based on the questions listed.

Box 4. HIV transmission from mother to child: The story of Rose

Rose is 24-years-old and married to John. They live in a small village and have two children. John goes to a nearby town each day to work. Rose works a plot of land and grows food for the family. Last year, Rose had a third child. Rose was healthy but the baby failed to thrive and doctors suspected AIDS. After 18 months the baby died of AIDS. Rose wants to have more children but fears they will also die.

Questions about HIV transmission from mother to child in regard to Rose's story:
1. How did the baby get AIDS?
2. Is Rose infected with HIV?
3. Should Rose try to get pregnant again?
4. Will Rose die of AIDS?
5. How did Rose get HIV infection?
6. What information does Rose need?

The group discusses transmission of HIV infection from mother to child; the facilitator provides factual information if needed.

Preparation

Much preparation is required with this method: the facilitator must refer to several sources of information to obtain a balanced view of the subject under discussion and often must prepare his/her own handouts for the participants. Once teaching notes and handouts are prepared, however, they can be used for a longer period of time with only minor changes to incorporate new knowledge. All of this means that a facilitator must have access to good reference sources and updated materials.

Teaching-learning process
In this method, the facilitator gives a short talk – about ten minutes – and allows learners to respond before continuing. The facilitator encourages learners to actively participate in the session. In informal situations the method can be used when the audience is large, when a new subject or topic is to be introduced, when much new material must be covered or when there is not enough suitable reading material available for the class.

Advantages and disadvantages
The advantages of the improved classroom lecture method are: much material can be covered in a short time, health workers are encouraged to participate, self-confidence among participants is promoted and large groups can receive instruction within a short time. The classroom method can be augmented with short lectures, discussions, activities and application of skills.

The main limitation of this method is cost, because participants often must travel from their respective health units to a faraway venue. This implies costs in terms of fares and daily subsistence allowances. There are also direct costs in terms of participants' transport time between their workplaces and the venue.

Evaluation
Evaluation of the improved class lecture method has shown it to be effective in terms of knowledge gained.

Method 5: the workshop

In many districts, workshops have been arranged through NGOs or donors to train different cadres on specific aspects of HIV prevention and AIDS care. This practice is decreasing, but workshops still have a role to play. Workshops which are often needed include:
- planning a district HIV prevention and AIDS care programme (an example from Ghana is given in Chapter 1, Box 2)
- training for STD management
- condom promotion, supply and social marketing (see Chapter 11)
- planning the set-up of a high-transmission area project
- training to improve health workers' communication skills.

Workshops which divide participants into groups to discuss specific issues provide a rich exchange of ideas, extending the learning/teaching process to include many viewpoints and perspectives. One method of proceeding is to have participants work in groups to discuss and write down constructive ideas or comments on a problem. These are then presented to the whole group, which also provides a record of ideas. Many

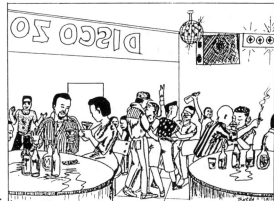

Risk behaviour: alcohol abuse often leads to unprotected sexual intercourse.

workshops are structured with modules including facts, stories, etc. but always with some aspect, problem or activity for participants to work on together.

Workshops can combine classroom lectures, group methods, independent learning, field trips and demonstrations. This possibility for using multiple methods is their great advantage. Also, they allow a fruitful interchange of ideas among people working in different places and practising different disciplines. Community members should be included in workshop planning.

Workshops require much preparation and experienced and specially trained facilitators if they are to be successful. The disadvantages of workshops are often related to cost. Also, a special meeting place may be needed, and participants attending a workshop often require accommodation. Facilitators may have to be brought from outside the district, which is another considerable expense. Furthermore, workshops often take key staff (who carry out the management functions of the health unit) away from their work.

Conclusion

This chapter surveys some of the wide range of methods and training strategies which can be adopted in HIV prevention and AIDS care programmes. Training is becoming crucial for health staff, patients, communities and their leaders, workers in other sectors, schoolchildren and teachers. The purpose of training is not only to assure that up-to-date knowledge is available, but also because the role of health workers is in flux. Communication skills, attitudes and the ability to work as facilitators continue to grow in importance. By examining different approaches to training we can learn which methods may be best suited to the wide range of situations in which health workers operate. A training component in the district HIV prevention and AIDS care programme is vital, and thus is mentioned in many other chapters of this book.

Further reading

AIDSTECH. *STD/AIDS peer educator training manual*, 1992. Can be ordered from: Family Health International, P.O. Box 13950, Research Triangle Park, NC 27709, USA; National AIDS Control Programme, Ministry of Health, P.O. Box 9083, Dar es Salaam, Tanzania; AMREF, P.O. Box 2773, Dar es Salaam, Tanzania.

Evian C. *Primary AIDS care: a practical guide for primary health care personnel in the clinical and supportive care of people with HIV/AIDS,* second edition by C. Evian, Jacana, (Private Bag 2004, Houghton 2041, Johannesburg, South Africa) 1995.

AMREF. *Manuals for health workers.* Independent learning programme for all levels of health workers. Mwanza, Dar es Salaam. (Five volumes.)

TANESA. *Syllabus for one week course on HIV/AIDS for health workers.* (P.O. Box 434, Mwanza, Tanzania.)

13 STD control efforts in health units

Heiner Grosskurth and Ezra Mwijarubi

- What are the potential consequences of STDs?
- Why is it important to offer STD patients immediate treatment?
- What is syndromic treatment?
- How can privacy and confidentiality be improved within health clinics for STD patients?
- How can STD control be integrated into antenatal care?
- How can sexual partners of STD patients be included in the treatment?
- How can health education be ensured?

Early and effective treatment of STDs (sexually transmitted diseases) is one of the most important ways to control the spread of HIV. STDs not only increase the risk of HIV transmission, but may also lead to serious complications, especially for women. This chapter describes efforts to control STDs at health units throughout the districts, including discussion of the clinical importance of STDs, case management, case finding, equipment, personnel and time requirements. Chapter 14 focuses on the efforts that need to be made at the district level to ensure an effective STD control programme.

Clinical importance of STDs

Prior to the global AIDS epidemic, classical sexually transmitted diseases (STDs) received little attention, neither in public health policy nor as a clinical subject. In health workers' training, STDs were often treated as a marginal issue. The onset of a new and deadly STD – HIV infection – has changed this situation dramatically.

Several years after the AIDS epidemic had established itself in East Africa, a correlation between HIV infection and classical STDs became apparent: individuals with a history of ulcerative lesions were more often found to be HIV-infected than those who reported no such sores (1). This was also true for STD patients without such sores, although to a lesser extent. While the association between STDs and HIV infection could in principle be explained by risky sexual behaviour, the different strength of this association for different STDs suggested that STDs in themselves represent an important reinforcing co-factor for HIV infection: ulcerative lesions and inflammation are believed to facilitate HIV transmission.

The existence of this co-factor effect has since been demonstrated and its implications have become widely accepted (see Chapter 14). Attempts are being made in many countries to improve the clinical management of STDs by providing better training for health workers and drugs that are effective in treating STDs. However, an additional problem is that advanced HIV infection may change the clinical course of STDs; for example, genital ulcers may become large and incurable.

STDs, however, are not a public health problem only because of their interaction with HIV/AIDS. STDs are a major health problem in their own right. Particularly for women of childbearing age, STDs are a major threat to health. Bacterial infections of the cervix uteri (the neck and the outer opening of the womb), mostly caused by *Neisseria gonorrhoeae* and *Chlamydia trachomatis*, are frequently asymptomatic, but have a great tendency to spread upwards and to lead to infection of the uterine cavity, the Fallopian tubes and the lower pelvic cavity. The consequences are frequently devastating. They include:

- acute pelvic inflammatory disease (PID), which is potentially lethal, as a consequence of generalized sepsis. PID also very often results in adhesions and scarification within the pelvic cavity, causing chronic pain;
- blocked tubes, resulting in ectopic pregnancy which, without intervention, may cause fatal internal bleeding;
- blocked tubes, which may cause infertility and lead to social stigmatization of women in many African societies;
- infections of the genital tract, which may ascend into the uterus following delivery and result in puerperal infection, high fever and death via sepsis;
- genital tract infections (infections of the cervix uteri) often cause eye infection (*ophthalmia neonatorum*) in newborn babies, which is still an important cause of blindness.

Syphilis is an extremely common infection in many African populations (2). The syphilitic ulcer usually heals within a few weeks, even if left untreated. However, the infection itself continues and may slowly destroy large blood vessels and parts of the central nervous system. In pregnancy this hidden infection (latent syphilis) often leads to spontaneous abortion, stillbirth, low birthweight or congenital syphilis in babies.

Although women carry by far the largest burden of STD sequelae, men may also face consequences such as infection of the epididymis or the testes, which is extremely painful and often results in infertility.

STD case management at health units

An essential task of dispensaries, health centres and hospital outpatient departments is to diagnose and treat patients with STDs effectively and without delay, and to seriously attempt to prevent future infection. STD patients – perhaps more than patients with other ailments – have a tendency to drop out of the official health care system and look for other, often less competent, sources of care if their expectations for immediate and effective treatment are not met in the first instance. For this reason it is vital that STD patients receive the required treatment when and where they first attempt to seek help.

The components of proper case management are:
- privacy and confidentiality;
- a caring attitude expressed by health workers;
- evidence-based diagnosis;
- syndromic treatment with effective drugs;
- health education to avoid future infection;
- provision and promotion of condoms;
- partner notification;
- recording and reporting;
- assessment of treatment outcome.

Privacy, confidentiality and health workers' attitudes
It is not rare to find adequately equipped health facilities with skilled staff who treat hardly any STD cases, even though attendance rates for other ailments are quite high. In such circumstances, surveys often reveal lack of privacy; or that health workers show a reproachful or moralistic attitude (3). These factors are of fundamental importance: they determine the rate at which STD services are utilized at the unit, and can therefore have an enormous impact on the sexual health of the entire community. Having an STD is embarrassing for most people, and patients do not like discussing private matters in the presence of other patients (see Box 1). Patients must be absolutely sure their private problems will not become a topic of gossip within the community. These points may seem obvious, but experience shows they are not always taken seriously.

Box 1. Privacy in health facilities

Privacy is usually easy to achieve: patients should be attended to one by one, and the door should always be closed when a patient is being seen by the clinician. This applies to all patients, not only for those with STDs.

Other staff walking in and out during an examination may also be perceived as a disturbance. To avoid this, a simple screen can be put up for privacy: even a sheet of cloth hung on a string may do the job.

In STD-related training courses for health workers, issues of privacy, confidentiality and a positive attitude towards patients should always be major topics for teaching and group discussion (see Chapter 14). STDs are extremely common in both men and women.

This has little to do with general promiscuity, and is more related to the insufficient availability of effective health care. It is time for health workers to regard STDs as 'normal' diseases, such as malaria. A reproachful and moralistic attitude will only scare patients away, and should be replaced with caring and reassurance.

Evidence-based diagnosis
In their daily routine, health workers often must see a large number of patients within a short span of time. The temptation is great to base prescriptions merely on patients' complaints. Not rarely, this approach will lead to wrong decisions causing serious mistakes. For example, a complaint of a sore will be treated as an ulcer, although the patient in reality may suffer from a different STD. However, experience shows that, to treat STDs effectively, certain minimal conditions must be met (see Box 2). An STD patient should *never* receive treatment without at least taking a brief history and receiving a quick genital examination.

Box 2. Practical steps in STD diagnosis

- Listen to the patient and be sure to fully grasp the situation: what does the patient really mean? A reported 'pain down there' may have many causes: a discharge, an ulcer, or even a pelvic inflammation. Two or three targeted questions will usually clarify the situation and in most cases can be completed effectively in less than a minute.
- Take a look: a brief examination usually reveals the crucial information: is there really a discharge? Many patients confuse various genital symptoms, with the result that the wrong syndrome may be treated. Might the symptoms suggest two concurrent underlying syndromes (e.g. an inflamed foreskin with an ulcer underneath? A vaginal discharge and lower abdominal pain?).
- Examine the patient on a bed or bench. This is also the only way to confirm mild discharge: in men, if the discharge is not obvious, the urethra can be massaged ('milked') by squeezing the penis once from the root to the tip. In women, the labia can be spread to diagnose discharge or an ulcer. A female patient also needs to be examined in lying position to verify lower abdominal pain.
- Speculum examination: Although effective STD case management in peripheral health units certainly does not depend on the capacity to perform speculum examination, it can be a useful tool. Health workers often lack the necessary skills and experience, and are hesitant to apply this diagnostic method. However, the nature of vaginal discharge, particularly if it is mild, can best be assessed by a speculum examination. This will show whether, for example, a reported mild discharge is suggestive of thrush; this will affect the treatment decision. It may also help to determine whether there is inflammation and discharge from the cervix. Furthermore, a speculum is needed to diagnose an intravaginal ulcer, which is occasionally seen in women coming in for treatment of another syndrome.

Syndromic treatment with effective drugs

The syndromic treatment of STDs is recommended strongly by WHO (4) and has been adopted by many African countries. What are the reasons and underlying principles? Contrary to common belief, STD symptoms and signs are rarely specific to particular causative agents. In other words, a health worker cannot tell just by looking whether a discharge is caused by gonococcal or chlamydial infection, or whether an ulcer is caused by chancroid or syphilis, and so forth. Several STD micro-organisms (e.g. chlamydia) can only be diagnosed by rather costly and sophisticated tests. Yet in most peripheral health units in African countries, laboratories are often not available (or not functioning). Even where laboratories do exist, regular quality control is often not practised. Further, dual infections are not uncommon. In women, a symptomatic vaginal infection is often accompanied by an asymptomatic (yet dangerous) cervical inflammation caused by a different organism. Both clinician and laboratory may often miss one of the causative agents. Lastly, when patients must return to the clinic for lab results before receiving treatment, they often fail to do so, particularly if they live far away.

Where reliable, cheap and fast laboratory testing is not feasible, it is best to base management of STDs on the diagnosis of syndromes. A syndrome is defined as a combination of symptoms and signs which may be due to various causative agents. Once the syndrome has been correctly diagnosed, based on a brief history and examination, a combination of drugs can be prescribed which cover the most frequently occurring aetiologies. The selection of drugs to be used in a particular country or region depends on three aspects: the causative organisms prevalent in the area, the susceptibility of these organisms to antibiotics and the cost of drugs.

Although a syndromic approach has disadvantages, they do not outweigh the positive aspects. This standardized approach will automatically overtreat patients in whom only one causative agent is present. This is particularly true for women: vaginal discharge syndrome is in no way a reliable predictor of a cervical infection. However, as these infections are frequent and serious, overtreatment may be justified. It is important to realize that in spite of the overtreatment the syndromic approach is still more cost-effective than a laboratory-based approach (16).

It has been argued that syndromic treatment can accelerate the development of antimicrobial resistance. However, the worst problems with resistance do not arise from unnecessary treatment of non-infected individuals, but from insufficient treatment of the infected, particularly if health workers prescribe too-low doses or if patients take antibiotics only until symptoms disappear. It is important that health workers convince their patients to adhere fully to the prescription and complete the course as given. Syndromic treatment involves taking a comparatively large number of tablets. This should be explained carefully, as otherwise patient compliance is often insufficient. The first dose should be taken in the presence of the health worker (directly observed treatment, or DOT). This is the major argument for keeping some STD drugs on hand (in a separate lockable box) in the clinic room. Health workers should also make a serious attempt to convince STD patients to return after seven days, and again thereafter to verify their cure. This is necessary to be certain that individuals are cured, as well as to determine the cure or failure rate for all patients in the STD programme.

Box 3. Flow charts for genital ulcer syndrome

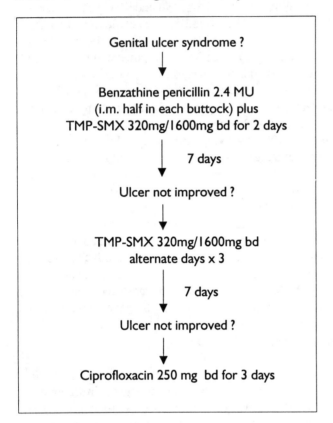

Genital ulcer syndrome ?

↓

Benzathine penicillin 2.4 MU
(i.m. half in each buttock) plus
TMP-SMX 320mg/1600mg bd for 2 days

↓ 7 days

Ulcer not improved ?

↓

TMP-SMX 320mg/1600mg bd
alternate days x 3

↓ 7 days

Ulcer not improved ?

↓

Ciprofloxacin 250 mg bd for 3 days

TMP-SMX = Trimethoprim-sulfamethoxazole; bd = twice per day

Clinical algorithms are available for various syndromes. An algorithm is a set of instructions used to guide decisions. Because they are organized according to a time sequence, algorithms often have the character of flow charts. The simpler and clearer such flow charts are, the easier it is for health workers to accept and use them. An example of a flow chart for genital ulcers used by AMREF in Mwanza Region is shown in Box 3. Current WHO recommendations for choice of drugs and flow charts can be found in recent publications of the World Health Organization (see 'Further reading').

Another factor in the choice of drugs is the aetiological pattern of various STD syndromes in a particular country or region. This should be established and monitored over time. The antibiotic susceptibility of *Neisseria gonorrhoeae* also requires regular surveillance. For responsible treatment it is therefore essential that at least one reference clinic and laboratory are available and operational within the country.

Health education to avoid future infection
In a busy clinic there is often little time for thorough health education, and experience shows that often none is given. However, there are some very convincing reasons for spending at least a few minutes getting the most important messages across.

STD patients have come to the clinic to seek help. In doing so, they are demonstrating concern for their health and are therefore more likely to be open to health education than people without STDs. With appropriate health education they may be the best candidates to become agents for change and allies in the struggle against AIDS and other STDs: they can have a substantial impact on others in the community.

STD patients are much more likely than others to return to the clinic with another STD in the future. This may be because their life-style places them at greater risk, or they may be reinfected by untreated spouses or other regular partners. Thus, health education can save a great deal of future work and costs. STD patients are also more likely than others to be HIV-infected. Because of this well-documented association (6), STD patients are an important target group for interventions against the further spread of HIV in the community (see Box 4).

Box 4. Three reasons to spend time on health education for STD patients

1   STD patients are highly motivated to listen. If they become peer educators, they may be the health worker's best allies in the struggle against AIDS and STDs.
2   Without health education, STD patients are likely to return with a new infection. Health education now will save time and money in the future.
3   STD patients are more likely than others to be HIV-infected. Providing education will help guard against the spread of AIDS in the community.

Time spent on health education, including risk reduction and partner notification (see below), is of great importance, and is bound to pay off. Health education means not just giving information: there must also be a chance to discuss it. A dialogue is far more likely to influence people than a list of 'don'ts'. However, in the face of the time pressures that are typical in many clinics, detailed discussions may simply not be possible. Clear information and convincing arguments are then preferable to no health education at all. Better, however, is to seek ways to make a discussion possible. Health education can, for example, be delegated to a skilled and motivated staff member, while the clinician continues with the outpatient routine. (This possibility is discussed briefly below under 'Integration into outpatient work'.)

The following topics should be covered, although they cannot be addressed in a single session:
- the infective nature of STDs;
- transmission through sexual intercourse;
- increased risks of infertility and other complications;

- increased risks of delivering sick children;
- the importance of completing treatment, even after improvement;
- reasons for reporting back to the clinic after seven days;
- the risk of reinfection by the partner;
- the advantage of and necessity of treating partner(s);
- how to use a contact slip (see section on partner notification);
- reduction of number of partners and/or condom use as preventive measures;
- the importance of sexual hygiene.

Health workers should also make an effort to convince STD patients to abstain from sex until the disease is cured and their partner has also been treated. Condoms should be offered as an alternative to bridge this interval.

Partner notification

Achieving partner notification is an essential part of the educational process described above. Its justification is clear, but implementation remains very difficult. Nevertheless some principles have become obvious. In the African cultural context, partner notification via the index case (the person presenting with an STD) is much more effective than contact tracing (finding the recent sexual contacts of an STD patient) by a health worker (7). However, to be motivated to notify their partners, index cases have to be convinced that treatment of their partners will benefit them as well.

Using contact slips is the best way to spare embarrassment for all involved, as well as to guide the process and save time. A contact slip may be simply a piece of cardboard containing the name of the health unit and the patient register number or a code indicating the diagnosis. Index cases should give a contact slip to each partner and urge them to report to the clinic. Based on this coded information, partners should be treated for the same syndrome as the index patient. For partners who come to the clinic, health education should be extended and an examination should be offered, but not as a precondition for treatment. If partners exhibit symptoms, they should also be encouraged to notify any other partners they may have.

Partner notification is a sensitive issue. It may lead to an embarrassing situation for both partners, and sometimes results in matrimonial conflicts and divorce. Health workers must also keep in mind that vaginal discharge does not always signal an STD: it is also often caused by *Candida albicans* (thrush) or bacterial vaginosis. Although these infections require treatment, they may occur on their own, without sexual transmission.

Recording and reporting

Health workers are accustomed to keeping patient register books, filling in tally sheets and/or producing monthly reports. The amount of paperwork to be done in peripheral health units is often enormous, while unfortunately health workers rarely receive the necessary feedback on the data they collect. However, health unit data can provide very helpful information, both for the district health management team as well as for the health workers themselves.

Keeping a separate patient register book for STDs will enhance the feedback process. Only absolutely essential data should be collected, such as the name and sex of the patient, the syndromic diagnosis, and the treatment given. A separate column should be used to enter follow-up data: date of return, clinical observations on return, and partners treated.

Assessment of treatment outcome

There are four possible treatment outcomes: cured, follow-up visits not completed, referred, definite treatment failure. Experience indicates that if the work is being done well and if the drugs in use are effective, the relative frequency of these outcomes will usually fall within certain limits.

Health workers can evaluate their own performance with respect to outcome (e.g. at monthly or quarterly intervals) using a simple monitoring form (see Box 5). Ideally this would be done in collaboration with the district STD coordinator, although it is not strictly necessary. The rates given in Box 5 may vary from community to community due to travelling distances, and seasonal and cultural influences. Health workers can establish their own targets in these areas, and work to attain them; this can serve as a motivating factor.

Box 5. Monitoring indicators

A monitoring form can be used to quickly calculate a few decisive indicators which can help a health worker to adjust or improve his/her work if necessary. These indicators include:

- trends in STD patient attendance over time;
- the rate of initial follow-up visits (should not be less than 50%);
- the rate of completed follow-up visits (those continued until a definite outcome has been noted – should not be less than 30%);
- the cure rate following first line treatment (should be above 85%; otherwise this may indicate the development of antibiotic resistance, which should be reported to the district STD coordinator);
- the condom 'acceptance' rate;
- the rate of partner treatment (should reach at least 30%, but a higher success rate can be achieved when high quality health education is extended to index cases).

Case finding

Neglected symptoms

A substantial proportion of patients with symptomatic STDs will take no action. This is apt to be true in up to 30% of genital ulcer cases and more than 50% of genital discharge cases. The phenomenon is more prevalent in women than in men (8), although the reason for this is not well understood, and may depend on several factors. In some societies genital discharge seems to be regarded as normal, reflecting how common the condition is. Frequent failure of health services to provide an effective cure may have contributed to this attitude. In addition, a woman may 'neglect' symptoms because she fears stigmatization if she seeks STD treatment. Other women may visit traditional healers, and feel they have been paying sufficient attention to their symptoms. But some STDs are simply ignored; health workers occasionally discover even rather large genital ulcers only by chance. Because STDs are associated with HIV infection and – particularly in women – many other complications, the detection and treatment of neglected STD syndromes should be regarded as an important aspect of health workers' routine duties.

Asymptomatic infections

A related problem is genuinely asymptomatic infection, in which neither symptoms nor signs are apparent. This problem is well known in women, where it may account for more than half of genital infections. For instance, most gonococcal and chlamydial infections of the cervix uteri are asymptomatic, but can be particularly dangerous. Asymptomatic infections are also common in men: in a large rural cohort about 85% of patients with urethritis had no signs or symptoms (9). In women, genital ulcers may remain undiscovered if situated within the vagina. A high proportion of men and women may be infected with chronic syphilis, but women often do not recall having had an ulcer (10).

It is not yet clear whether asymptomatic infections directly increase the risk of HIV transmission. Nonetheless, they are very likely to contribute greatly to STD prevalence in the community, because they represent a constant reservoir for reinfection. Therefore, reducing the frequency (prevalence) of asymptomatic infections is an important goal. One possible solution – in addition to screening, as discussed below – is the provision of mass treatment: treating all adults in a country within a short time, regardless of whether they have STD symptoms or not. This option is still controversial, but research is being carried out.

Simple screening options for detection of STDs

Ideally, screening options that would reliably detect neglected syndromes and asymptomatic infections would be available. Unfortunately, at present there are no simple laboratory tests which can provide this for all patients in a cost-effective way. Some screening options for women do exist: though far from optimal, they are simple, not difficult to implement and able to detect at least a substantial portion of STDs in these patients. Two such options are described below.

1. Women attending an antenatal clinic, under-five clinic or family planning service can be routinely asked whether they have symptoms such as vaginal discharge or other genital ailments. In addition, a simple genital inspection can be routinely performed, not necessarily including a speculum examination. All women reporting symptoms and all those with signs of an STD are treated, using the relevant syndromic algorithm. Although vaginal symptoms are not direct predictors of

cervical infections, treatment for these infections should always be provided because of their high prevalence and their enormous potential for complications.

This procedure requires a degree of privacy. While it may be argued that this is not easy to obtain at a busy antenatal clinic, simple solutions (such as the string and cloth mentioned in Box 1) can be quite effective. Experience has shown that these arrangements are easily accepted by health workers, and much appreciated by women receiving treatment (11). Midwives and nurses working in antenatal, under-five and family planning clinics are often not used to such procedures. They will need additional training: this should include the importance of STDs to women's health, syndromic management of STDs and STD-related health education. The partner notification that is recommended when STDs are found may be a difficult issue requiring special consideration in the training phase (for details, see Chapter 14).

2.   Another option is to combine screening for asymptomatic cervical infections with the above approach. These infections are frequently associated with the presence of certain risk factors (see Box 6). During a short interview, the health worker asks a small number of questions to see which risk-related factors are present. If the 'score' (for example, at least two positive answers to four questions) indicates it, the woman may be treated for both gonococcal and chlamydial infections. Questions should be worded and asked in a neutral way, to avoid embarrassment. This method has been evaluated in pregnant women, and proved to be a useful detector of STDs, while being well-accepted (11, 12). Although the sensitivity and the specificity of this approach are not very high, it remains presently the only feasible option to detect asymptomatic cervical infections in the absence of simple laboratory tests for screening.

Box 6. Risk factors associated with asymptomatic cervical infection

The factors listed below have been shown to be associated with gonococcal or chlamydial infection of the cervix uteri:
- age of woman below 21 years/25 years
- single, separated, divorced or widowed
- present partnership shorter than three months
- more than one partner in the last 12 months
- partner frequently absent from home
- partner symptomatic
- a history of lower abdominal pain
- last child delivered more than five years ago
- painful urination (dysuria)
- painful sexual intercourse (dyspareunia)

The association of such factors with STD risk obviously depends on the cultural and sociological environment. A particular factor may or may not be associated with increased STD risk in a particular geographical area. In the absence of area-specific research results, STD control programme managers can work with their staff to choose from the above list to arrive at a set of questions that is suitable to their region. It is important that the set of questions and the decision flow chart (what to do, based on the score of the patient) are kept short and simple to ensure feasibility. Carrying out the procedures for both of the options above can be accomplished with a total time investment of less than three minutes per woman – which, even in a busy antenatal clinic, should be an affordable time investment.

Screening options for urethritis in men

The leukocyte esterase dipstick test is cheap and simple to perform. A positive result obtained from first void urine is suggestive of urethral infection, and frequently associated with asymptomatic gonococcal or chlamydial infection in men (but much less so in women) (13). The positive predictive value of this test for asymptomatic urethritis in men depends on the prevalence of urethral infections; in Tanzania it was found to be in the range of 25–50% that is, up to half of men with a positive leukocyte esterase dipstick test had an urethral infection (9, 13).

The test is rarely used in screening the general population, and its positive predictive value is too low to recommend such an approach. However, in the context of providing health care at peripheral units, the test may be used to screen for urethritis in men who come to the unit with other STDs (e.g. genital ulcers), as dual infections are not uncommon. If the test is positive, treatment should be given according to the guidelines for urethral discharge.

Screening for and management of serosyphilis

The 1993 World Development Report recommends screening and management of serosyphilis in pregnant women as one of the most cost-effective public health intervention presently available (14). In spite of this, regular screening is still carried out in only a few locations.

In untreated syphilis, after syphilitic ulcers have healed spontaneously, the infection may cause secondary symptoms such as *condylomata lata* on the genitals, or generalised skin alterations, but the infection most often leads to latent (asymptomatic) syphilis. If left untreated in pregnant women, this infection often results in spontaneous abortion, stillbirth or the delivery of seriously ill children (congenital syphilis).

The rapid plasma reagin (RPR) test is a low-cost screening method which does not require specialized laboratory personnel. It can be adequately performed by a midwife or nurse, making it feasible for peripheral health units, although some training and experience are required (see Chapter 14).

The test is performed on venous or capillary blood. Centrifugation is advisable, but not essential: the separation of serum and blood cells can also be achieved through simple sedimentation, though waiting time is increased by 30–60 minutes. In the test, a calibrated drop of test liquid is added to a small amount of serum on a test card. The card must then be shaken rather vigorously for several minutes before the test result can be read. This is best done with the help of an automatic shaker, if electricity is available. However, in some places patients have been employed to shake their own test cards.

The RPR test has some pitfalls, of which the health worker should be aware. The test may produce false positive results under a number of conditions: malaria and pregnancy are major examples. Furthermore, if the patient has had syphilis previously for a long period before receiving treatment, the results of the RPR test will not always be negative, even after effective treatment. This means that overtreatment may occur. However, this seems justifiable when the complications of syphilis are taken into account. Meanwhile, health educators need to realize that a positive RPR test does not necessarily mean that the patient has an STD.

At health units with functioning laboratories, where the RPR test can be titrated (giving a titre rather than just a positive or a negative result), additional useful information can be obtained. A titre of 1/16 or higher most likely indicates acute syphilic infection, while titres of 1/1 to 1/8 may be the result of previous infection.

A positive RPR in a pregnant woman, however, should always be treated, regardless of the titre. It is extremely important to treat syphilis in pregnancy as early as possible; otherwise stillbirth or neonatal syphilis may be inevitable. Syphilis is treated with injections of 2.4 MU Benzathine penicillin i.m., half into each buttock. In some STD control programmes two repeat doses are given, although no clear evidence is yet available on whether this method is more effective.

Ophthalmia neonatorum

Bacterial infection of the maternal genital tract frequently results in infection of the newborn baby. These infections usually affect the eyes and lead to more or less severe conjunctivitis. While *Chlamydia trachomatis* is the most frequent causative agent, *Neisseria gonorrhoeae* is the most dangerous. Gonococcal conjunctivitis usually involves both eyes and is marked by an abundant production of pus. The infection usually occurs within a few days of delivery, and may rapidly progress to destruction of the cornea, resulting in blindness. Although precise data are lacking, ophthalmia neonatorum is considered an important cause of blindness in sub-Saharan Africa (15). A newborn baby with purulent eye infection should be treated as an emergency case. Waiting even a few hours may result in irreversible eye damage (see Box 7).

Introducing or re-introducing regular chemoprophylaxis of ophthalmia neonatorum is highly recommended. This simple and very cost-effective procedure can easily be performed at all health units (see Box 8). Its use has been discontinued in several countries because it sometimes causes chemical conjunctivitis. However, this complication is reversible, and rarely occurs when procedures are properly carried out.

Box 7. Treatment of ophthalmia neonatorum

Systemic treatment using effective antimicrobial injections are preferred. WHO recommends the following drugs: Ceftriaxone, 50 mg/kg i.m. as a single dose, to a maximum of 125 mg, or Kanamycin, 25 mg/kg i.m. as a single dose, to a maximum of 75 mg, or Spectinomycin 25 mg/kg i.m. as a single dose, to a maximum of 75 mg (4). It should be noted that Kanamycin may damage hearing. Alternatively, Erythromycin syrup (50 mg/kg per day orally, divided over four doses, to be given for 14 days) may be tried. Penicillin injections (e.g. PPF) are obsolete, as 80% or more of gonococcal strains are resistant to this drug in many areas.

In addition, pus should be removed and the eyes frequently rinsed with clean water. Health workers must take all precautions to protect themselves: the purulent eye discharge is highly infective. Moreover, large amounts of pus tend to accumulate beneath the eyelids, sealing them. This pus is usually under high pressure and will spurt out when the lids are opened. The eyelids should be opened with caution, preferably under a cover of gauze, and gloves should be worn.

Only if no systemic antibiotics are available an attempt should be made to treat the eyes with antibiotic eye drops or ointments. These should be applied at least hourly, after cleaning the eyes. However, this treatment is not always sufficient to rescue the affected eyes.

The mother (and her partner) should also be treated, using the algorithms for genital discharge syndrome.

Box 8. Prophylaxis of ophthalmia neonatorum

Soon after delivery, newborn babies receive a drop of 1% silver nitrate (a solution of 0.1 g of silver nitrate in 10 ml of saline) in each eye. Proper storage of this solution is vital (it should not be exposed to light or kept in particularly warm places in the clinic); the bottle must be securely closed after use. Otherwise, as water evaporates from the solution, the concentration of silver nitrate may become high enough to result in toxic effects on the eye. For the same reason, the solution should be replaced at least every six months.

Alternatively, tetracycline eye ointment (1%) or erythromycin (0.5%) can be used. This method seems to work reliably as a prophylaxis, even in areas where systemic tetracycline treatment is no longer effective against gonorrhoea.

Organization of STD work at the clinic

Integration into outpatient work

Where personnel and financial resources are very limited, specialized STD clinics are not affordable. Nor are they feasible where rural populations are widely scattered. More important, STD services labelled as such may be counterproductive: most patients do not want the rest of the community to know they have attended such a clinic. Special STD clinic hours are inappropriate for the same reason. Consequently, the management of patients with STDs should be included in the routine work of outpatient clinics.

The importance of health education for STD patients has already been emphasized above. However, as noted, in a very busy outpatient clinic, health workers often find it very difficult to provide the necessary health education in the short time they have available for each patient. One way to solve this dilemma is to have a separate health worker (e.g. a nurse or well-trained auxiliary staff member) perform this crucial task. (The training necessary for staff members serving as health educators is discussed further in Chapter 14.) This same person may also be supplied with a limited amount of STD drugs, which can be dispensed to STD patients during the educational session. Then the first dose can be taken under supervision and the importance of full compliance emphasized.

Practical aspects of STD work at antenatal clinics

At a busy antenatal clinic, screening for STDs and serosyphilis should be integrated into the usual routine in a practical manner. Women attending the clinics can be channelled through a number of contact points:

- *initial group health education:* information about STDs can be given to all women present; the importance of screening to the health of both mother and baby should be emphasized, and procedures should be explained. All this is particularly important when STD control efforts are introduced at a health unit, as otherwise mothers might be surprised and scared of the new procedures.
- *individual registration:* antenatal clinic cards or personal records should be filled out by the health worker and kept by each woman.
- *blood sampling:* this should be done at least once per pregnancy. The blood can also be used for other tests if possible, e.g. the determination of haemoglobin level. For practical reasons, a health worker will perform an RPR test when a sufficient number of serum samples are collected, e.g. from eight women. Women later return to this contact point as the last step of their clinic visit.
- *interview and examination:* women are seen individually by a clinician (nurse/ midwife). Routine questions are asked about pregnancy-related problems, along with screening questions for symptomatic STDs and risk factors (see Box 6). A routine antenatal examination is carried out (checking for oedema, fundus, blood pressure, bodyweight and so forth), as well as a brief examination of the genitals as described in the section on screening options (see above). The STD risk score is assessed, and a diagnostic code entered on the card (for example, VDS would indicate vaginal discharge syndrome, and RS+ would mean 'risk score positive').

- *individual health education:* if possible, individual health education should be given to women with genital infections. This should preferably be provided by a separate health educator (but may be given by the clinician or the tester/treatment provider at the end of the visit).
- *notification of the RPR result, syphilis treatment or other STD treatment:* at this stage women return individually to the syphilis screening point to receive test results (see 'blood sampling' above). If treatment is required, it should be given at this contact point, without sending the women anywhere else (e.g. to the injection room), since this may mean additional waiting time – and a marked loss of seropositive pregnant patients if women become impatient and leave the clinic. All other STD-related treatment can also be provided at this point, with the first dose taken under the supervision of the health worker. The necessity of full compliance must be emphasized.

Integration of an STD component into under-five clinics

Because of the high prevalence of STDs, and their enormous implications for women's health, all women who come into contact with the health system should be screened for STDs. In addition to integrating STD work into the context of antenatal clinics – which should be regarded as essential – under-five clinics offer another chance to identify many women with STDs.

The importance of STDs should be explained to mothers when they attend MCH clinics with their children. Otherwise, particularly when such a service is first introduced at the health unit, mothers may not understand why attention is directed not only at their children but towards their own sexual health.

A simple procedure can be used, quite similar to that described for antenatal clinics: mothers should routinely be asked whether they suffer from genital discharge, an ulcer or any other genital problem. Risk can be assessed as described above (although this has not yet been evaluated scientifically) and a brief examination should be offered. The same physical arrangements are required here as in the antenatal clinic: a simple partition is needed where questions are asked and the examination carried out, to allow some privacy and confidentiality. Without this, the suggested procedure will be unacceptable to many mothers.

Integration of STD services into family planning clinics

Compared to the large number of women attending antenatal and MCH services, family planning clinics cover a much smaller portion of the female population. However, family planning clinics provide comparatively favourable conditions for STD screening, as women usually expect a genital examination.

Furthermore, women who request the insertion of an intrauterine device (IUD) – if these devices are available – must be checked carefully for cervical infection. If present, treatment (following the guidelines for vaginal discharge) should be given a few days before the IUD is implanted. If this is not done, the IUD insertion may lead to endometritis or pelvic inflammatory disease. In areas where gonococcal or chlamydial infections are highly prevalent, giving this treatment routinely may be justified, as the cervical infection is often asymptomatic.

Equipment and consumables

The following equipment and consumables are needed to provide STD services:

- Curtain or screen (see Box 1).
- Examination bed or bench to perform an appropriate genital examination. This can be produced locally, and should be situated so that light from a window can be used.
- Torch to provide light for examination: a necessity when a speculum examination is to be done.
- Gloves: a simple genital inspection at antenatal/MCH clinics can be done without gloves if STDs are unlikely to be present, but gloves must be worn when examining patients who present with symptoms of STDs. Otherwise, a thorough inspection of the penis or anal region, as well as spreading the labia or a speculum examination, may be hazardous to the health worker.
- Speculum: not essential in the context of STD case management at peripheral units. If used, it should be placed in a plastic bowl with antiseptic solution for at least 15 minutes following each examination, before receiving its final cleaning for re-use. It should be stored in a clean place, packed in a clean and sturdy box or wrapped in a piece of clean cloth.
- Complete set of treatment algorithms: these documents should be easily accessible on the clinician's desk. Ideally, they should be kept in transparent plastic covers for durability.
- Drug storage: STD drugs may be stored in a separate lockable box in the clinic room within reach of the clinician. Such an arrangement not only supports drug accountability, but also patient compliance, as drugs can be taken under supervision (Direct Observed Treatment – DOT).
- Plastic mug and drinking water for DOT.
- STD drugs, cotton wool, methylated spirit, needles and syringes are needed. If these are to be reused they must be properly sterilized: remember that the prevalence of HIV infection is usually higher in STD patients than in the general population.
- Emergency package in case of anaphylactic reactions after treatment with Benzathine penicillin: such reactions are extremely rare, but do occur. It is therefore advisable that patients remain in the clinic for a few minutes after treatment, so that emergency aid can be provided if necessary. For such situations, an emergency package should contain two bottles of a saline drip (or preferably a plasma expander), a set for giving infusions, fixation plaster, a vial of adrenaline, vials with sterile water for injection, and a few sterile disposable syringes with needles.
- Condoms: these must be properly stored (not exposed to heat or sunlight). Expired condoms should be discarded. If the quality of condoms is not up to standard, patients and other users will become disheartened, and even the best condom promotion programme may be thwarted.
- Condom demonstrator: to provide health education on condom use, a condom demonstrator should be used. This can be a round piece of wood, the size of an erect penis, mounted on a small wooden board.
- Register book: an STD patient register book is needed, and monitoring and reporting forms should be at hand, stored in a file.

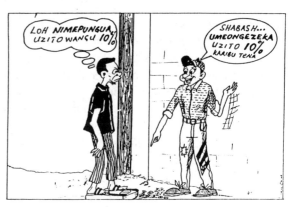

A flourishing business in Mwanza. Many people are concerned about weight loss. The man on the scale knows he lost several kilograms, but the owner of the scale says he gained and should come again.

Personnel and time required

Even in a high STD prevalence area, the number of new STD patients presenting will rarely exceed one to three per day. The number may be higher in cities, once good STD services have been established at a particular outpatient clinic and become well known by the population. With no more than five new cases per day, it should be feasible for the clinician to allocate at least 10–15 minutes to each STD patient.

If more time is available, it is certain to be beneficial for both the patient and the community, but under the actual conditions in a busy outpatient clinic this may not be realistic. In such a situation, it may be possible for a separate health worker to provide health education, reducing the clinician's contact time to five to ten minutes. Taking a short history, performing a brief examination, providing the most essential explanations about the patient's condition, giving directly observed treatment and making the necessary brief notes in the register book are indispensable elements of professional care.

When STD care is incorporated with ongoing antenatal and MCH clinic work, additional time for health education will always be required. The most practical way to provide this is to have a health worker meet with several women at once (10–15 minutes per group). The additional direct contact time for the clinical procedure is in the range of three minutes for a healthy woman and may go up to ten minutes if an infection is diagnosed or suspected. Again, most of this time will be for health education which could be delegated to another staff member, serving as a health educator; as mentioned above, this person should receive the necessary training.

If syphilis screening and treatment is established at antenatal clinics, a second additional health worker may be needed, depending on the number of new ANC (antenatal care) attenders per day. The additional contact time required will depend on experience and routine, but on average should be about 15 minutes per woman.

In total, for a programme including STD services for patients and screening as outlined above, there should be at least two outpatient clinic workers and at least one (two are better) antenatal/MCH nurses per health unit who have training and competence in STD case management. If family planning clinics are separately staffed, at least one of these workers should also be trained.

Collaboration with district health personnel

Inevitably, there will be situations when the clinician needs help or advice. This can be provided by the district STD coordinator, who should visit the clinic at least once per month initially (when STD services have just been started). This can later be lengthened to bi-monthly or quarterly intervals.

Health workers should discuss problematic cases with the coordinator. Ideally, such cases can be seen jointly: the coordinator's visit should be planned in advance so that any patients needing special attention can be invited to attend at that time.

Conclusion

The connection between STDs and HIV has increased attention to STD prevention and control: STDs increase the risk of HIV infection and often lead to other serious complications, especially for women. But STDs are also a major health problem in their own right. Effectively treating and preventing the spread of STDs is a major task for health workers in outpatient and MCH services. Good case management consists of several vital components, which should be integrated into existing services. Simple, cheap and sufficiently sensitive screening tests are not yet available, except for syphilis, and the syndromic management of STDs has proved to be superior to more classical approaches. Since many patients with STDs are asymptomatic or may neglect their symptoms, screening at antenatal, MCH and family planning clinics may present the best opportunity to identify women with STDs. History-taking, genital examination and risk assessment are useful in this regard. Health education is essential; risk reduction and partner notification should be emphasized.

Acknowledgement: We are very grateful to Professor David Mabey, London School of Hygiene and Tropical Medicine, for his advice and comments.

Further reading

Holmes KK, Mardh PA, Sparling PF, Wiesner PJ eds. *Sexually transmitted diseases*. New York, McGraw-Hill, 1989.

Nduba J, Mabey D. *Self-instructional manual on sexually transmitted diseases*. Nairobi, African Medical and Research Foundation, 1992.

World Health Organization. *WHO model prescribing information: drugs used in sexually transmitted diseases and HIV infection*. Geneva, 1995.

World Health Organization. *Global Programme on AIDS. Management of sexually transmitted diseases*. WHO/GPA/TEM/94.1. Geneva, 1994.

References

1. Cameron DW, Simonsen JN, D'Costa LJ et al. Female to male transmission of human immunodeficiency virus type 1: risk factors for seroconversion in men. *Lancet* 1989, 2(8660): 403–7.

2. De Schryver A, Meheus A. Epidemiology of sexually transmitted diseases: the global picture. *Bulletin of the WHO* 1990, 68: 639–54.

3. Lwihula G, Grosskurth H. People's perceptions on STDs, their health care seeking behaviour and attitudes towards AMREF integrated STD clinics, Mwanza Region, Tanzania, including policy implications. Presentation at the VIIIth International Conference on AIDS in Africa, Marrakesh 1993.

4. WHO. Management of patients with sexually transmitted diseases. Report of a WHO Study Group. *WHO Technical Report Series* 1991, 810: 1–103.

5. Mayaud P, ka-Gina G, Grosskurth H. STD case management. In: *Prevention and management of sexually transmitted diseases in Eastern and Southern Africa: current approaches and future directions. Naresa Monograph,* no. 3. Nairobi, Naresa, 1994.

6. Pepin J, Plummer FA, Brunham RC et al. The interaction of HIV infection and other sexually transmitted diseases: an opportunity for intervention. *AIDS* 1989, 3: 3–9.

7. Wellington M. Detection of asymptomatic carriers and partner notification. In: *Prevention and management of sexually transmitted diseases in Eastern and Southern Africa: current approaches and future directions. Naresa Monograph,* no. 3. Nairobi, Naresa, 1994.

8. Mulder D. Disease perception and health-seeking behaviour for sexually transmitted diseases. In: *Prevention and management of sexually transmitted diseases in Eastern and Southern Africa: current approaches and future directions. Naresa Monograph,* no. 3. Nairobi, Naresa, 1994.

9. Grosskurth H, Mayaud P, Mosha F, et al. High prevalence of asymptomatic gonorrhoea and chlamydial infection in rural Tanzanian men. *British Medical Journal* (in press).

10. Mosha F, Nicoll A, Barongo L, et al. A population-based study of syphilis and sexually transmitted disease syndromes in north-western Tanzania. 1. Prevalence and incidence. *Genitourinary Medicine* 1993, 69: 415–420.

11. Mayaud P, ka-Gina G, Cornelissen J, et al. *Validation of a new WHO algorithm for the clinical management of vaginal discharge in Mwanza, Tanzania.* Submitted to Bulletin of the WHO.

12. Vuylsteke B, Laga M, Alary M et al. Clinical algorithms for the screening of women for gonococcal and chlamydial infection: evaluation of pregnant women and prostitutes in Zaire. *Clinical and Infectious Diseases* 1993, 17: 82–88.

13. Mayaud P, Changalucha J, Grosskurth H et al. The value of urine specimens in screening for male urethritis and its microbial aetiologies in Tanzania. *Genitourinary Medicine* 1992, 68: 361–365.

14. World Bank. *World Development Report 1993: investing in health.* New York, Oxford University Press, 1993.

15. Fransen L, Klauss V. Neonatal ophthalmia in the developing world. Epidemiology etiology, management and control. *International Journal of Ophthalmology* 1988, 11: 189–96.

16. Mayaud P, Grosskurth H, Changalucha J et al. Risk assessment and other screening options for gonorrhoea and chlamydial infections in women attending rural Tanzanian antenatal clinics. *Bulletin of the WHO* 1995, 73: 621–630.

14 District STD control efforts

Heiner Grosskurth and Ezra Mwijarubi

- How can STDs affect HIV transmission?
- What is the Piot-Fransen model of STDs in the community?
- How can sufficient drug supplies for treating STDs be ensured?
- What do politicians have to do with STD control?
- What is the core group concept?
- How can the district health team organize an effective STD control programme?

The importance of sexually transmitted diseases (STDs) at the individual patient level, as well as their possible complications, is clear (see Chapter 13). But what are the consequences of STDs for the community at large? Furthermore, what financial burden do STDs place on district health services and the economy as a whole? What can be done by the district team to control STDs effectively? This chapter includes information on primary prevention; improving treatment-seeking behaviour; training; drug supply; support and supervision; monitoring; the concept and importance of core groups; collaboration with reference centres and management of the programme.

Public health importance

Control of HIV infection

The fact that STDs enhance HIV transmission implies that effective control of classical STDs should lead to a substantial reduction in new HIV infections. This was first established among a selected group of urban commercial sex workers in Kinshasa (1). A routine intervention programme for the general population was later shown to be both feasible and highly effective. This programme (carried out in Mwanza, Tanzania, with support from the European Union) reduced the rate of new HIV infections by 40%, as demonstrated by a trial comprising a rural cohort of 12,000 individuals (2). In addition, mathematical modelling applied to data from another large rural population strongly suggests that classical STDs have been a major factor in allowing the HIV epidemic in Africa to reach such a serious level (3).

Today, efforts to reduce STDs should form a vital component of AIDS control at the district, regional and national level in all countries. Together with attempts to reduce risky sexual behaviour, STD control should be given high priority by health managers, administrators and political leaders.

STDs: a major public health problem in their own right
STDs deserved great attention even before the AIDS era, as they place a huge burden on the health of millions of people (especially women) particularly in countries with very limited resources. However, health programme planners have not understood and appreciated this sufficiently in the past.

The World Development Report of 1993 very clearly demonstrates the importance of STDs to public health in Africa (4). Among diseases causing the highest loss of healthy life years, STDs (excluding HIV infection) rank among the top ten for adults. For women of childbearing age, STDs are nearly the heaviest burden on health, second only to maternity-related disorders. Other very serious conditions such as tuberculosis, respiratory tract infections or injuries clearly rank below STDs for this group.

Both STDs and HIV infection are marked by a particularly high rate of new infections (incidence) in the vulnerable group of young women. The problem starts as soon as young people become sexually active, and by the age of 25 very high prevalences of STDs and HIV infection are recorded (5).

Economic burden caused by STDs at district level
The economic burden caused by STDs may best be illustrated by an example from Mwanza Region in Tanzania. A typical district has a population of 300,000 people or roughly 130,000 sexually active adults. In a population-based survey conducted in 1991, about 10% of men and 3% of women in the general population reported having suffered at least once per year from an reproductive tract infection (RTI. RTIs include infections like bacterial vaginosis and Candida albicans infection which are not always transmitted through sexual intercourse but can occur spontaneously) (5). If these figures are extrapolated to one district, and assuming that 25% of the patients have more than one episode, they suggest that at least 10,400 STD episodes occur per average district and year.

About 70% of the patients reported that they attended a formal health unit, but 40% sought help from other sources.

These figures tie in well with observations from the STD intervention trial in Mwanza Region. After STD services had been improved in 26 health units serving a population of 85,000 adults, 5,800 patients with reproductive tract infections were treated per year (2). If extrapolated this suggests that about 8,800 RTI episodes were treated per average district and year.

It costs about US$ 17,600 per district each year to cover drug costs alone. When adding the costs of training, equipment, supervision, fuel and the opportunity costs of health workers' time, the total costs per average district will be in the range of at least US$ 70,000 (16).

The economic burden for the population must also not be neglected. Patients often have to pay informal user fees at health units, and it can be assumed that the 40% of the patients seeking help from traditional healers and other sources have to spend the equivalent of at least another US$ 10,000 in cash or in kind.

It is more difficult to estimate the economic costs of treating STD *sequelae* (e.g. surgery performed on women with ectopic pregnancies, treatment of chronic pelvic pain, attempts to treat infertility, care of disabled children) and costs caused by loss of productivity due to death or illness. The total economic burden caused by STDs and RTIs may well come to more than US$ 100,000 in an average district each year.

Elements of STD control at district level

The elements of STD control at the district level include:
- primary prevention;
- improvement of treatment-seeking behaviour;
- facilitation of improved STD case management at health units;
- STD control in core groups;
- collaboration and interaction with the STD reference clinic and laboratory.

Primary prevention

In the context of STD control, primary prevention includes all measures taken by an healthy individual to protect him or herself from getting infected. It is far better to prevent diseases than to cure them, and STDs are no exception to this rule. However, this is no easy task, because preventing STDs is about adjusting people's behaviour, a most difficult achievement (see Box 1).

Box 1. Achieving changes in sexual behaviour

Obviously it takes time for people to adapt their behaviour. It is therefore not surprising that this is also the case with sexual behaviour. We should not expect quick and dramatic changes as an outcome of behavioural interventions; both programme managers and donors should be realistic in their expectations.

This does not mean such interventions are useless, ineffective and therefore not justified. It does mean that they should be well targeted and accurately planned, and that implementation should be a long lasting effort.

All of us working in this field should learn to be patient. Let us take a very obvious example from industrialized countries: although anti-smoking campaigns started many years ago, a significant reduction in smoking has only recently been observed in the USA, along with some indications of reduction in Europe.

The objective is to design and implement district-based intervention activities which help individuals to adjust their sexual behaviour and thus to prevent STDs. Safe sexual behaviour includes some or all of the following:

- postponement of first sexual experience-based on an informed decision;
- reduction of the number of sex partners;
- always using condoms for casual sexual contacts;
- using non-penetrative sexual techniques.

Interventions to encourage these behaviour changes consist of various information, education and communication (IEC) activities, as outlined below.

Targeting behavioural interventions

Time, personnel and funds are limited, in a district health programme as well as anywhere else. It is not realistic to try to reach everyone; instead efforts should be selectively targeted. It is therefore necessary to identify those portions of the population who may find it easier to undergo a behavioural adaptation process, as well as those who are most at risk. It is also important to identify what type of intervention is feasible with the personnel and financial resources available.

Various groups may be possible candidates for efforts to achieve primary prevention (see Box 2). The list is not exhaustive, and additional groups may also be identified. The district health management team can identify one or two of the most promising groups in a district and concentrate efforts on them.

Box 2. Potential target groups for primary prevention activities

- school pupils and students
- youth groups and out-of-school youth
- community development associations
- women's groups
- factory workers
- plantation workers
- miners
- police force
- military personnel

Adolescents

This group deserves special consideration, as IEC activities targeted at young people may influence patterns of sexual behaviour before they are fully established, and may therefore be more effective than in adults. Adolescent girls are often more concerned with the implications of unwanted pregnancies and infertility than with the risk of HIV infection. An HIV/STD control strategy which addresses these concerns may therefore be very effective. Many countries in Africa have officially adopted HIV/AIDS prevention and sexual health education as an objective for the educational sector. However, implementation has hardly begun.

Addressing primary prevention of STDs should not be seen as a task of the health sector alone. It concerns many other sectors as well: for example, it can also be considered an issue for schools, transport companies, armed forces and prisons, just to name a few. However, in many cases health personnel have played a catalyst role to begin a process which otherwise would not have been started (see Box 3).

Box 3. Discussing sex with adolescents

Talking about sexual matters with school pupils and other young people is often perceived as a difficult undertaking. Many professionals in the education sector are reluctant to broach the issue.

However, those who try are usually rewarded with a great deal of positive feedback. Adolescents are very interested in discussing sexual matters, and parents are usually relieved when someone else takes on the subject. When district health workers have facilitated discussions on sexual health aspects at school, headmasters and teachers have usually been very supportive.

Options

It is well known that increased knowledge and even changes in attitude do not necessarily lead to changes in practice, as these are often influenced by many additional factors. On the other hand, increasing the level of problem awareness and modifying attitudes are preconditions for any substantial change toward safer sexual behaviour. Again, adolescents may be more capable than adults of actually putting into practice what they know and believe, particularly when the whole peer group participates in the process.

How to achieve problem awareness and attitude modification? Group discussions, peer health education and classroom teaching at schools are among the options available.

Group discussions: the facilitator gives a short introductory overview of the frequency and importance of STDs and their complications. He/she helps the group to engage in a lively discussion as quickly as possible. 'Starters' can be of great help here. These may be pictures or posters highlighting a particular problem, e.g. a drawing of a schoolgirl being approached by a young man on her way home from school. The starter should not offer solutions or messages, but only help trigger group discussion.

Groups should not be too large, including no more than 20 participants at most, but results are better with smaller numbers, e.g. 8 to 12, if feasible. Otherwise many will be left out of the discussion. The facilitator serves as a resource person, and should guide but not dominate group discussion. This means that he/she should not give a lecture, but act as moderator and provide facts when necessary.

Peer health education: a peer educator is a knowledgeable member of the target group who influences other members through his/her own attitude and behaviour. Peers are probably the most effective educators – if well selected and trained – and are therefore excellent allies for the district AIDS programme coordinator. Peer educators are themselves school students, factory workers, etc. They should not receive any regular rewards or allowances for their efforts, since this would set them apart from the rest of the group.

During group discussions it may become clear which individuals seem well suited to the task of peer educators. This can help the AIDS programme coordinator to identify candidates. The group may also be asked for their suggestions. Peer educators should be well accepted by the group, ideally opinion leaders, and ready to commit themselves to the task. The district AIDS programme coordinator should train peer educators carefully and meet with them often to get feedback and to give them additional training and motivation. One coordinator can supervise about ten peer educators, depending on the time available. See also Chapter 12 for more information on training peer educators.

Classroom teaching at schools: this is a much less effective method: while it can usually increase factual knowledge, it rarely creates personal concern. However, larger numbers of young people can be reached, and classroom teaching is therefore certainly of value. Ideally, this option should complement group discussion and peer education.

In many countries, good teaching materials on AIDS prevention can be obtained from the respective Ministry of Education or from NGOs. STD-specific materials are not yet available in most countries, but can be prepared locally, e.g. a poster explaining major STD complications. (See also Chapter 12 for more information on classroom teaching.)

Support from politicians and other leaders

Sexual health and the prevention and treatment of STDs are usually not on the agenda of politicians or other influential individuals. However, we need their understanding, concern and support in the struggle against AIDS and STDs.

At district level, this means discussing the problem with key people in the local government and other important institutions, both at the district headquarters and in larger communities within the district. Direct personal contact is a good way to approach this; these individuals might also be invited to attend short seminars.

Besides merely dispensing information, it is often necessary to positively influence the attitude of opinion leaders towards certain groups. Stereotypes such as: 'young people should not have sex' or 'prostitution should be forbidden' must be addressed. It is not always easy for older people to give up such views and accept unpleasant realities. However, this is an important step to ensure that STD control efforts will find the necessary tolerance and support from influential persons in the community.

Box 4. The Piot-Fransen model for STDs (taking a rural female population as an example)

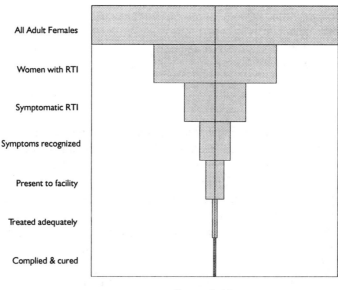

All Adult Females

Women with RTI

Symptomatic RTI

Symptoms recognized

Present to facility

Treated adequately

Complied & cured

Percent of adult women

RTI = reproductive tract infection

Improving treatment-seeking behaviour

The Piot-Fransen model
There is a common belief that STD control is mainly a matter of training and drugs. This belief disregards the fact that the majority of those with STDs never attend a health unit. This may best be illustrated using a model originally developed to describe what happens to tuberculosis patients in a population (14).

This model has recently been redesigned to explain the epidemiology of STDs at the community level (see Box 4, ref. 15). Let us consider STDs in women as an example: the model describes a typical situation in many African communities. About 50% of all sexually active women in the community may be infected with a reproductive tract infection (RTI), most with a genuine STD. Only about half of these may be symptomatic (7). Again, only half of symptomatic women with STDs may seek help (8), and of these only about 65% are likely to find their way to a health unit (6).

That is, in general, 85% of those infected will have dropped out of the system by this point, leaving only the remaining 15% to report to a health unit. Lacking improved

STD case management, only one-quarter of these may actually get sufficient treatment, and not all of these will fully comply. It is then not unrealistic to assume that only about 2% of all women with an infection will eventually be cured. Improving case management may increase this percentage to about 15%. Obviously it is at least equally important to motivate behavioural change, to increase the number of those who seek treatment, and to screen for those who are asymptomatic or who do not recognize their symptoms.

Some screening options for asymptomatic or neglected cases were discussed in Chapter 13, as this goal can at least partly be achieved by health units. This chapter discusses the district team's options to improve people's treatment-seeking behaviour. The objective is to conduct district-based activities which increase the utilization of STD services.

Public health education

Apart from gaining and maintaining a good reputation, health units themselves cannot directly improve people's treatment-seeking behaviour. This can however be achieved through educational campaigns involving the community as a whole. This again involves efforts by the district health team.

The sexually active population needs to be convinced that STDs present a serious problem in their particular community, that STDs can do much harm and that treatment is possible and available. People especially need to be convinced to seek treatment as soon as they observe an STD symptom. Therefore, they also need to know which symptoms indicate an STD.

How can this best be achieved? A public health campaign should be started by those with the most experience. In many districts this will be the district AIDS programme coordinator, working in collaboration with other persons or institutions. The district coordinator should act primarily as a facilitator to inspire influential members of the community to address the population, either publically or via various groups or associations to which people belong. It should be noted that this type of health campaign is easier to effect and more straightforward than the efforts toward primary prevention described above.

- Educational materials: some NGOs have developed a set of educational materials to instruct people about STDs and the need for early treatment. These can be purchased and utilized if funds are available, but campaigns can also be conducted with little financial input.
- Billboards: mobile billboards can be used on market days to attract attention. Pictures help to provide information and to sensitize the population. At least two health educators are needed for such a public session, e.g. to answer questions. A portable loudspeaker may also be helpful.
- Videofilms: open-air showings could be given in the evenings, followed by discussions and information presented by district personal.
- Talks/leaflets: as a more modest solution public health talks can be given, during which leaflets with STD information can be distributed. Such leaflets are available from some health ministries and NGOs (9).

Again, existing formal groups and schools can be utilized to address individual target groups. Help from opinion leaders can also be sought: the impact of the campaign will be strengthened.

When using any of these approaches, it is also essential to improve STD services at nearby health units at the same time, so that the campaign has credibility.

Interaction with pharmacists and traditional healers

Despite efforts to improve treatment-seeking behaviour, some STD patients will still seek treatment from other sources, for example, directly from pharmacists or drug vendors. In most countries, pharmacists are not authorized to prescribe drugs. In reality, however, they treat a substantial number of STD patients, particularly in towns and cities, usually without any clinical examination. Ideally, pharmacists should refrain from selling antibiotics without a medical prescription, and refer the patient to the health unit. The same applies to drug vendors. This expectation, however, is unrealistic.

There is a pragmatic solution to this dilemma. The district health team can ensure that pharmacists and drug vendors are informed (e.g. through short seminars) about why and how doctors treat STDs, using the new syndromic approach, based on national and WHO algorithms. There is nothing wrong in providing information about correct medical treatment as it should be given by *official prescribers*. Some of those who sell drugs may improve their methods of treating STDs after attending such seminars, but also they may become more willing to refer cases to health centres. Likewise, it may be helpful to provide up-to-date drug susceptibility data on *Neisseria gonorrhoea*, and to explain the meaning of these data: it is important to strongly discourage pharmacists and vendors from selling ineffective antibiotics, as well as the frequent practice of selling a partial dose of antibiotics to customers who cannot afford a full treatment. From an epidemiological point of view, as well as from a clinical and ethical point of view, it is far better not to offer anything at all than to sell inadequate treatments, particularly if full and effective treatment is available at the local health facility.

In many areas, traditional healers also treat STDs. Many people seek treatment from both systems, often simultaneously. Traditional healers usually claim they can cure STDs, although few traditional remedies have been scientifically researched. However, the extremely high prevalence of STDs in many areas in Africa despite a dense net of traditional medical services does not support the assumption that there are highly effective traditional drugs for treating these diseases.

It has occasionally been possible to convince traditional healers to refer STD patients to health units. It is worthwhile to encourage this, and to work toward a fruitful dialogue. Collaboration could benefit both sides. There are situations where Western medicine cannot offer cheap and effective treatment for STDs, while traditional medicine can alleviate the problem to a certain extent (e.g. in patients with herpes genitalis infection or with therapy-resistant genital ulcers due to advanced HIV infection).

Improved case management

Detailed information on how to diagnose and manage STDs at dispensaries, health centres and hospital outpatient departments is given in Chapter 13. This chapter deals with the role of the district health team in enabling and supporting health units so they can perform their tasks effectively. Within this context the district health team has four equally important tasks:

- training of health workers;
- provision of STD drugs;
- support and supervision of peripheral units;
- monitoring, evaluation and feedback.

Formal training of health workers
Learning new concepts: Until recently, STDs did not receive much attention in the training of health workers. The enormous importance of STD control was not yet understood, and STD-related epidemiological knowledge as well as practical experience in STD control at peripheral health facilities were not yet available. Most current health staff were trained prior to the development of modern STD-control concepts. Now they are not only expected to acquire additional knowledge and skills, but to depart from previous concepts and accept a new method of case management (see Chapter 13). Of course this is no easy task. Consequently, careful training and retraining are needed, as well as patience and perseverance on the part of supervisors and programme managers for many months after the training period.

Structure and contents of STD training: STD training can be organized at district or regional (provincial) level. Trainers should be recruited from staff members experienced in STD case management and in health education, and who have skills and interest in teaching. At least two trainers are needed for each course. (For more information on training methods and determination of content, see Chapter 12).

Good STD training consists of two parts: classroom learning and the provision of practical experience. The following topics should be covered in the course: the importance of STDs to public health; the causes, the complications and the treatment of important STD syndromes; the psychological situation of STD patients and the correct attitude of health workers; health education of patients including partner notification and training on condom demonstration.

Classroom learning: Classroom learning should always comprise teaching and a substantial amount of group exercises (see Box 5). Good STD management cannot be learned by just listening to a teacher. For example, repeated practising involving role plays is required in order to learn the necessary counselling and health education skills. Such skills are very important for health workers to treat STD patients effectively.

Practical experience can be gained at a busy outpatient department which frequently treats STD patients. Alternatively, learners could be attached to an STD reference clinic for a brief period. Similarly, if antenatal care or MCH personnel are to be trained, they can be attached to clinics with a well-functioning STD component.

Teaching materials: A training manual based on the syndromic case management concept should be used. These are available from the national AIDS/STD control programmes in various countries. Distributing manuals to trainees for private study a month before the course begins has been shown to improve course results. A self-instructional manual is available both in English and Swahili (11). Each trainee should have a set of treatment flow charts to use during the course and to take back to the health unit afterwards.

Box 5. STD training for health professionals

Many health workers find it difficult to sit in a classroom for a whole day. Listening with full concentration for more than an hour without a break should never be requested from students. Listening should therefore alternate with discussions, role plays, group work and other exercises.

Duration of training: How long should STD training last? Clearly more time will be needed for training lower cadres or those who have long been away from learning and teaching. In the Mwanza STD control trial, good results were obtained with one week of classroom learning, but efforts to shorten it to three days have not been very successful in our experience.

The duration of practical training depends on the number of STD patients treated at the training health unit. At minimum, each learner should be able to observe all major syndromes being treated by his tutor clinician twice, and handle another two cases of each syndrome him/herself, under supervision. This is roughly equivalent to handling 30 new STD cases, the number of cases treated in many health centres over a two-week period.

Participants: Who should be trained? The guiding principle is: train those who do the job. Often courses and seminars are used as incentives to reward individuals for previous work, even when the training is not necessary to their present job. But granting favours is not the issue at hand. Resources are scarce, and only those who already work as clinicians at their health units and who definitely will treat STD patients should be sent for training.

In some cases very pragmatic decisions have to be taken: we sometimes need to train less-qualified staff, as there may be units where much of the daily routine is managed by nurses or auxiliary personnel. In most countries, these staff members are not officially permitted to prescribe treatment. But in reality they are the ones who keep things going in many of the more remote dispensaries. It is certainly better to provide additional training to less-qualified individuals than to keep them uninformed because of official principles.

Drug supply

Centralized drug supply with standardized kits: Drugs for STD treatment may be supplied in ready-made kits, either as part of an essential drug programme, or by a special STD control programme using special STD drug kits. In both cases, drugs arrive in standard quantities without taking community size or local STD frequency into consideration. District personnel then have two tasks: to see to it that the kits reach the peripheral health units when needed and to ensure that drugs are utilized sensibly and cost-effectively.

Centralized drug supply based on actual needs: In some programmes drugs are made available based on consumption at individual health units. The advantage of this approach is that the supply is adjusted to actual needs, and ideally there is neither a surplus nor a shortage. In this case, district personnel have the additional tasks of monitoring consumption in detail, providing drugs accordingly and ordering timely replacement drugs for the district stock, based on the consumption data compiled.

Revolving funds: In some areas, there is no centralized drug supply or else some essential needs are not being met, and drugs for STD treatment may not be available. Local pharmacies are often nonexistent in rural areas, or may not have the necessary effective drugs; they often sell drugs at rather high prices. In such cases, drug supply initiatives at regional or district level may be tolerated or even encouraged by the authorities. The strategy often used is a revolving fund system, which may cover more than just STD drugs. Such revolving funds can be used to generate an income for community development projects (see Box 6).

Box 6. Revolving funds and profit margins

Both communities and the project should resist the temptation to maximize the profits earned by the fund, even when intended for very useful development purposes. Treatment for STDs, like that for tuberculosis, should ideally be available at very low cost or even free of charge to ensure high coverage and compliance.

User fees, particularly when substantial, may lead to a significant decrease in STD patient attendance rates, and thus to an increase of untreated STDs with potentially serious long-term health implications (12), especially if the population is poor.

However, if patients consider STDs to be a leading health problem and have sufficient cash at their disposal, willingness to pay is often high. Fishermen in Lake Victoria ranked STDs as their number one health problem and were content to pay for health services delivered to their islands by boat. The project could thus recover all running costs without reducing attendance.

How does a revolving fund work? The principle is that an initial investment is made, a basic drug stock is purchased and part of it is supplied to all participating health units. This is done by a local institution (called the project in this chapter) which may be an NGO, a religious institution or a cooperative. The project may be located in the district or at a regional centre. Financial means to cover the initial investment might come from various sources, such as participating communities, development programmes, NGOs or charity organizations.

Health units sell the drugs to their patients at standardized low prices. By doing so they accumulate funds, which are used to buy new drugs from the project to refill their stocks. Because the project buys in comparatively large quantities and has access to cheap non-profit suppliers, and because both the project and the health units operate with very low profit margins, drugs are much cheaper than at commercial pharmacies. However, prices must cover transport costs, remuneration of the project staff (usually one person per district), depreciation of any necessary investments (e.g. furniture) and should be calculated taking the inflation rate into account.

The crucial issue is how the funds and stocks are controlled, supervised and accounted for. It has proved worthwhile to engage an independent third institution to do this, as long as it is not involved in the actual handling of funds and drugs. This structure minimizes conflicts of interest. Such an independent institution could, for example, be a commission chosen by and working under the district medical officer. At community level, it may also be possible to involve community health committees in the financial supervision of their respective health units.

Revolving funds are also vulnerable to high inflation rates and to devaluation of the local currency, as replacement drugs usually have to be bought with foreign currency.

Drug utilization and accountability

Responsibility of the district health team: The purposeful and responsible use of drugs is essential in any health unit. This is true for all types of drugs supplied. However, because STDs are not only an individual health problem but also have a strong public health dimension (as with tuberculosis or leprosy), it is particularly important that drugs for the treatment of these diseases are consistently available, correctly prescribed, and used for their intended purpose. To ensure this is one of the most crucial tasks of the district health management team.

Constraints on reliable access to drugs from the patients' point of view: Which are the most frequent problems encountered in this context? There are three interlinked issues: drug shortages, underdosages and artificial inaccessibility. Improving planning and management can help to ensure a reliable supply of drugs, in so far as this is within the capacity of the district staff. Sections below on support, supervision and training, and on monitoring and evaluation, address ways to improve these areas. However, first some background information must be provided.

Shortage of drugs in centralized supply systems is a frequently heard complaint from patients and peripheral health workers. Difficulties may occur at different stages:

- Genuine supply problems between the drug factory and delivery to the district. This is related to management capacity above the district level. Accumulating substantial drug stocks at district level is often the only remedy against such shortages. The stock can be used as a buffer in case of delays from the central supplier.
- Difficulties in getting drugs from the district headquarters to the peripheral health units. This is a frequent problem in areas with lack of regular transport and with limited resources. Ensuring a constant and punctual drug supply is a definite challenge for the district health team. Close interaction with health workers at peripheral units is required. If the district medical officer and person responsible for STD control in the district are inventive and ready to improvise, they can usually solve the problems. Again, it may be helpful to accumulate buffer stocks at the health units.
- From the patient's point of view, shortages may occur even when the supply to the health unit is well organized due to the efforts of the district team.

In 1995, a survey was conducted in rural Tanzania. Several hundred patients were visited at home a few weeks after they had sought STD treatment from local health units which had access to a fully reliable drug supply. Patients were interviewed about service satisfaction, drugs received, compliance and other related issues.

Results clearly showed that the majority of patients had been diagnosed and treated correctly. However, far too many (about one-third of the patients) had obviously experienced one or more of the following. They were:
- told drugs were not available;
- given underdoses (20% to 50% of the recommended doses);
- forced to pay for all drugs (which were officially supplied free of charge);
- forced to pay to complete a treatment, and thus did not always complete it.

Cross-checking of the respective health units revealed that drug stocks were sufficient, and in most cases records showed that a full drug treatment had been given.

In many resource-poor countries, health workers live under very difficult economic conditions, and can only make ends meet with an additional income. It is against this background that we should interpret such study observations, and find ways to overcome the difficulties. While district health professionals cannot solve the economic problems of their country (and usually suffer under these conditions themselves), strict supervision can ensure that their efforts to control infections disease like STDs are not in vain.

From a purely epidemiological point of view, illegally enforced payments for drugs are tolerable as long as they do not keep people from seeking or completing treatment. On the other hand, treating with underdosed amounts of drugs is clearly equivalent to grievous bodily harm, particularly in view of the association between STDs and HIV infection.

Checking drug utilization
At the health unit: The supervising officer (routinely the district STD control coordinator, and occasionally the district medical officer) should check the drug utilization of health units regularly. How can this be done effectively?

In principle, the number of STD syndromes treated over a certain period of time must tally with the drugs consumed during that period. Because STD syndromes are treated using standardized flow charts, it is easy to calculate the amount of drugs which should have been issued by a health unit since the last supervisory visit.

This calculated consumption can be compared to genuine consumption by taking a physical inventory of the drugs present at the health unit and subtracting it from the previous balance. Differences will immediately become apparent. Although some small differences will always exist, major discrepancies are cause for concern (see also Box 8).

The procedure described above is useful in all types of drug supply systems. Not only does it enhance drug accountability, but also helps to identify any methodological mistakes in the prescription practice of health workers. In centralized supply systems which work according to actual need, as well as in revolving fund systems, these consumption data also provide the information needed to replenish stocks. The whole process can be administered with the help of a few simple forms.

At the individual patient level: A number of patients should occasionally be visited and interviewed about the drugs they received and their compliance with the recommended treatment. To facilitate this, drug specimens may be shown, to make sure interviewer and patient have the same drug in mind. This task can be performed by the district STD control coordinator or by another person from the district management team.

For the district STD drug stock: The same procedure used for health units (see above) can also be used to monitor drug consumption at the district headquarters itself (except when drugs are supplied in standardized kits; if so, monitoring at district level is not needed).

For example, in centralized drug supply systems working based on actual consumption, the district pharmacist provides drugs for the various health units to the district STD control coordinator, who delivers them to the respective units. The district pharmacist can use the collated drug consumption forms from the various health units to quickly get an overview of drugs supplied during one supervisory visit. This procedure ensures the supervision of the district STD coordinator and also enables the district pharmacist to order new drugs and give feedback to national or regional authorities.

Use of drugs for diseases other than STDs: Aside from the above considerations, a question remains about whether drugs which may have been supplied particularly for the treatment of STDs should also be used for other diseases; for example, as treatment for a child with pneumonia. This is of particular concern when other drugs are out of stock and STD drugs are the only antimicrobial medicines available. Generally speaking, there is no justification – ethical, medical or economic – for withholding potentially life-saving therapy from a patient. However, these drugs should only be used when the situation is serious, and the case should be well documented. Experience has shown that such situations do not occur frequently, even where the general supply of essential drugs is grossly insufficient.

Support, supervision and in-service training

Regular support and strict supervision are of utmost importance for any STD control programme. Several projects which neglected these essential elements have collapsed completely. Why are these elements of such enormous importance?

1. Training provided during a course needs to be reinforced and skills have to be consolidated. This is the case particularly in the first year improved case management is introduced at a health unit. Without this *consolidation* health workers have a tendency to depart from the syndromic approach after some time and readopt previous ways of managing STDs.
2. Health workers need *feedback* (and get it far too rarely). Supervision visits – if done well – satisfy this demand, which in turn will maintain the *motivation* of health workers.
3. Supervision visits are the only way to enforce *drug accountability*, without which the programme is likely to eventually fail.

Box 7. The importance of support and supervisory visits

-   Regular and effective support and supervisory visits are the backbone of the district STD control programme.
-   Without them, the programme is likely to fail.

Who should provide support and supervision? This is the classical task of an experienced clinician, the district STD control coordinator. Additional supervisory visits by the district medical officer will also be very beneficial, and the district AIDS programme coordinator may act as a replacement during leave periods, etc. In health units which already have an STD component in their antenatal or MCH work, the district MCH coordinator should also participate.

How often should supervisory visits be made? Assuming that STD services have recently started in a particular health unit, the first visit should be conducted as soon as possible. Even the best training is no guarantee that the new service will get started smoothly. Health workers often feel unsure of how to apply their freshly learned knowledge and skills, so the earlier this first visit is made the better. Thereafter, supervisory visits should be made at monthly, and later at quarterly, intervals. Supervision at longer intervals is an invitation to failure.

Supervision checklist: Various points should be considered when providing in-service training and supervision. A checklist has proven to be a helpful guideline (see Box 8).

Box 8. Supervision checklist

- Staff availability: Are any problems anticipated due to illness or leave?
- Equipment: Is it complete? Are repairs needed?
- Patient register book: Is the information complete and consistent?
- Treatments given: Have algorithms been followed?
- Clinical discussion: Did the health worker see any interesting or difficult cases?
- Selected topic for revision: What would the health worker like to discuss?
- Statistics: How many patients? Which syndromes? Cure rates? Any trends or changes as compared to the usual pattern? Why?
- Feedback: Discuss performance and statistics, compare with rest of the district.
- Drug consumption: How much has been consumed in relation to cases treated?
- Stock taking: Does the physical stock tally with calculated consumption?
- Reporting: Have forms for the district and higher authorities been forwarded?
- Replenishment of drugs.

Support of STD control at antenatal/MCH/family planning clinics
The tasks and activities of antenatal care and MCH workers are described in detail in Chapter 13. Again, it is the responsibility of the district team to ensure that these tasks can be and are fulfilled. Obviously, good support can only be provided if the district team has the necessary support skills. The training of the district MCH coordinator in STD management is therefore a priority. Furthermore, he/she should acquire a substantial amount of practical experience before training others and launching STD control efforts in peripheral units.

Checklists and forms such as those mentioned above for the supervision of the outpatient clinician can also be used for STD work at antenatal care/MCH clinics.

Monitoring, evaluation and feedback
Each health unit can monitor important data such as clinical cure rates or partner treatment rates on its own. The principal methodology is described in Chapter 13. However, health workers at a peripheral unit often need the help of the district STD control coordinator for this task. The district STD control coordinator should complete the monitoring form together with the health worker. The district STD control coordinator then compiles the data from the various units and arrives at quarterly treatment effectiveness tables for the whole district. Discussion with the respective health workers can compare data from a particular unit with district averages. Marked differences should be discussed in detail and – if necessary – advice for improvement given.

The district STD control coordinator should also share his/her observations with the district AIDS programme coordinator and the district MCH coordinator (if STD control has already been introduced at MCH/antenatal care clinics). Once per quarter the district STD control coordinator should report to the district medical officer on the STD situation in the district and discuss the performance of the various clinics.

A drop in the cure rates should be reported to the STD reference laboratory and national AIDS/STD programme. Such a drop may indicate development of antimicrobial resistance, which – if confirmed – may call for a change in the treatment strategy. Likewise, low attendance, return or partner treatment rates call for action by the district medical officer and district STD control coordinator. In this case, refresher training for the health workers may be necessary.

STD control in core groups

Preventing and treating STDs in high-transmission risk groups is an important element in any STD control programme. There are strengths in this approach but also limitations which should be understood.

The core group concept

In this context, the terms 'core group', 'high-risk group' or 'high frequency trans-mitters' are not social science concepts, and definitely do not describe a moral assess-ment. Instead, they are purely epidemiological terms. 'Core group' has a statistical meaning: a core group is a subset of the population made up of a critical number of individuals who have many more than a certain number of different sex partners in a given time period, for example, five or more per year. In this, they differ from the population at large, who generally have fewer than five different partners per year.

Obviously commercial sex workers are not the only ones who fall under this defini-tion. Other such groups may be migrant workers, semi-nomadic fishermen, truck drivers, soldiers and perhaps others. But single individuals who fulfil the definition are also included in the core group.

The core group concept postulates that certain epidemics can only occur and continue to exist in a general population if a core group exists. (Another example of the effect of such a threshold is a certain minimum amount of mosquitoes, without which malaria would disappear from an area. In other words, a small number of infected mosquitoes will be insufficient to maintain the infection in a community.)

This means that:

- Treating one STD case in a member of the core group may prevent many more new STD infections (including new HIV infections) than treating one infected person from the general population. For example, for gonorrhoea this may be in the range of an additional 30-fold prevention or more (13). The exact figure will depend on the transmission probability per single sexual contact between an infected person and an uninfected partner.
- Effective STD case management in the core group can drastically reduce STD prevalence in a community, as well as HIV incidence (the rate of new infections per time unit).
- If most core group members were to reliably use condoms for most sexual inter-courses, a high preventive impact would be achieved for the general population.

The cost argument is also quite appealing: treating one core group case is likely to prevent multiple transmissions of the STD. Thus, considered in terms of prevention of new cases, it is more cost-effective to treat core group cases than to treat STD patients in the general population.

Limitations of core group interventions

Core groups can be found in most communities. However, while commercial sex workers can easily be identified, belonging to the core group is much less obvious for many other individuals. This is the case, for example, for many women who occasionally engage in paid sex because of economic hardship, but who do not operate from bars or brothels. It is very difficult to reach such individuals through intervention programmes. Particularly in rural communities, it is often almost impossible to identify and target the high-risk portion of the population.

In conclusion, the core group concept is appealing, and therefore district STD control programmes should include a core group component, targeting interventions to the easily accessible part of the core group population. This is likely to be a very useful and cost-effective public health intervention. However, it is difficult to cover the core group entirely, and interventions for the general population remain a necessity.

STD prevention and management among commercial sex workers

STD services within the formal health sector – even if completely integrated into out-patient services – are often not accepted and utilized by commercial sex workers, which makes implementation of STD control for them rather difficult. To solve this dilemma, several options may be used, depending on the availability of funds.

IEC for bar and guesthouse managers: One or two short seminars can be conducted, inviting owners and managers of all high-risk establishments in the community. The objectives are to provide information and to create acceptance for a peer education initiative.

IEC through peer education: During a focused group discussion with commercial sex workers about their professional situation and about the risk of STDs and HIV infection, interested and capable women can be identified for training as peer educators. Training proceeds through orientation seminars on STDs and other related topics. The women then receive condoms and leaflets from district personnel. This helps them to reduce their own risks and to educate their colleagues to do so as well. They should promote condom use among their peers and encourage them to seek treatment for STDs at out-patient clinics with improved STD services. Condom dispensers are mounted in bars and guesthouses and refilled by the peer educators. Peer education can be backed up by additional group meetings for all commercial sex workers, during which sexual health topics are discussed. Peer educators are not paid for their work but receive regular technical support from district personnel. A certificate and other small incentives may be provided to enhance motivation (T-shirts, etc.).

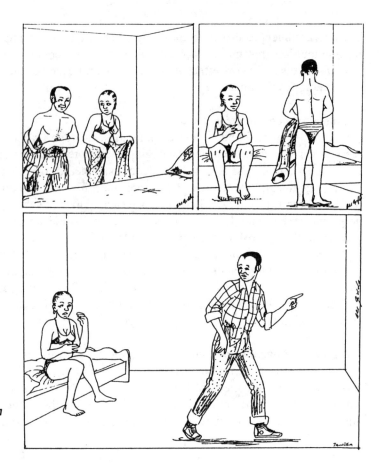

The woman insists on a condom, and the man agrees to go get one.

Mobile STD case management: a community nurse with training and experience in the syndromic management of STDs visits commercial sex workers at bars and guesthouses regularly. Health education and group discussions take place. She or he offers examination and treatment of symptomatic STDs at the women's workplaces and also routinely supplies condoms. Preferably this approach should be combined with IEC activities using peer educators.

Mobile STD screening: in addition to providing treatment for symptomatic patients, the community nurse screens all commercial sex workers once per month at their workplaces, using a speculum. If a functioning laboratory is available at the district hospital, cervical swabs may be taken routinely from all women for gram stain and microscopy. Patients with symptoms or signs of infection are treated syndromically. Those with gonococcal infection of the cervix should be treated for both gonococcal and chlamydial infection.

Static women's health centre: commercial sex workers (and other women) can visit a drop-in centre close to their workplaces. This centre, staffed by two nurses or a medical assistant and a nurse, can provide family planning services, antenatal care and MCH care, as well as STD treatment. Monthly screening for STDs and treatment for other minor ailments may be offered. Health education sessions are also given at the centre or elsewhere.

STD control in other core groups

STD-related health education may be targeted at other groups (e.g. plantation workers, soldiers, truck drivers, etc.) depending on the priorities of the district health team. This should involve group discussions, and peer educators should be identified and trained. Condom promotion and early treatment for STDs should be strongly emphasized.

If funds are available, a health worker from the respective institutions (plantation camps, barracks, trucking companies) should be invited to attend STD training at the district hospital. STD treatment services should then be offered regularly within the institution. The district STD control coordinator should conduct support visits on a regular basis. If possible, drugs can be provided by the company or service concerned, as well as transport for the district STD control coordinator. Progress should be regularly discussed with the management of the relevant institutions.

Collaboration and interaction with the STD reference clinic and laboratory

The role of the reference clinic

Routine laboratory services are not necessary and may even be counterproductive in a syndrome-based STD control programme, as described in Chapter 13. However, a reference clinic with a laboratory serving the wider area is needed to monitor the following parameters:

- the pattern of STD aetiologies for all major syndromes;
- the possible development of resistance of *Neisseria gonorrhoea* to antibiotics;
- the clinical and microbiological cure rates of STD patients

Specialized staff with expertise in STD control are usually available at such institutions. The reference clinic can also be used to train health workers.

Utilization of services

In the day-to-day work of the district STD control programme, routine collaboration with the reference clinic is unnecessary. However, a good working relationship is very helpful in several ways. For example, if the development of drug resistance is suspected at any health unit within the district, this should be reported to the reference institution without delay. A field team including a microbiologist from the reference centre may be detached to the district to investigate the field situation.

If the reference clinic is within convenient reach, special problems or difficult cases in the district may be discussed with the reference clinic staff, either occasionally or as part of a regular clinical conference (e.g. on a quarterly basis).

The clinic staff may be invited to district-based STD training courses to strengthen the district team by acting as facilitators.

Limitations

The reference clinic should *not* be used as a referral institution. STD patients exhibit a strong tendency not to follow referral instructions but to drop out of follow-up completely. Therefore, if at all possible, options for giving second line and even third line treatment should be available at the health unit of first contact, or at least within the district.

STD control at district level: a management task

Although the concept of STD control is straightforward, its implementation is not simple. We have to think in various dimensions: time, geographical area to be covered, available staff and their capacity, means of transport, possible collaborators, etc. We have to set priorities and make cost-effective choices. We need to ensure that the right type of inputs are provided at the right time. This presents an interesting managerial challenge. The following observations may help:

Personnel: Who are the actors in a district STD control programme? Which roles can they play? The distribution of tasks may be organized as follows:

- The *district medical officer* carries the institutional responsibility and is the programme manager of the district AIDS/STD control programme. He/she may delegate most of the technical work, but the district medical officer's leadership and guidance is extremely important during the planning process and in the supervision of the programme. The STD programme can only succeed if the district medical officer is genuinely interested in it and takes a supportive attitude. Time is scarce, and STD control will only be one of the district medical officer's many tasks. However, field supervision visits by the district medical officer can make all the difference in the quality of work in the peripheral health units.
- The *district STD control coordinator* is the field manager of the district STD control programme. The district STD control coordinator's routine task is to make regular support and supervision visits to health units, including drug supply. He/she must be an experienced clinician, preferably a medical assistant. The district STD control coordinator would typically be trained at the reference clinic in a neighbouring district which already has a functioning control programme. He/she should be sufficiently senior to be accepted by the officers in charge of the various health units. On the other hand, the district STD control coordinator must be flexible and ready to conduct long field trips on a regular and punctual basis. A good working relationship with community authorities should be developed. Not infrequently, the district STD control coordinator should plan and participate in preventive activities in the community, so some public-speaking qualities are helpful. Enthusiasm is necessary to do the job well!
- The *district MCH coordinator* is usually a nurse/midwife. Typically, MCH work has been her task for many years, and ideally, as its coordinator she has acquired substantial managerial skills. As district MCH coordinator, her job will be to introduce

an STD component into the existing MCH and antenatal care clinic routine. She should first develop her own competence in STD case management. Thereafter she can lead the process, starting in a few clinics. Training and supervision of health workers are major tasks. The district STD control coordinator and MCH coordinator need to collaborate closely.

- The *district AIDS programme coordinator* has the task of an IEC officer: information, education and communication targeted at the general public and at existing groups in the community is his/her main field of activity. Although AIDS control and STD control programmes overlap to a certain extent, the promotion of primary prevention of STDs and efforts to improve treatment-seeking behaviour are typical tasks of the district AIDS programme coordinator, as these tasks cannot routinely be fulfilled by the district STD control coordinator (who mainly has a clinical function, as described above). The district AIDS programme coordinator needs some understanding of modern STD case management. Many field activities cannot be performed alone, and at least one part-time health educator should be available to work with the district AIDS programme coordinator. The district AIDS programme coordinator, the part-time health educator and the district STD control coordinator will occasionally conduct joint activities.

- The *district pharmacist* has a key role to play: he/she assists the drug supply process from the central level to the district, and is accountable for drug storage and administration. The pharmacist regularly provides drugs to the district STD control coordinator for the various health units, and supervises the district STD control coordinator as far as drug consumption is concerned.

- The *training team for STD courses* should comprise at least two facilitators. Ideally, a training course should be planned by all the officers listed above, and organized by the district STD control coordinator and district AIDS programme coordinator as a collaborative effort. An experienced clinician from a peripheral clinic as well as the district MCH coordinator may contribute as trainers. Support can also be obtained from the STD reference clinic or from a neighbouring district.

All in all, introducing a new programme to the district health system is like getting a heavily loaded wagon moving by physical force. A group of people is needed, but just having these individuals on hand is not sufficient. They all need to push or pull in the same direction with enthusiasm and great effort. In the beginning, movement will be slow. But once a start is made, less effort is required to keep things going.

Setting priorities

As we have seen, STD control has several components. Not all of these can be launched at the same time. Likewise, STD control cannot be established throughout a whole district overnight. Therefore, it must be decided what the most important issues are and what should be done first.

An important principle is to start new activities on a small scale. Being over-ambitious leads to disappointment, frustration and failure. It is vital to establish the programme in small steps or modules! Making mistakes is inevitable, but it is better to make these mistakes in a pilot situation, where they can be easily corrected. The scope of the programme and its coverage should only be expanded after gaining competence and self confidence.

Making plans and carrying them out
The scenario described in Box 9 describes one way of setting priorities and getting the programme off the ground.

Box 9. Establishing district STD control: example of a master plan

Preparation phase (six months): train the district STD control coordinator and the district AIDS programme coordinator (this may be done at already-operational STD services outside the district). Organize an STD training course for a small group of selected health workers. Organize the basic drug supply on a modest scale. Prepare the strategy and the means for a first IEC campaign.

Pilot phase (one year): establish improved STD services in the outpatient department of the district hospital and at two health centres or dispensaries in communities. Make frequent supervision and support visits. Hold campaigns to improve treatment-seeking behaviour in the respective communities. Establish primary prevention activities at one primary or secondary school in the place where district headquarters are located. Ensure adolescents' access to STD services at the pilot health units. Organize STD training for the district MCH coordinator (externally or in the district hospital outpatient department).

First implementation phase (one year): establish improved STD services in another six peripheral health units. Perform IEC campaigns in the respective communities to improve treatment-seeking behaviour. Hold a training course for antenatal care/MCH staff. Introduce STD treatment into antenatal care/MCH clinics at the district hospital and two other pilot units (initially without syphilis screening). Extend IEC activities to another two schools.

Second implementation phase (two years): add more peripheral health units and establish STD services in one or two local institutions (barracks, factory, plantations and so forth). Start a peer education programme with female bar workers at the district centre or at a high-transmission area, and provide STD services. Extend STD services to the remaining antenatal care/MCH clinics. Introduce syphilis screening at the three pilot health units. Repeat campaigns in the same communities and schools as above, and expand these activities to a few more schools.

Third implementation phase (two years): ...

Throughout – remember: small is beautiful, at least in the beginning. Gain competence and self confidence before you take the next step.

Around the middle of the pilot phase a more detailed master plan will be needed (based on experience collected up to that point). This can be developed during a short workshop lasting a day or two. Such workshops are most effective if the participating group is small (no more than 10–12 participants). However, the quality of planning will be enhanced by input from potential users and collaborators (interested health workers, community leaders or school headmasters).

Detailed *operational plans*, such as supervision itineraries, are needed to implement the programme effectively. It is of great importance that peripheral health units know when the district STD control coordinator and the district MCH coordinator are expected to visit. Only then can health units plan their own work appropriately, allocate the necessary time, avoid conflicting commitments and invite patients with special problems to a joint clinic to be held with the supervisors. The collaborating health units and communities should be absolutely sure that itineraries are adhered to. Reliable and predictable supervision visits are the key to success.

Management structure

As with most aspects of district health services, good planning and management are required to get STD control started effectively. But how should responsibilities be organized? There is no set managerial structure to guarantee success, but team meetings combined with direct dialogue between the district medical officer and the various actors has proved to be an effective approach.

Intersectoral cooperation is needed, particularly with the educational sector. It may be useful to form a steering committee comprised of relevant district officers or heads of collaborating institutions who meet once or twice per year to provide the official framework for this cooperation. The routine collaboration is best accomplished through the direct interaction of those involved in the practical work, e.g. the district AIDS programme coordinator, the district STD control coordinator and the head teachers of participating schools.

Clear task allocations are required. A realistic operational work plan needs to be designed for each officer concerned. The district medical officer should frequently check that work plans are adhered to. Progress of the programme should be monitored quarterly, comparing it to the master plan.

Equipment and consumables needed

Training materials: the need for a training manual and a complete set of flow charts has been mentioned above (see Formal training of health workers). Samples of contact slips, monitoring forms and a register book should also be available (see Chapter 13). Other essential items are: a good blackboard (to be re-painted before the course starts, if necessary), chalk, writing pads and pens. An overhead projector with transparencies and markers is not essential but very helpful. Video equipment (if available) may be used to watch films and to record and review role plays.

Supervision and drug supply: the district STD control coordinator (and possibly the district MCH coordinator as well) needs a sturdy lockable box (about 50 x 30 x 30 cm) to transport medicines and other consumables to peripheral units. Box files for empty supervision forms, records and data sheets are also required. The district STD control coordinator, the MCH coordinator and the district AIDS programme coordinator should be suitably equipped for field activities (e.g. gum rubber boots, umbrella, etc.).

Public health educational campaigns: billboards are very useful, if available and affordable (can perhaps be obtained in collaboration with an NGO). Otherwise leaflets, condoms and simple condom user instructions will suffice. A portable loudspeaker is often helpful and can possibly be borrowed from other projects.

School and youth activities: educational materials such as discussion starters (pictures such as the cartoons that illustrate this book) can be self-prepared or obtained from the educational department and/or from relevant NGOs. Small incentives for active peer educators (badges, T-shirts and the like) are also needed.

Core group interventions: routine equipment consists of a drug box or case, drugs and other consumables, gloves, a speculum, a metal bowl, antiseptic solution, an electric torch, a register book. If collaboration with a lab is possible, materials for cervical swabs (microscopic slides, a slide box, swabs, a spirit-lamp, cotton wool) and for syphilis serology (syringes, needles, vacutainers, tourniquet, cotton wool, methylated spirit, a marker pen) will be needed.

Transport

Transport capacity is a crucial precondition for all the components described above: support and supervision visits, drug supply and community-based IEC campaigns. In principle, one or two vehicles should be available for district health services. But demand on these vehicles will be high, and often includes demands from other sectors. Not rarely, the vehicles may break down. As a result, in reality, reliable means of transport are often not available. Furthermore, the fuel budget may be far too small to cover needs.

There is no easy remedy for this problem. But there is also no reason for becoming frustrated and lethargic. Much can be done with imagination, perseverance and good planning. Some ideas include:
- start by establishing a range of STD control activities where transport is not essential, e.g. within the district headquarters itself;
- include communities where other district services operate regularly, and get permission for co-utilizing their transport systems;
- coordinate field visits: the same official service vehicle can be used jointly and simultaneously by a tuberculosis/leprosy coordinator, an MCH coordinator, an STD coordinator, an AIDS coordinator and other extension workers. This of course requires careful planning, preferably on a quarterly basis;

- seek support from NGOs operating in the same district. Even if their programmes are not health-related, they may be willing to share their means of transport;
- negotiate with the management of trading companies or other commercial suppliers (e.g. Coca Cola) to take the district STD control coordinator with them on their regular routes. Commercial supply lines are often very regular and reliable, and most people are happy to help;
- provide STD services to institutions with their own transport: military barracks, factories, plantation camps, mining companies. These institutions should guarantee transport for the district STD control coordinator before their workers are trained and their services start.

Conclusion

STDs represent an immense burden, not only on the health of individual patients (particularly women of child-bearing age) but also on the health care system and the economy at large. Effective STD control can in turn greatly reduce the rate of new HIV infections. STD control should become a compulsory element in AIDS programmes.

The task of the district health management team is to ensure four essential components of STD control: promotion of primary prevention, induction of improved treatment-seeking behaviour, facilitation of proper case management at health units and establishment of effective control activities in high-risk groups.

To ensure effective case management at peripheral health units, regular and detailed support supervision visits are of utmost importance. These should be provided by an experienced clinician (referred to as the district STD control coordinator in this book) and, after STD activities have been extended to antenatal care/MCH and family planning clinics, by the district MCH coordinator as well. The district STD control coordinator may be involved in the initial training of health workers, which should consist of both classroom teaching and practical sessions; furthermore, the district STD control coordinator helps to ensure a reliable supply of drugs to health units and cost-effective utilization of drugs.

Primary prevention efforts should focus on adolescents, while efforts to promote early treatment-seeking behaviour should be targeted towards the whole sexually active population. Such activities should be initiated by an experienced IEC officer using both peer educators and other approaches. Often this can be done by the district AIDS programme coordinator, who may collaborate with NGOs or other institutions to achieve this target. To establish a core group intervention among commercial sex workers, a community nurse should provide regular screening and treatment of STDs and facilitate peer health education.

Acknowledgement
We are very grateful to Professor David Mabey, London School of Hygiene and Tropical Medicine, for his advice and comments.

Further reading

Holmes KK, Mardh PA, Sparling PF, Wiesner PJ, eds. *Sexually transmitted diseases.* New York, McGraw-Hill, 1989.

Nduba J, Mabey D. *Self-instructional manual on sexually transmitted diseases.* Nairobi, African Medical and Research Foundation, 1992.

Prevention and management of sexually transmitted diseases in Eastern and Southern Africa: current approaches and future directions. Naresa Monograph, no. 3. Naresa, P.O. Box 11771, Nairobi, 1994.

Vuylsteke B, Laga M, Alary M et al. Clinical algorithms for the screening of women for gonococcal and chlamydial infection: evaluation of pregnant women and prostitutes in Zaire. *Clinical and Infectious Diseases* 1993, 17: 82–88.

World Health Organization. *WHO model prescribing information: drugs used in sexually transmitted diseases and HIV infection.* Geneva, 1995.

References

1. Laga M, Alary M, Nzila N et al. Condom promotion, sexually-transmitted diseases treatment, and declining incidence of HIV-1 infection in female Zairian sex workers. *Lancet* 1994, 344: 246–248.

2. Grosskurth H, Mosha F, Todd J et al. The impact of comprehensive management of sexually transmitted diseases on the incidence of HIV infection. *Lancet* 1995, 346: 530–536.

3. Robinson J, Mulder D, Auvert B, Hayes R. Modelling the impact of alternative HIV intervention strategies in rural Uganda. *AIDS* 1995, 9: 1263–1270.

4. World Bank. *World Development Report 1993: investing in health.* New York, Oxford University Press, 1993.

5. Mosha F, Nicoll A, Barongo L et al. A population-based study of syphilis and sexually transmitted disease syndromes in north-western Tanzania. 1. Prevalence and incidence. *Genitourinary Medicine* 1993, 69: 415–420.

6. Newell J, Senkoro K, Mosha F et al. A population-based study of syphilis and sexually transmitted disease syndromes in north-western Tanzania. 2. Risk factors and health seeking behaviour. *Genitourinary Medicine* 1993, 69: 421–426.

7. Mayaud P, Grosskurth H, Changalucha J et al. Risk assessment and other screening options for gonorrhoea and chlamydial infections in women attending rural Tanzanian antenatal clinics. *Bulletin of the WHO* 1995, 73: 621–630.

8. Mulder D. Disease perception and health-seeking behaviour for sexually transmitted diseases. In: *Prevention and management of sexually transmitted diseases in Eastern and Southern Africa: current approaches and future directions. Naresa Monograph,* no. 3. Nairobi, Naresa, 1994.

9. AMREF Mwanza and Kuleana Mwanza. *Sexually transmitted diseases.* Leaflet, 1993.

10. Wynendaele B, Bomba W, Mganga W et al. Impact of counselling on safer sex and STD occurrence among STD patients in Malawi. *International Journal of STD and AIDS* 1995, 6: 105–109.

11. Nduba J, Mabey D. *Self-instructional manual on sexually transmitted diseases.* Nairobi, African Medical and Research Foundation, 1992.

12. Moses S, Manji F, Bradley J et al. Impact of user fees on attendance at a referral centre for sexually transmitted diseases in Kenya. *Lancet* 1992, 340: 463–466.

13. Hethcote HH, Yorke JA. *Gonorrhea transmission dynamics and control. Lecture notes in Biomathematics.* New York, Springer, 1984.

14. World Health Organization. *Technical information WHO/TB/*67.53, 1967.

15. Fransen L. Can the control of STDs contribute to AIDS prevention in developing countries? Oral presentation at the IX International Conference on AIDS, Berlin, June 1993 ('Meet the experts' symposion).

16. Gilson L, Mkanje R, Grosskurth H et al. Cost-effectiveness of improved STD treatment services as a preventive intervention against HIV in Mwanza Region, Tanzania. Oral presentation at the XI International Conference on AIDS, Vancouver, July 1996

15 HIV testing at district level

Arnoud Klokke

- What is needed to set up HIV testing facilities?
- What is the difference between rapid assays and ELISA?
- Can pooling of samples be used to reduce costs?
- What should be done if the first test result is positive?
- How can an infected person have a negative test result?

The most commonly used method to find out if someone is infected with the human immunodeficiency virus (HIV) is by testing for the presence of HIV antibodies in their blood. Routine testing for the virus itself is not yet possible. In a district, HIV testing is mostly done in a hospital laboratory, and may be carried out for various reasons: to screen blood units and blood donors, to test in- or outpatients (diagnostic testing), to carry out voluntary testing among healthy persons or to monitor the epidemic through sentinel surveillance, for example among antenatal women. Each group requires a different testing strategy.

This chapter describes the minimum requirements for proper HIV testing at the district level in terms of laboratory needs and counselling services. Subsequently, the various testing strategies for different purposes are discussed. HIV testing is relatively expensive and is an additional burden on the limited resources of a district or hospital. There are, however, methods to reduce the costs of HIV testing, such as the re-use of tests and pooling of samples, which are presented in the final section of this chapter.

Requirements

Minimum requirements

Before starting HIV testing at a health facility, a few basic conditions should be met, such as adequate space and trained staff. Distilled water should also be on hand, if possible. Sometimes all reagents, including distilled water, are provided with the test kit. Trained staff and a clean room, however, are indispensable for proper testing, plus a sound administration system which can guarantee confidentiality.

HIV testing is only feasible if enough samples are anticipated. For instance, if fewer than ten units of blood per week have to be tested, it is better to refrain from testing blood units at all. The staff will not gain enough experience with HIV testing and errors are more likely to be made through inexperience. A better solution is to purchase safe blood units from a larger neighbouring blood bank, if this is feasible.

Diagnostic and voluntary testing require appropriate counselling services and individuals should never be tested against their will. *Informed consent* is vital: this means that a person understands what the test involves, what the result may mean to him or her, and voluntarily agrees to testing. Prior to giving a blood sample, patients and volunteers should participate in a pre-test counselling session with a qualified staff person; they should then be asked if they consent to being tested. Informed consent is always necessary, unless testing is for screening or surveillance purposes and the results are not linked in any way to an individual. Blood taken from blood donors can be tested without permission of the donor. If feasible, however, pre-test counselling should also be carried out; if the donor wishes to be informed about test results, post-test counselling is also necessary.

In all cases, confidentiality of the results of HIV testing is an absolute necessity. All testing for HIV antibodies should be done exclusively under code number. Only the medical doctor and/or the counsellor should be able to link individuals with their code numbers, which should be kept in a special register in a locked cupboard. Laboratory staff should not know the names of individuals to be tested nor work with named samples. It is obvious that a sound registration system is required to guarantee confidentiality and to avoid serious errors caused by mixing samples and code numbers.

Samples for testing

Tests for HIV antibodies can be done on serum, saliva, urine or blood eluate. Most commercially available test kits require serum. To get serum, whole blood is taken from the individual by venous puncture, using a syringe, a needle and a clean container of at least 5cc. If other body fluids can be used for the test, this should be indicated by the test kit. Saliva (not sputum) should be spat into a plastic container and stored at 4°C. Urine samples can be collected in a container. Blood eluate, collected by skin piercing (finger or heel prick), is spotted onto special filter paper, dried at room temperature and stored at room temperature in a plastic bag, preferably with some desiccant (1). If properly stored, the sample may be held for testing for a year or more.

HIV test kits

Many test kits are available for HIV antibody testing, differing in principle, methodology, price and quality. The quality or accuracy of a test is expressed as sensitivity and specificity.

- **Sensitivity** describes the chance that a test result will be positive when HIV antibodies are present. In other words, if test A has a sensitivity of 98%, then it can be expected to identify 98 of 100 truly HIV-infected individuals, with no more than 2 false negatives.
- **Specificity** describes the chance that a test result will be negative if HIV antibodies are not present. For instance, if test B has a specificity of 95%, then it can be

expected to identify 95 of 100 truly HIV-negative persons, with no more than 5 false positives.

However, in the field the sensitivity and specificity of a test is generally lower than the manufacturer's results (see Box 1).

Box 1. Performance of HIV antibody tests in field conditions

The performance of a test depends on the quality of the environment in which the test is performed. A test often performs better in a qualified reference laboratory than in the field. The performance of rapid assays and ELISA HIV tests was evaluated in eight district hospital laboratories in Mwanza Region. The results showed considerably higher levels of false positive and false negative tests in the rural laboratories than in the reference laboratories. For instance, while Organon EIA (an ELISA) has a sensitivity and specificity of 100% and 99.4% in reference laboratories, at these eight peripheral laboratories the same EIA had 93.5% and 90.0% sensitivity and specificity respectively. The sensitivities of three rapid assay tests (HIVCHEK, Test Pack and Immunocomb) dropped from 98–100% in the reference laboratories to 84–98% in the rural laboratories, while specificities of 96–100% decreased to 69–93% in the rural laboratories (2, 3).

Test kits can be divided into four groups: rapid assays, enzyme linked immunosorbent assays (ELISA), IgG antibody captured particle adherence tests (GACPAT) and Western blots.

Rapid assay: Some examples are HIV-SPOT, HIVCHEK, Test pack, ImmunoComb, Serodia HIV, and Recombigen HIV. The main characteristic of rapid assays is that the tests are easy to use, testing takes only a few minutes and may be done one by one. Sensitivity and specificity, however, are reduced as speed increases: in general, the quicker the test, the lower the sensitivity and specificity. These single tests are relatively expensive. Costs per test vary from US$ 1.10–4.80, and are typically in the range of US$ 2–3.

Enzyme linked immunosorbent assay (ELISA): There are many different types of ELISA for HIV, such as Wellcozyme, Enzygnost and Organon. ELISA tests have better sensitivity and specificity than rapid assays, not only in highly qualified institutions in developed countries such as the reference laboratories of the World Health Organization (WHO), but also at the peripheral level in developing countries. Testing is done by batch. The larger the batch, the lower the price per test will be. Costs per test vary from US$ 0.90 to $ 2.60, but generally average US$ 1.00, when obtained in large quantities.

IgG antibody captured particle adherence test (GACPAT): GACPATs are a modification of the commercially available Serodia HIV test (a rapid assay). A GACPAT is comparable with an ELISA as far as sensitivity and specificity is concerned, but is about ten times less costly (about US$ 0.10 per test). This test requires locally prepared micro-well plates and overnight incubation.

Western blot: A Western blot detects specific viral antibodies by combining with their respective viral proteins. This technique, which requires experienced personnel, is not a routine test and is used only for research purposes. This test is expensive (US$ 10–20 per test) and not practical for use by districts.

Equipment

Tests vary with respect to the equipment they require. Commercial rapid assays (such as HIV-SPOT) do not require additional equipment. Other test kits require a pipettor with variable volumes, as specified in test kit instructions (such as 0.5–10, 10–50, 50–200, or 200–1,000 uL) (price about US$ 150). Using a manual washing procedure for ELISAs and GACPAT, a twelve or eight multi-channel pipettor is needed (about US$ 750). These pipettors also require disposable tips (yellow for a volume less than 200 uL and blue for volumes over 200 uL). If large batches of ELISA tests must be performed, a machine for washing (US$ 3,000) saves time, but requires maintenance and supervision. Most test results can be read with the naked eye. However, weak reactive ELISA tests require either a strip reader (US$ 700) or a plate reader (US$ 3,000–7,000).

Testing strategies

WHO recommended strategy

A single test of a sample for HIV antibodies may not be sufficient to give a reliable result. WHO (4) has recommended the test strategies outlined in Box 2, which vary depending on whether the subject is a blood donor, a symptomatic patient or an asymptomatic person, and the HIV prevalence in the area. Obviously, the more tests required (strategies II and III), the higher the costs per sample will be.

One test is sufficient for blood donors. If the sample is negative the blood can be used, if the sample is positive or non-negative the blood needs to be discarded; if testing is done with a rapid assay prior to bleeding the donor, and the test result is positive or non-negative, the donor is deferred. It is important that a test with high sensitivity is used, that is, one that produces as few false negatives as possible. For surveillance purposes one test is adequate, if HIV prevalence is high (greater than 10%). If HIV prevalence is 10% or less a second confirmatory test is required.

A patient with symptoms of HIV infection does not always need to be tested; but if testing is done, a confirmatory test should be performed, irrespective of the prevalence of HIV. Asymptomatic individuals require a confirmatory test if reactive in the screening test; if HIV prevalence is 10% or less and both the first and second test results are non-negative, a third test is required before diagnosing HIV infection.

Box 2. WHO recommended strategies for HIV testing

Reason for test	All/in accord with HIV Prevalence	Strategy
Blood donor	All	I
Surveillance	Prevalence > 10%	I
	Prevalence 10% or less	II
Diagnosis (symptomatic)	All	II
Diagnosis (asymptomatic)	Prevalence > 10%	II
	Prevalence 10% or less	III

Strategy	N of tests		
I	One	+ -	
II	Two	+	-
III	Three	+	-

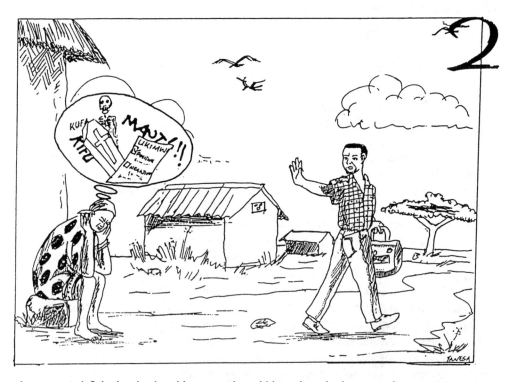

A woman is left by her husband because she told him that she has tested HIV-positive.

Type of tests

When testing according to strategy I, samples should be screened using a test kit with the highest possible sensitivity. False positives are acceptable, but false negatives should be avoided as far as possible. GACPAT and any ELISA can be used for this purpose. Rapid assays should be used for blood unit screening only. Tests with high specificity are the first choice for testing individuals, to minimize the chance of giving false positive results (i.e. telling people they are HIV-positive when in fact they are not).

Confirmatory testing requires a test with a principle which is essentially different from the principle of the screening test. This may be a second type of rapid assay or an ELISA. The WHO proposes a second ELISA as the confirmation test of choice. If confirmatory testing is necessary but not feasible at a district laboratory, the sample may be forwarded (on filter paper) to a central regional laboratory for confirmatory testing.

Window period

A negative test result does not necessarily mean that the individual is not HIV-infected. A recent infection (less than three months before testing) often cannot be detected by the currently used HIV tests, because it usually takes 4–12 weeks after infection with HIV for HIV antibodies to appear in the blood. The time between the infection and the detection of antibodies is called the window period. During the window period, a person who is HIV-infected will still test negative in an HIV antibody test (see also Chapter 17).

Reducing cost per test

As noted above, the costs of the available tests (rapid assays and ELISA tests as the most common ones) range from US$ 1–5 per test. If additional (confirmatory) testing is required, costs may be doubled. Such expenses are often beyond the limited budget of district health facilities, especially if the high demand for testing blood units and patients, testing for sentinel surveillance and requests for voluntary testing are taken into account; for the latter, however, a cost-recovery system may be applied. Fortunately, testing costs can be reduced without loss of sensitivity and specificity, making this laboratory service possible at peripheral level. There are at least three ways to reduce costs: pooling, re-use of tests and GACPAT use.

Pooling

In a population with low prevalence, pooling samples may reduce the cost per test by 50% or more (5, 6, 7). However, the higher the prevalence, the lower the number of samples that can be pooled. Box 3 describes the process of pooling, and gives an estimate of the percentage of tests that can be saved.

Re-use of HIV-SPOT device

The single testing device, as used by HIV-SPOT, can be used twice in some cases (8, 9): if a sample is non-reactive, the device can be re-washed at the end of the testing procedure and kept at 4°C for a period up to 14 days. It should be used at the first opportunity within this period. If this is done in combination with pooling, costs are reduced even further.

Box 3. Pooling samples

Mix equal volumes (50 ul) of consecutive samples in a clean test-tube and handle this as one 'sample'. If the test result is negative, all individual samples are negative; if the test result is not negative, all individual samples must be retested individually. Fear of diluting the antibody concentrations to below the detection level of the test in use should not prevent using this cost-reducing tool, since only very high dilutions make a normal positive sample weak reactive; for an ELISA this may be 1:10,000, while for a rapid assay such as HIV-SPOT the equivalent figure could be 1:1,000. Eluates may be pooled, but no studies have been done on pooling saliva.

Percentage of tests saved by pooling samples

	HIV prevalence			
	2.5%	5%	7.5%	10%
Proposed pool size (number of samples)	5–10	4–6	3–5	3–4
Estimated percentage of tests saved by pooling	65%	55%	44%	35%

GACPAT

The GACPAT reduces the cost per test (10) to about US$ 0.10 and maintains sensitivity and specificity at the ELISA level; however, it requires overnight incubation (see Box 4). If distilled water is available, the test is easily manufactured locally at the district laboratory; if not, the GACPAT can be produced at a central regional laboratory and issued to districts. The GACPAT has the advantage that it allows testing of either serum or blood eluate. Testing urine and saliva with GACPAT is not recommended.

Choosing the best strategy

Each hospital should choose the HIV test which suits it best, taking into account the following conditions:
- reason for testing: blood units, voluntary testing, diagnostic testing, sentinel surveillance;
- test strategy;
- HIV prevalence in the population;
- available budget.

Table 1. Overview of HIV testing suggestions and possible combinations

Test	Subject	Cost reducing activity	Equipment	Material	Normal cost per test (US$)	Reduced cost per test[1]
Rapid assay	Donor	Pooling Re-use	Pipettor	Serum	2.00	Less than US$ 1.00
GACPAT	Donor Patient Voluntary Sentinel	Pooling	Pipettor Multichannel pipettor	Serum Eluate	0.10	Less than US$ 0.10
ELISA	Donor Patient Voluntary Sentinel	Pooling	Pipettor Multichannel pipettor Washer / Reader	Serum Eluate Saliva	1.00	Less than US$ 1.00

[1] If cost reducing strategies (e.g. those shown in column three) are applied.

Box 4. HIV testing using GACPAT

The GACPAT method was field tested for detection of HIV in district hospitals in Mwanza Region. Plates were prepared at the reference laboratory, and kits with 96 tests (each consisting of wash buffer, reagent, and coated microwell plate) were issued to three peripheral hospitals, where 1054 serum samples were tested in single using GACPAT. The samples were transferred to the regional laboratory and the HIV status of each sample was again determined by testing with GACPAT and an ELISA, with confirmatory testing using a second ELISA or Western blot.

There was 97.6% agreement between the GACPAT tests results of the district hospitals and those of the regional reference laboratory. In 95.9% of cases, GACPAT test results in the district hospitals agreed with the HIV status determined by more expensive tests. In the district hospitals, the GACPAT's sensitivity and specificity were 92.6% and 98.7% respectively. GACPAT is thus a cheap HIV test which can be easily used at peripheral hospitals for donor screening and diagnostic testing. As with any test, additional HIV testing may be required if the test result in not negative (see Box 2 and reference 11).

Low-budget testing is made possible by using:

- filter paper sampling;
- pooling, depending on prevalence;
- screening with GACPAT (and confirmation with an ELISA that accepts blood eluate, possibly at the central regional reference laboratory).

Conclusion

The WHO-recommended testing strategy in Box 2 should be followed, no matter what laboratory facilities are available in a district. Appropriate counselling and strict confidentiality are absolutely necessary. The choice of the type of HIV test may depend primarily on the financial position of the health facility. A health facility with a poor laboratory and restricted financial resources should completely refrain from testing. A health facility with a poor laboratory but some financial resources should first improve its laboratory. Then HIV testing can begin, using rapid assay, GACPAT or ELISA methods (depending on the availability of skilled personnel) for screening blood units and individuals. In many situations, activities such as pooling or re-use of devices can help to keep testing costs to a minimum.

Further reading

AHRTAG. *Practical issues in HIV testing.* AHRTAG Briefing Paper. London, 1994. Available from: AHRTAG, Farringdon Point, 29–35 Farringdon Road, London EC 1M 3JB, UK (free to developing countries, US$ 5.00 elsewhere).

Bugando Medical Centre. *Practical steps using GACPAT for HIV testing.* Available free of charge from: Head, Pathology Department, Bugando Medical Centre, P.O. Box 1370, Mwanza, Tanzania.

Constantine NT et al. *HIV testing and quality control: a guide for laboratory personnel.* Durham, NC, Family Health International.

Medical Mission Institute. *Policy paper on HIV antibody tests.* Würzburg, AIDS and International Health Department, Medical Mission Institute.

UK NGO AIDS Consortium. *Preconditions for providing HIV testing.* London, UK, AIDS Consortium, 1993.

World Health Organization. *Can mandatory HIV testing stop the AIDS epidemic?* Geneva, 1994.

World Health Organization. *WHO guidelines for standard HIV isolation procedures.* WHO/GPA/RID/VAD/94.2. Geneva, 1994.

References

1. Klokke AH et al. Evaluation of HIV testing of blood spotted paper samples. *Tropical Doctor* 1991, 21: 120.

2. Heessen F et al. *Performance of rapid anti-HIV assays for screening of donor blood under field conditions in Africa.* VIIIth International Conference on AIDS. Amsterdam, 1992.

3. Dolmans WMV et al. *Feasibility and costs of ELISA versus rapid assays for HIV screening of donor blood in rural hospitals in Tanzania.* VIIIth International Conference on AIDS. Amsterdam, 1992.

4. World Health Organization. Recommendations for the selection and use of HIV antibody tests. *WHO Weekly Epidemiological Record* 1992, 67: 145–149.

5. Emmanuel JC et al. Pooling of sera for human immunodeficiency virus (HIV) testing: an economical method for use in developing countries. *Journal of Clinical Pathology* 1988, 41: 582–585.

6. Parry JV et al. Are seroepidemiological surveys for human immunodeficiency virus infection based on tests on pools of serum specimens accurate and cost-effective? *Clinical and Diagnostic Virology* 1993; 1: 167–178.

7. Mortimer JY, Saving tests by pooling sera – how great are the benefits? *Journal of Clinical Pathology* 1980, 33: 1120–1121.

8. Svendsen J et al. Re-use of 'HIVCHEK' in developing countries (Letter). *Lancet* 1990, 336: 1198–1199.

9. Wannan GJ et al. How many bloods will a 'HIVCHEK' Multiple tests for HIV antibody for a single screening kit. *Tropical Doctor* 1992, 22: 151–154.

10. Parry JV et al. An Immunoglobulin G antibody capture particle-adherence test (GACPAT) for antibody to HIV-1 and HTLV-1 that shows economical large-scale screening. *AIDS* 1989, 3: 173–176.

11. Klokke AH, Berege ZA. Reducing the cost of HIV testing through the use of the IgG antibody captured particle adherence test (GACPAT) in district hospitals. *Tropical and Geographical Medicine* 1995, 47: 296–299.

16 Medical care-related transmission

Balthazar Gumodoka, Isabelle Favot and Wil Dolmans

- How important are poor injection and sterilization practices to the spread of HIV?
- How can injection and sterilization practices be improved in a district?
- What occupational HIV risks do health workers face?
- What can a district do to reduce the occupational risks of HIV?

Giving and receiving medical care – whether along a road, at home or in a clinic, health centre, private consulting room, dentist's chair or hospital – has always carried risks. Now these risks have become greater because of HIV. In some cases the giver takes greater risks than the receiver; in others the receiver risks more than the giver. There are four situations in which HIV transmission may occur during medical care: from patient to patient (mostly by injections), from donor to patient (in blood transfusions), from health worker to patient (rare, but documented cases do exist), and from patient to health worker.

In countries with high HIV prevalence, medical care-related HIV transmission is relatively important, but sexual transmission still remains by far the most significant mode of transmission, and it is here that emphasis on preventive measures should be placed. Nonetheless, health workers have a special responsibility to make sure their patients are not put at risk of HIV infection.

This chapter will focus on two aspects: reducing the risk of patient-to-patient HIV transmission due to inadequate injection and sterilization practices; and dealing with the occupational risks faced by health workers, who may be infected by patients. In both cases the focus will be on what can be done at district level to reduce medical care-associated transmission. Blood transfusions are dealt with in Chapter 17.

Injection and sterilization practices

Transmission of HIV via contaminated needles and syringes or reused invasive equipment in health care settings has been reported in several countries. In a district, the risk of transmitting HIV by injection depends upon the HIV prevalence, how commonly

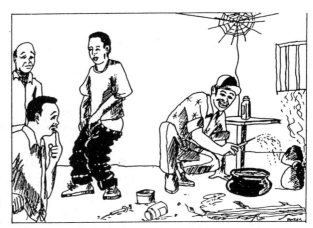

Unsafe medical practices: injections are a popular method of treatment, and their use is not limited to official health facilities.

injections are given, whether needles and syringes are reused and the adequacy or inadequacy of injection and sterilization practices. In Burkina Faso, the number of intramuscular injections given varied greatly among four dispensaries, indicating that health staff behaviour may be a decisive factor (1).

A detailed study was conducted in Mbeya Region, Tanzania, on the relationship between HIV transmission and injections (2). HIV prevalence was estimated at 30% among adults attending the health facilities, each adult patient had on average one to two injections per year and injections were considered safe in 97.5% of cases. It was concluded that with an established AIDS intervention programme supporting the health system less than 0.4% of the total incidence of 4,500–8,500 HIV-infections in that region was attributable to medical injections. Outside such an intervention programme, however, injections could be considered a more significant mode of HIV transmission.

It should also be noted that this study did not include injections outside the formal health sector (nor did any other known study). Traditional healers and unlicensed practitioners may not be well-trained in hygienic practices but still use modern technology such as antibiotics and injections to enhance their treatments. This may be a major mode of transmission in some districts.

Improving practices
A small survey of health facilities can provide information on current injection and sterilization practices. Box 1 gives the results of one such study. A survey may include an assessment of:

- knowledge of health workers on indications for treatment by injection, plus prescribing practices;
- patient demand for injections; in many places, popular demand for injections is high and leads to overprescription of injections (3);
- responsibility for sterilization: who does the sterilization and how is it done?;
- equipment availability: needles (disposable or not), syringes, sterilization equipment; reasons for possible shortages;
- injection practices: how many times are 'disposable' needles used, how are needles disposed of, are needles reused without sterilization?

Box 1. Injection and sterilization practices

In 1991 a baseline study of 66 randomly selected health facilities in Mwanza Region found that:
- The relationship between knowledge available at a specific health unit and prescribing practices at that unit was minimal. Therefore it seems that increasing the staff's knowledge may not reduce unnecessary injections.
- 70% of injections given for common conditions were avoidable.
- Patient demand for injections was high and probably led to overprescription of injections.
- The overall percentage of contaminated syringes and needles was 40%.
- 66% of the facilities' injection practices were unsatisfactory.

After injection and sterilization practices have been assessed, interventions can be developed. These may include:
- *Reduce the number of injections given*: by issuing prescription guidelines for common conditions and promoting orally ingested drugs rather than injections.
- *Improve sterilization practices*: sterilization guidelines need to be well known. A sheet with simple instructions can be prepared and posted in the health facility.
- *Reduce the demand for injections*: community awareness about the effectiveness of oral drugs and the side effects of injections can be raised through posters, educational talks and leaflets; not only via health services but also via other channels such as schools.
- *Improve supervision*: via the implementation of routine, formalized supervisory visits including a checklist to be used by the district medical officer or nurse.
- *Improve supplies*: stock reusable syringes and needles, time clocks, sterilizing equipment and sufficient oral drugs; stocks should be monitored.

These interventions can be introduced through training workshops for health workers, held locally in health centres or schools. This type of workshop is not costly and does not require staff to be away from their health facilities for more than one day. Box 2 shows how this was done in Tanzania and what was learned in the subsequent evaluation.

Sterilization is often delegated to the lowest cadre of a health facility, who are usually untrained. The evaluation in Box 2 emphasizes the importance of training all health facility staff, instead of limiting training to senior staff. All staff from the dispensaries attended the training, but for the health centres only the senior staff were involved. The staff attending the workshops may not disseminate the newly acquired knowledge, so the effect of the training is limited, as was the case in the health centres described in Box 2. It is therefore important for all staff cadres to attend such training sessions. If this is not feasible, training should focus on the staff actually doing the sterilization and their supervisors in the health facility.

Box 2. Evaluating the effects of training

In early 1992, one-day training workshops were held in all health centres in the districts of Mwanza Region, Tanzania, for the senior staff of the health centres and all staff of their four to six satellite dispensaries. Posters were displayed and educational information was also given to people attending the health units. Trainers came from the region and the district. Four months later an evaluation was carried out which showed that:

- Avoidable injections dropped from 70% in 1991 to 55% in 1992.
- The percentage of patients receiving injections dropped from 24% in 1991 to 11% in 1992.
- Contamination of syringes dropped from 44% in 1991 to 22% in 1992 at dispensaries. No changes were observed in the hospitals and health centres.
- Knowledge of indications for injections had improved for nurses and nursing assistants, but not for medical officers.

Once the staff have been trained and the health facility is equipped with sufficient needles and syringes and appropriate sterilizing equipment, regular supervision is still essential. If not, the effect of the training will be short-lived. This is illustrated in Box 3, which gives an evaluation of such an intervention two years later. In this case study supervisory visits were not increased following the intervention. In addition, most of the trained health staff had been transferred. The data show that regular supervision on issues related to prescribing practice and sterilization is crucial, and that staff retraining will be needed every two to three years.

Occupational risk for health workers

Although the occupational risk of health workers acquiring HIV infection is currently considered to be small (4), that risk will rise as the number of HIV/AIDS patients increases in the coming decade. Providing medical care to HIV-infected patients will become a major activity for many health workers in high-prevalence developing countries. The occupational risk of HIV infection among health workers depends on three factors: the prevalence of HIV infection among patients, frequency of accidental exposure to HIV and the chance of transmission after occupational exposure to HIV.

The number of HIV/AIDS patients in clinics, health centres and hospitals is high, and rising in many districts. HIV prevalence among people in clinical settings is considerably higher than in the general population. In a hospital in Mwanza town 45% of admissions to the general medical and tuberculosis wards aged 15–44 years were HIV-infected, while HIV prevalence was 12% among the general urban population aged 15–54 years (5).

Box 3. Injection and sterilization practices in 10 health facilities in Magu District, Tanzania, two years after training in injection and sterilization practices

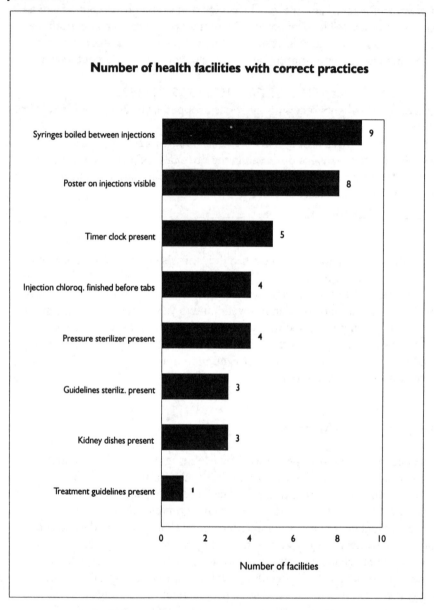

Number of health facilities with correct practices

Practice	Number of facilities
Syringes boiled between injections	9
Poster on injections visible	8
Timer clock present	5
Injection chloroq. finished before tabs	4
Pressure sterilizer present	4
Guidelines steriliz. present	3
Kidney dishes present	3
Treatment guidelines present	1

Number of facilities

The occasions on which health workers can be exposed to HIV-infected fluids include needle stick injuries, skin punctures during surgical procedures, splashes of blood or body fluids (e.g. in obstetrics). In developing countries, supplies of hygienic and protective equipment are often inadequate and working conditions more difficult, which increases the likelihood of incidents involving possible exposure to HIV. Studies in Africa have shown that accidental exposure to body fluids is not uncommon (see Box 4). A surgeon may have one or more percutaneous accidents per year, and a nurse probably less than one.

Box 4. Occurrence of pricks and splashes in African health care settings

- In Mwanza Region, Tanzania, the number of pricks and splashes recalled in the last month by health workers in 9 hospitals corresponded to a per health worker average of 5 prick and 9 splash incidents per year (6).
- In a Nigerian hospital health workers suffered 0.6 accidents with sharps per year (7). Surgeons had 2.3 accidents per year.
- In Zambia, 12 prick accidents occurred in treating 1161 consecutive surgical patients: 8 among surgeons and 4 among other personnel (about 1 per 100 operations) (8).
- In Tanzania, surgeons reported a prick accident in 0.7% of 488 procedures. An examination of 1667 used gloves, however, showed that 22 gloves had a total of 27 perforations, or in 5.5% of the procedures; among surgeons this figure was 9.7% (6).

The risks associated with occupational exposure to HIV through percutaneous injuries from needles or other instruments is thought to be low: transmission may occur in about 0.2–0.25% of cases or 1 for every 400–500 accidents involving exposure to HIV-contaminated blood (9). In reality, very few doctors, nurses or laboratory workers have become infected during their work (10). HIV is most likely to be transmitted by a penetrating injury, usually from a hollow-bore needle. This means that the chance is very small that workers will become infected after most common injuries. Until now, no studies in developing countries have shown additional HIV risks for health workers. Studies from the early years of the epidemic found equal seroprevalence rates among health workers and the general population in both Zaire and Senegal (11, 12). But the larger proportion of beds now being occupied by HIV patients and low efficiency in preventing injuries is likely to have increased risks since then. Preventive measures are imperative, particularly in surgical, obstetrical and laboratory departments.

Traditional birth attendants (TBAs) may be at risk of HIV infection due to lack of protective practices. A survey on occupational blood contact and HIV infection among traditional birth attendants in Rwanda showed a high frequency of blood-skin contact, indicating a need for attendants to learn infection control precautions (13). However, the TBA's risk of HIV infection was found to be small.

Assessment of protective measures for prevention

Protective measures not only protect against HIV, but also against other infections such as hepatitis B. However, the costs of providing protective equipment and training for all staff in a district may be prohibitive. If training all staff is not feasible, a less-costly alternative is to train only staff involved in high-risk procedures, such as surgical, obstetrical, and laboratory intravenous and clean-up procedures.

Three steps to improve protective practices are: first, a brief assessment of short-comings in terms of preventive practices in health facilities (an example of such an assessment is shown in Box 5). Second, based on that assessment, a list of equipment, supplies and activities needed to protect workers should be compiled and ordered. Third, the health workers should be trained on HIV/AIDS and how to improve their practices and use equipment and supplies correctly. The second and third steps are discussed below.

Box 5. Problem assessment in health facilities

A study was undertaken in Mwanza Region in 1993 to ascertain the extent of health facility shortcomings in preventive practices and the risks faced by workers. The topics and some of the findings at the time of the assessment are listed below.

- *General hygienic facilities and equipment*: water supply, presence of soap and disinfectant, use of sharp-proof containers for disposal of needles, use of proper waste pits, plastic or canvas bags for soiled linen. In Mwanza Region, very few health units had an adequate water supply or proper waste disposal.
- *Specific protective wear and gear*: availability and use of uniforms and aprons, gloves, long-sleeved gloves, forceps to remove needles from syringes, rubber boots, masks in operating theatres, protective eye gear in operating theatres and labour wards, mouthpieces for resuscitation, etc. Shortages of gloves were a recurrent problem in Mwanza Region, and disposable gloves were reused until worn out.
- *Care practices*: in Mwanza, only 16% of staff in nine hospitals used gloves consistently for venepuncture and 30% for wound dressing. Glove use by laboratory staff for venepuncture was only 6%. Only the labour room staff consistently used gloves for delivery and vaginal examination. Used needles were not always properly recapped – that is, the cap was held in the hand, rather than putting it on a table. In only two of the nine hospitals in Mwanza Region were long rubber gloves used consistently for the manual removal of a retained placenta.
- *Knowledge of health workers*: most health workers had fairly adequate knowledge about which body fluids can be infective.

Measures to reduce occupational exposure

Although occupational exposure of health workers to HIV cannot be eliminated, it can be reduced. Fulfilling certain conditions and providing facilities can reduce risks, but in practice risks will only be decreased if health workers consistently adhere to a number of protective practices. Should exposure still occur, a protocol for dealing with the situation should be at hand. The required conditions and facilities include adequate general facilities and specific protective wear and gear. Further, health workers should apply both technical and behavioural/organizational protective practices.

General facilities:
- clean water, immediately available;
- simple soap for hand-washing; antiseptic soaps or solutions (iodine, chlorhexidine or cetrimide) if resources allow;
- safe containers, fixed in place, for sharp instruments (puncture proof with a cover), with a portable container to transport sharps to and from the patient;
- covered containers such as dustbins; simple buckets to collect placentas;
- a pit or incinerator for waste disposal;
- thick canvas or plastic bags (a better option) for soiled linen;
- plastic covers in good condition for mattresses in operating theatre or labour room;
- means to boil water (e.g. a kerosene stove) and a container to sterilize instruments; an autoclave, if resources allow;
- 2% glutaraldehyde solution or 10,000 ppm hypochlorite for sterilization of instruments (soak 30 min.). If unavailable household bleach can be used (two tablespoons to two cups of water);
- in hospitals: a manual ventilator (eg. ambu bag) to avoid direct mouth-to-mouth contact during resuscitation.

Specific protective wear and gear:
- uniforms for medical staff;
- provisions to cover cuts or abrasions of health workers;
- domestic gloves and a sufficient amount of sterile medical gloves (disposable if finances allow);
- long-sleeved gloves in labour wards (for removal of placentas);
- forceps (to hold needle covers when needles are re-sheathed) or sheath-holders;
- aprons, gowns, rubber boots, masks and protective eye gear (glasses or goggles) in operating theatres and labour wards (also in general wards if finances allow).

Technical protective practices:
- safe re-sheathing and discarding of needles;
- used sharp instruments and body tissues or fluids should be transported and/or discarded in closed containers labelled as bio-hazardous material;
- gloves should be worn when handling blood or other potentially infected body materials and when caring for bleeding patients or patients with open wounds;
- surgeons should preferably use double-gloving (14, 15). If not enough gloves are available, at least the non-dominant index finger, which sustains most prick accidents (8), should have extra protection.

Behavioural and organizational protective practices:
- display guidelines;
- observe strict attention and working discipline, particularly during complicated procedures;
- reserve the performance of complicated and especially risky invasive procedures for more experienced staff members;
- ensure that the above-mentioned required conditions are met and facilities and supplies are available at all times, as far as possible. This includes, for instance, procedures that assure gloves will be ordered on time and broken equipment will be repaired or replaced as soon as possible.

A protocol for dealing with accidents where exposure to HIV may have occurred should include at least emergency measures after accidents, such as:
- allow the wound or needle prick to bleed for a few minutes; then wash the area with a disinfectant or soap;
- amply rinse mucous membrane splashes with clean water;
- check the HIV status of the patient; if unknown request the patient's permission to determine it;
- check the HIV status of health workers and repeat at three and six month intervals if negative. Provide appropriate counselling support (16);
- the prophylactic properties of anti-retroviral drugs is not clear. (Further, the current costs of combination therapy with multiple drugs are very high and beyond the budgets of many health facilities in developing countries.) Therefore, these drugs cannot presently be recommended.

This suggested protocol can be carried out by a medical officer or other staff member charged with the task. In larger hospitals this task may be taken up by a 'nosocomial infections committee', if such a body is in place.

Training
Health workers should be trained, based on the needs and shortcomings identified and the resources available. Knowledge of the occupational risks of HIV transmission may need to be strengthened. More important, health workers should take better precautions to protect themselves. Training health workers could be part of a one-week general course on HIV/AIDS which also includes medical care for AIDS patients and tuberculosis (see Chapter 12). Training can also be done in the context of short one-day workshops on injections and sterilization, held in the health facilities. A third option is an independent learning programme which involves all health workers and associated staff (see Chapter 12).

Compliance
Unfortunately, adherence to standard procedures is often low, even after training. One commonly sees lab assistants doing venepunctures without gloves, even though they are on hand, or a surgeon using a single pair of gloves when a double pair is available.

Factors that contribute to low compliance with precautionary measures may include (17):
- unavailability of protective materials;
- dislike of precautions (e.g. wearing gloves or other protective wear);
- personal underestimations of risk;
- lack of routine in undertaking precautions;
- lack of a role model (someone who consistently takes precautions);
- lack of routine enforcement procedures for supervision.

To improve compliance, materials should be available and accessible, and continuing education and supervision are needed to establish appropriate use. Protocols or standard procedures for dealing with injuries should be available at each health facility, and a nosocomial infections committee can be formed within the hospital to help ensure that these procedures are followed. Such a committee receives reports of any infectious disease contracted within the hospital, so they can monitor incidence; supervises health workers concerning their hygienic and preventive practices; and manages the condition and the supply of equipment and protective gear (18). In addition, protective measures and compliance with them should become a regular agenda item at staff meetings (e.g. bi-monthly).

The implementation of protective practices can also be enhanced by inter-professional counselling, whereby health workers of the same professional level discuss current practices and problems encountered in their own working environments among themselves on a regular basis.

Conclusion

Medical care-associated transmission in a district comprises a small but not insignificant proportion of all HIV transmission. Districts should ensure a safe blood supply at all times (see also Chapter 17). Safe injection and sterilization practices are also a vital part of a reliable health care delivery system. The number of HIV infections transmitted by injection can be greatly reduced by a few basic measures, including brief training of the staff involved in sterilization, and strengthening supervision. Ensuring an adequate supply of disposable needles (and assuring they are actually discarded after one use) is a potentially effective way to reduce HIV transmission, but may be too expensive for many districts in Africa.

Although the occupational risk faced by health workers is small, and for most health workers considerably smaller than the risk of HIV transmission through sexual contact, it is nonetheless an important concern among many health workers. Therefore, a district health programme should see to it that the knowledge of its health workers is up to standard. In addition, basic protective equipment needs to be made available and used. Solutions should be sought for cost-related problems; for example, supplying large numbers of expendable items such as gloves may be too large an expense for a district. In some districts, patients are requested to bring gloves for an operation or delivery. In other places, funds generated from user fees may be used to purchase gloves for health workers. These realities need to be discussed and options explored by staff committees.

Further reading

WHO, Global Programme on AIDS. *Preventing HIV transmission in health facilities.* GPA/TCO/HCS/95.16. Geneva, November 1995.

World Health Organization. Guidelines on sterilization and disinfection methods effective against human immuno-deficiency virus (HIV). *WHO AIDS Series,* no. 2. Geneva, WHO.

World Health Organization. *HIV prevention and care: teaching modules for nurses and midwives.* Geneva, 1993.

World Health Organization. *AIDS in Africa – a manual for physicians.* Geneva, 1992.

World Health Organization. *Guidelines for the clinical management of HIV infection in adults.* Geneva, 1991.

References

1. Vincent-Ballereau F, Lafaux C, Haroche G. Incidence of intramuscular injections in rural dispensaries in developing countries. *Transactions of the Royal Society of Tropical Medicine and Hygiene* 1989, 83: 106.

2. Hoelscher M, Riedner G, Hemed Y et al. Estimating the number of HIV transmissions through reused syringes and needles in the Mbeya Region Tanzania. *AIDS* 1994, 8: 1609–1615.

3. Reeler AV. Injections: a fatal attraction? *Social Science and Medicine* 1990, 31: 1119–1125.

4. Marcus R, Kay K, Mann JM. Transmission of human immunodeficiency virus (HIV) in health care settings. *Bulletin of the WHO* 1989, 67: 577–582.

5. Kalluvya S, Ishengoma M, Mkumbo EN et al. HIV/AIDS in the medical wards of an urban referral hospital Tanzania. *TANESA Working Papers,* no. 9. Mwanza. January 1996.

6. Gumodoka B, Favot I, Berege Z, Dolmans, W. *Occupational risk of health workers in Mwanza region.* Accepted Bulletin WHO.

7. Adegboye AA. The epidemiology of needle stick and sharp instrument accidents in a Nigerian hospital. *Infect Control Hosp Epidem* 1994, 15: 27–31.

8. Consten E, van Lanschot J, Henry P et al. A prospective study on the risk of exposure to HIV during surgery in Zambia. *AIDS* 1995, 9: 585–588.

9. Ippolito G, Puro V, De Carli G et al. The risk of occupational human immunodeficiency virus infection in health care workers. *Archives of Internal Medicine* 1993, 153: 1407–1408.

10. Henderson DK. HIV transmission in the health care environment. In: Broder S, *Textbook of AIDS medicine,* 1994.

11. Mann JM, Francis H, Quinn T et al. HIV seroprevalence among hospital workers in Kinshasa, Zaire. *JAMA* 1986, 256: 3099–3102.

12. Sow I et al. HIV-1, HIV-2 and HBV serologic status among Dakar hospital workers. In: *Program Abstract from IV International Conference on AIDS,* Stockholm, 12–16 June 1988. (Abstract)

13. Habimana P, Bulterys M, Usabuwera P. A survey of occupational blood contact and HIV infection among traditional birth attendants in Rwanda. *AIDS* 1994, 8: 701–704.

14. Bennett B, Duffy P. The effect of double gloving on frequency of glove perforations. *Obstetrics and Gynaecology* 1991, 78: 1019–1022.

15. Quebbeman EJ, Telford GL, Wadsworth K et al. Double gloving: protecting surgeons from blood contamination. *Archives of Surgery* 1992, 127: 213–217.

16. Gerberding JL, Henderson DK. Managing occupational exposures to blood-borne pathogens: Hepatitis B virus, hepatitis C virus and human immunodeficiency virus. *Clinical and Infectious Diseases* 1992, 14: 1179–1185.

17. Korver A, Blok L. *HIV infection and occupational risk factors. Discussion paper.* AIDS Coordination Group, Amsterdam, September 1995.

18. Evian C. *Primary AIDS care.* Johannesburg, Jacana publishers, 1993.

17   Reducing HIV transmission via blood transfusion: a district strategy

Zachariah Berege and Arnoud Klokke

- When should a district have a blood bank?
- Why is a system based on voluntary donors better than using relative donors?
- How can donors with high-risk behaviour be identified early and deferred
- Can guidelines for blood transfusion reduce the number of unnecessary transfusions?

Blood transfusion is one of the most powerful life-saving interventions in modern medicine. The need for blood transfusions is relatively high in Africa, particularly among young children and women, because of the high prevalence of severe anaemia caused by malaria and other anaemia-causing disorders, and poor maternity services (1, 2). It is essential that standard procedures are followed to ensure a safe blood and blood products supply. This pertains to ABO-blood group and Rhesus typing, cross-matching, use of sterile equipment, recording, storage of blood and sound quality control procedures. Blood transfusion also carries the risk of transmitting hepatitis B and C, syphilis and malaria (3). Recently, the risk of transmitting HIV has been added to this list. Recognition of the blood-borne character of HIV early in the onset of the AIDS epidemic led to immediate changes in transfusion practices in the developed world. In less-developed countries, however, only limited resources are available for health care, and blood transfusions are no exception. Blood which is not screened for HIV antibodies before being transfused accounts for an estimated 10–15% of HIV infections in sub-Saharan Africa. Among children, blood transfusions may be the cause of about one-quarter of HIV infections.

District and national estimates of annual needs for blood transfusions depend on the prevalence of the medical conditions mentioned above and the criteria used to decide whether a transfusion will be given. In Tanzania, the number of blood transfusions is estimated at 6 per 1,000 persons per year (4); half of these transfusions are given to children under five. Applying strict criteria to blood transfusions should lower this number: in a district with a population of 500,000, about 3,000 units of blood will be needed annually.

A blood transfusion can be regarded as a organ transplant, and its benefit to the patient must be weighed against the many risks such as viral or other infections, transfusion reactions or irregular antibody formation which may hamper future transfusions. To reduce these risks, all components of a blood bank must be well organized: location, equipment, personnel, reagents and consumables. Therefore, this chapter starts with a description of a blood bank and its requirements. Many district hospitals have relied on blood supplied by relatives on an emergency basis. This practice has several disadvantages, including an increased risk of transmitting HIV infection. A voluntary donor system offers a better alternative. Such a system has been set up in Mwanza, and that experience is presented here. Finally, other methods used to reduce transfusion-associated HIV transmission are discussed, including minimizing the use of blood and facilitating autologous blood transfusion.

The blood bank at district level

A blood bank is a medical facility which handles and stores blood units from donation to transfusion. When blood is needed for transfusion, safe units of blood compatible with that of the patient should be available at the blood bank. All steps and measures taken to guarantee the safety of the blood unit are part and parcel of the blood bank's work: blood collection, storage at 4°C, screening for HIV, HBV and syphilis, blood grouping and cross-matching. These steps must be properly administered.

In most districts, the district blood bank is part of the laboratory. Examination of the donor, collection of the unit of blood, screening, grouping and cross-matching of the unit are performed by laboratory staff. Blood must be properly stored: it is inappropriate to store units in multi-purpose refrigerators among test kits, reagents and drugs.

A blood bank is a specific organization in which sensitive material (blood), equipment and expensive reagents play an important role; skilled personnel is therefore essential. If a blood bank does not perform at least 50 transfusions per month, or cannot maintain its organization, it is better to refrain from blood banking. A neighbouring hospital may be able to provide assistance.

Organization
In the body, red blood cells have a lifespan of 120 days at 37°C; in a ACD bottle whole blood may survive 21 days at 4°C, if well preserved, and in a CPD-A blood bag may be viable for up to 35 days. Once a unit is collected, conservation must begin and the organization must be ready for the task: refrigerators must be maintained continuously at 4°C, and serological screening tests and skilled personnel should be available. The unit must be used before its expiry date. At the time of transfusion, the blood unit has typically already cost US$ 20–30, not including labour (5, 6). To ensure that a blood bank is prepared for emergencies, a full-time staff should be present: dedicated and skilled people, including the attendant who keeps the blood bank clean, and the nurse who is in charge, takes blood, handles the administration, and checks the refrigerators. A donor recruiter is also needed to find donors.

Box 1. Minimum essential equipment and consumables requirements for a hospital-based blood transfusion service with an established laboratory

Collection of blood
- separate blood collection place; should be comfortable and pleasant for donors.
- blood collection beds: number depends on how much blood is needed. A minimum of two beds is required for simultaneous collection from two donors.
- blood bags. Single bags are US$ 1 each. Once a regular voluntary blood donors' panel is established, multiple bags can be introduced for making packed cells and smaller volumes for children. A double blood collection bag costs US$ 2, a triple US$ 4.
- disposable lancets
- scales for weighing collected blood
- domestic scales for weighing donors
- registration books
- forceps, disinfectant, cotton, thermometer
- refreshments for donors
- test tubes
- stripper

Laboratory
- colorimeter and reagent for Hb measurement
- refrigerator: 130 litre model, preferably solar energy powered: about US$ 5,500
- minimum/maximum thermometer
- waterbath/incubator
- LISS solution
- coombs
- reagent for blood grouping
- HIV test, RPR/VDRL test
- plasma extractor
- tube sealer
- test tubes 12x75 mm
- timers
- separate registration: blood grouping, cross-matching, control system for blood release, HIV/RPR screening, blood removed from blood bank
- blood request forms
- blood giving sets
- colloid/crystalloid (commercially purchased or self-made).

Equipment
A blood bank must be able to conserve blood units for 21–35 days at 4°C: thus, refrigerator(s) are the heart of a blood bank. Moreover, blood should be screened before transfusion, requiring a refrigerator for keeping test kits at 4°C and other equipment and

clean consumables. Cleanliness is essential, and so clean water must be available. Most equipment requires electricity; if not available, alternative power sources (solar, kerosine) should be furnished continuously. Minimum requirements are listed in Box 1.

Reagents

Screening blood units for HIV and syphilis antibodies and hepatitis B surface antigen (HB$_s$Ag) requires expensive test kits. Although screening costs for HIV antibodies may be reduced (see Chapter 15), screening for HIV, HB$_s$Ag and RPR remains an expensive but obligatory procedure. Determining the ABO and Rhesus group and performing the cross-match require expensive reagents which are not readily available. Testing for irregular antibodies requires commercial test panels which expire within 21 days; such cell panels are not yet available in most hospitals in Africa.

Donors

A blood bank without donors is like a hospital without patients; once they appear, they should be handled with care. Blood donors can be divided into three categories:
- relative donor: a family member who is donating because the patient needs to be transfused;
- paid donor: earns money for his/her blood donation;
- voluntary donor: donates regularly (2–3 times per year) without payment.

Family donors are as likely as any other community members to be infected with diseases which are prevalent in the community. Therefore, prevalence figures for HIV, HBV and other sexually transmitted infections are high among this type of blood donor when these infections are common in the community. The most desirable donor is a voluntary blood donor. There are several advantages in using voluntary donors rather than relative donors:
1   The risk of transfusing false negative units is likely to be lower among voluntary blood donors than among relative blood donors (7).
2   A stock of blood can be kept if voluntary donors are used. Blood can therefore be provided more rapidly in case of emergencies.
3   Collecting blood from voluntary donors is more cost-effective than from a patient's relatives or paid donors; the practice of paid donors must be avoided, according to the National Guidelines on Blood Transfusion in Tanzania. The loss of units due to the high infection rate among blood donors can be markedly reduced if a regular blood donor population is created and those known to be infected are barred from further blood donation. This means fewer infected units will be collected, only to be discarded.

Therefore, especially because of the risk of HIV transmission through blood transfusion, systems relying on relative donors should be dropped if possible, in favour of ensuring a stock of screened blood from voluntary blood donors, and excluding individuals and groups at higher HIV risk from donating blood.

Recruitment of voluntary donors
Donor recruitment is an integral activity at a modern blood bank: establishing a blood bank with voluntary donors is necessary to ensure a safe blood supply, and thus increase the effectiveness of blood transfusions in terms of saving lives. The Tanzanian Guidelines on Blood Transfusion are available from the Ministry of Health; copies could be distributed by TANESA.

The public relations officer of the blood bank is called the donor recruiter; his/her job is to actively approach low-risk groups within the community, to convince potential voluntary donors to come forward for donation, and to ensure that voluntary donors turn up regularly at the blood bank for donation. A blood donor recruiter should have a background in medicine, good interpersonal and organizational skills, and communication abilities.

Institutions in the neighbourhood of the blood bank with a large supply of potential blood donors can be identified. Secondary schools are a good source of voluntary donors (7) and an active programme should be set up to encourage students to volunteer for blood donation. Religious organizations and the like are additional possibilities. The preferred voluntary donor population is males aged 15-20 years, since this group has been shown to have a lower HIV prevalence (7). The donor recruiter should provide information on different aspects related to blood transfusion (8). Therefore, prior to approaching the target population, a seminar on blood transfusion should be held for school authorities and others concerned, to clear up misconceptions and to ensure support for the recruitment. Box 2 suggests topics to be discussed during these seminars and recruitment lectures.

Box 2. Topics for a donor recruitment session

- Brief explanation of 'what is blood?'
- Who needs blood and why: different patient groups and underlying diseases causing anaemia.
- Who can give blood: emphasizing that a physical examination is conducted to see whether the person has enough spare blood to donate.
- How blood is collected: use of sterile disposable equipment and confidentiality.
- Regeneration of blood elements after donation.
- What happens to the blood.
- Who cannot give blood and why.
- Medical and other benefits for the voluntary donor.

Donor deferral
In order to keep the costs of a safe blood supply as low as possible, population groups at increased risk for HIV infection need to be excluded, using a short risk score questionnaire to identify risk factors (9). Potential donors who do not satisfactorily

answer one or more of the questions (see examples in Box 3) need to be deferred and replacements recruited. It is important to explain to voluntary donors that their blood may not be suitable for use, and that while this does not necessarily mean they are infected with HIV, they may be. Counselling blood donors will not be required as this may discourage individuals from blood donation. If a blood donor wants to know his/her HIV status, they will be approached as an individual requesting voluntary HIV testing. Then he/she will be given pre-test counselling, a separate blood sample drawn and tested, and the result disclosed to the individual during post-test counselling.

Box 3. Risk factor identification of donors

A study in Zimbabwe examined the cost-effectiveness of different approaches to risk factor identification (9). The most cost-effective strategy was deferral of donors who did not pass screening, followed by HIV antibody testing for donors who had passed. The following questions were used:
- Have you had a genital ulcer during the last year?
- Have you had an STD during the last year?
- Have you paid for sexual intercourse during the last year?
- Have you had more than one sex partner in the last year?

Anyone answering 'yes' to any of these questions was deferred. In addition to these questions on STDs and sexual behaviour, additional questions may be used: for example, a history of tuberculosis or working at a high-risk occupation, such as bar worker, truck driver, miner or fisherman. The choice of questions depends on local circumstances.

Regular donors
It is safer to use blood donors who donate regularly than first-time blood donors (8, 9). Because it takes considerable time and effort to create a steady donor population, incentives may be a useful way to retain donors: for example, if the donor agrees to return for a second donation within 4–5 months, he/she is entitled to free treatment and consultation for any diseases (excluding pre-existing conditions) during that five-month period. This benefit is only valid for that period and may be renewed by making another donation within an established time period. It is important that the staff of the blood bank provide high-quality services and adequate information on blood donation to the donor, and are also able to locate the donor to ask for the next donation (10). To prevent donors becoming infected by HIV or other blood-transmittable pathogens, they should receive information on how to avoid HIV and other infections.

Screening blood for HIV antibodies

Screening blood for the presence of HIV antibodies prior to transfusion allows the elimination of the majority of infected units. However, the HIV antibody test has two limitations. First, an HIV test will be negative if the blood donor is in the 'window period' of the infection. The window period is defined as the time between HIV infection and seroconversion during which there are not sufficient circulating antibodies against HIV to obtain a positive HIV test. The window period has a duration of about three months. The actual risk that a donor is in the window period depends on the incidence of HIV. Assuming that all blood is collected from first-time donors with a 1% annual HIV incidence, the risk that a donor is in the window period at the time of donation is 2.5 per 1,000.

Secondly, test sensitivity – the probability that the test will be reactive in an HIV infected and seroconverted person – is less than 100%. Specificity and sensitivity differ from test kit to test kit and from laboratory to laboratory (see Chapter 15). Test kits never have a sensitivity nor specificity of 100%; moreover, the situation and the skill of the technician giving the test also affect whether the accuracy stated by the manufacturer will be met. Thus, some units will test false negative; how many depends on HIV prevalence in the donor population and the sensitivity and specificity of the test kit used. For instance, if HIV prevalence is 10% and the test sensitivity and specificity are 95% and 99% respectively, 5.6 per 1,000 units will test false negative and may infect a patient with HIV. This reason alone is an important argument for establishing reliable blood banks with skilled staff and limiting the number of transfusions to the very minimum, by using guidelines and autologous blood transfusion techniques. Moreover, the window period and test insensitivity also provide important reasons to collect blood from donors who are at less risk of HIV infection, especially steady voluntary blood donors, as mentioned above.

Finally, administrative errors may cause transfusion of HIV-infected units. A number of steps must be taken to avoid such errors:
1. Number the blood units and samples prior to drawing blood from the donor to avoid administrative mistakes.
2. Record donor data, serology data and cross-matching in separate books.
3. Always store screened and unscreened units separately, whether in the same or different refrigerators.
4. Upon completion of serology testing, mark, remove and destroy immediately all units which are positive for HIV or HBV; units with a positive RPR test should be kept at 4°C for 72 hrs before transfusion. Negative units transferred to their respective shelves, refrigerator or compartment must be recorded in a control book which indicates the date, test result for the transferred unit, action undertaken and signature of the laboratory technician.

Minimizing unnecessary blood transfusions

Because of the potential hazards related to blood transfusion, it should be reserved for use in only the most serious cases: the risks involved may outnumber the benefit to the patient, and may even threaten his/her survival. Rarely should blood be used for the management of haemorrhage, which can be controlled with volume expanders, and it should never be used for elective surgery (see 'Autologous blood transfusion' below). In addition, costs must be considered.

Since the majority of blood transfusions are performed on children under five, special attention should be given to this group. The main criteria for giving blood transfusions to young children are haemoglobin concentration (Hb) and clinical status. In one study child survival chances increased only when the transfusions were given within 48 hours (11). A 25% decrease in blood transfusions among severely anaemic children, with no increase in mortality, has been obtained by introducing a transfusion protocol (12). This protocol proposed treating cardiac failure and anaemia by means other than blood transfusion, observing the child at hourly intervals for 8 hours and transfusing if the condition did not improve after initial treatment. An example of the problems associated with introducing blood transfusion guidelines is given in Box 4.

Box 4. Avoiding unnecessary blood transfusions

Criteria to avoid unnecessary blood transfusion has been developed in Mwanza Region. Initially, it was estimated that between 23% and 39% of blood transfusions in the region's eight hospitals were avoidable. Three quarters of these avoidable blood transfusions were carried out on children under five years (1).

The results of the situation analysis were discussed with regional senior staff and resulted in consensus on guidelines for the prescription of blood transfusions. These guidelines were then introduced through training workshops to all blood transfusion prescribers in the region. An evaluation study carried out one year later showed a significant decrease in avoidable blood transfusions in children (from 52% to 33%) (13). However, this was offset by an increase in avoidable blood transfusions among adults. Overall, there was very little improvement. It was concluded that development and introduction of guidelines alone is not sufficient to change blood transfusion practices. Additional measures appear to be necessary, such as regular clinical meetings or strict supervision by the senior medical staff.

Box 5. Guidelines for safe blood transfusion

I. CHRONIC ANAEMIA
Children under five
1.1   Hb <= 40 g/L, complicated by any disorder which may aggravate the symptoms
1.2   Hb > 40 g/L, complicated by congestive cardiac failure (CCF) or hypoxic spells

Pregnant women
1.3   Hb <= 50 g/L, even without clinical signs of CCF
1.4   Hb > 50 g/L and < 70 g/L in presence of CCF, pneumonia or other serious bacterial infection, malaria or pre-existing heart disease
1.5   If pregnancy exceeds 36 weeks and Hb <= 60 g/L or Hb > 60 g/L and < 80 g/L with presence of condition(s) mentioned under 1.2b

Patients older than five years
1.6   CCF regardless of Hb concentration
1.7   Hb < 50 g/L with CCF, hypoxia, severe infection or haemolytic sickle cell crisis

2. PATIENTS WITH ACUTE BLOOD LOSS
Give initial treatment:
2.1   Efforts to stop bleeding
2.2   Volume replacement with crystalloid solution (saline up to 50 ml/kg) followed by colloid for the first 12 hours

Give blood if:
2.3   There is hypovolemic shock after initial treatment
2.4   Blood loss is > 25% of total blood volume and bleeding continues

3. ELECTIVE SURGERY
3.1   Hb >= 100 g/L, no contraindications and major blood loss is anticipated: perform acute isovolaemic hemodilution
3.2   Hb < 90 g/L and expected blood loss is > 500 ml: postpone surgery, examine patient for cause(s) of anaemia and treat If anaemia cannot be corrected, homologous blood transfusion is indicated
3.3   Blood transfusion is indicated prior to surgery if the patient has sickle cell disease and a Hb < 70 g/L

4. EMERGENCY SURGERY
4.1   Patient with acute blood loss: see point 2
4.2   Patient with chronic anaemia in need of general anaesthesia: transfusion is indicated if signs of shock or CCF
4.3   Hb >= 100 g/L, blood loss anticipated: perform acute isovolaemic hemodilution

Unnecessary blood transfusions can be reduced by:

1. Introducing *guidelines* for a limited and well identified number of qualified persons ordering blood transfusions. Box 5 presents a summary of sample guidelines.
2. Using a *blood request form* which contains sufficient information to decide if a potential blood transfusion candidate meets the criteria: patient's name, hospital identification number, age, sex, indication for transfusion, previous transfusion history and name of the requesting physician. If the criteria for blood transfusion are not met, the request should be reconsidered.
3. Establishing a *hospital blood transfusion committee* in line with national guidelines on blood transfusion. Such a committee should meet monthly, provide continuing education on blood transfusion, critically review transfusion practices on site and institute corrective actions when necessary.

Plasma substitutes such as sterile pyrogen-free saline, although largely under-utilized, are a cheap alternative to blood for the management of patients with acute haemorrhage (14).

Autologous blood transfusion

The safest blood a patient can receive is his or her own. Such a transfusion is called an autologous blood transfusion: the collection and subsequent re-transfusion of the patient's blood. The most common methods of autologous transfusion are:

1. Intra-operative blood salvage for ectopic pregnancies.
2. Pre-operative blood deposit for elective surgery whereby the patient donates one unit at least three days before surgery. This method requires that the planned surgery is carried out in a timely manner, and separate recording and storage facilities. This method cannot be used in emergency surgery.
3. Acute isovolaemic hemodilution, whereby blood is collected and simultaneously replaced by volume expanders prior to surgery. If the patient's Hb is 100 g/L or more, major blood loss is anticipated and no contra indications are present (sickle cell, severe respiratory and cardiac disease, renal impairment or sepsis), the patient should undergo acute isovolaemic hemodilution. This method is also suitable for patients scheduled for caesarian section (15). The advantages of acute isovolaemic hemodilution are that blood is on hand in the operating theatre and that it allows greater flexibility in the use of scarce homologous blood. Blood collection units, sterile pyrogen-free saline and blood giving sets are the only requirements.

Prerequisites for developing a successful autologous blood transfusion programme are consensus by the blood transfusion committee on which methods should be applied in which settings, and educating surgeons on the topic. This education should include:
- advantages of autologous blood transfusion;
- management of acute blood loss by volume expanders;
- types of patients for whom autologous blood transfusion may be appropriate.

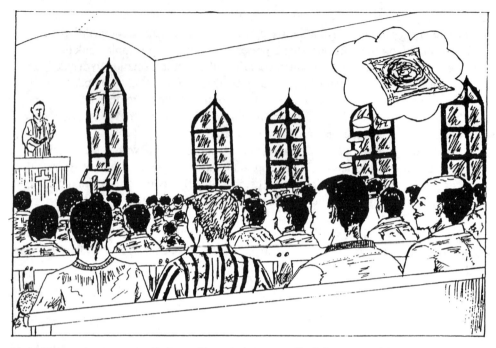

Many men and women are facing a dilemma because of religious opposition against condom use.

Conclusion

There is a high demand for blood transfusion in Africa, especially among children and women of childbearing age. The risk of HIV transmission through blood transfusion can be reduced by:

- establishing a well-organized blood bank based on a voluntary donor system;
- recruiting blood donors among low risk groups such as secondary school students;
- using screening questions to defer voluntary high-risk donors;
- testing blood units for HIV;
- minimizing the number of blood transfusions by adherence to blood transfusion guidelines, and supervising the implementation of such guidelines;
- using autologous blood transfusion when possible.

Further reading

TANERA. *Guidelines for blood transfusion*. Bugando Medical Centre, Mwanza. Available free of charge from TANESA, P.O. Box 434, Mwanza, Tanzania.

World Health Organization. *Safe blood and blood products*. Document WHO/GPA/CNP/ 932. Distance learning materials, including five volumes: guidelines and principles for safe blood transfusion practices; safe blood donation; screening for HIV and other infectious agents; blood group serology; trainer's guide.

World Health Organization. *Guidelines for blood donor counselling on HIV*. Geneva, 1994.

References

1. Gumodoka B, Vos J, Kigadye FC et al. Blood transfusion practices in Mwanza Region, Tanzania. *AIDS* 1993, 7: 387–392.

2. Addo-Yobo EOD, Lovel H. How well are hospitals preventing iatrogenic HIV? A study of the appropriateness of blood transfusion in 3 hospitals in the Ashanti Region, Ghana. *Tropical Doctor* 1991, 21: 162–164.

3. Mhalu FS, Ryder RW. Blood transfusion and AIDS in the tropics. *Clinical Tropical Medicine and Communicable Diseases* 1988, 3: 157–166.

4. Ministry of Health (Tanzania), National AIDS Control Programme (1994). *NACP Report*, no. 9, Dar es Salaam.

5. Van Dam CJ, Sondag-Thull D, Fransen L. The provision of safe blood-policy issues in the prevention of human immunodeficiency virus transmission. *Tropical Doctor* 1992, 22: 20–23.

6. Watson-Williams EJ, Katahaa PK. Revival of the Ugandan blood transfusion system 1989: an example of international cooperation. *Transfusion Science* 1990, 11: 179–184.

7. Jacobs B, Berege ZA, Schalula PJJ et al. Secondary school students: a safer blood donor population in an urban settlement with high HIV prevalence in East-Africa. *East African Medical Journal* 1994, 71: 720–723.

8. Jacobs B, Berege Z, Attitudes and beliefs about blood donation in Mwanza Region, Tanzania. *East African Medical Journal* 1995, 172: 345–348.

9. McFarland W, Kahn JG, Katzenstein DA et al. Deferral of blood donors with risk factors for HIV infection saves lives and money in Zimbabwe. *Journal of AIDS and Human Retrovirology* 1995, 9: 183–192.

10. WHO Global Blood Safety Initiative. *Consensus statement on how to achieve a safe and adequate blood supply by recruitment and retention of voluntary, non-remunerated blood donors.* WHO/GPA/INF/93.1. Geneva, 1993.

11. Lackritz E, Campbell CC, Reubush II TK et al. Effect of blood transfusion on survival among children in a Kenyan hospital. *Lancet* 1992, 340: 524–528.

12. Craighead IB, Knowles JK. Prevention of transfusion associated HIV transmission with the use of a transfusion protocol for under fives. *Tropical Doctor* 1993, 23: 59–61.

13. Vos J, Gumodoka B, Van Asten HA et al. Changes in blood transfusion practices after the introduction of consensus guidelines in Mwanza region, Tanzania. *AIDS* 1994, 8: 1135–1140.

14. WHO Global Blood Safety Initiative. *Use of plasma substitutes and plasma in developing countries.* WHO/GPA/INF/89.17 and WHO/LAB/89.9. Geneva, 1989.

15. WHO Global Blood Safety Initiative. *Autologous blood transfusion in developing countries.* WHO/GPA/91.1 and WHO/LBS/91.2. Geneva, 1990.

Part five
Consequences
of the epidemic

18 Care and counselling

Eric van Praag, Veronica Schweyen and Japheth Ng'weshemi

- Can AIDS care help in HIV prevention activities?
- How can district health services cope with the increasing number of people living with HIV/AIDS?
- What are the needs of AIDs patients?
- What is the role of the family and the community?
- How can NGOs and government join hands in AIDS care?

Globally, around 14 million adults and 1 million infants and children are infected with HIV, according to 1995 estimates. Eastern, southern and central Africa account for three-quarters of all current infections, with on average slightly more females than males infected in these countries. Age distribution analysis shows that mainly younger, more productive age groups are affected, and that females are infected at a younger age than males (1).

This high level of HIV infection means that large numbers of people require or will require care and counselling. For example, in a district of 300,000 people, with a stable HIV prevalence rate of 5%, between 600 and 1,000 adults will develop AIDS each year. If all require admittance to district hospitals and stay two weeks on average, this implies 2–3 AIDS admissions per day and 25–40 beds occupied by AIDS patients throughout the year. In addition to the lack of resources to cope with the sheer numbers involved, the real differences in most districts hospitals between HIV/AIDS and other chronic fatal illnesses in young adults (such as leukaemia, cancer of the cervix, sickle cell anaemia or chronic liver damage) are the attitudes and stigmatization involved.

The expressed needs of people living with HIV/AIDS (PLHAs) include access to common drugs and emotional support, consideration of their families, household help, financial assistance and empathy from health staff. A comprehensive approach to care is thus required, including more than clinical care.

Such care involving many sectors, such as clinical, nursing, social welfare, religious and community groups, contributes to lessen the burden of AIDS on the health system and on society. It opens communication opportunities to strengthen prevention activities and to identify infectious opportunistic infections such as tuberculosis at an early stage and to properly manage them. Moreover, at the district level, these various sectors can easily plan and complement their activities together through functional existing collaboration mechanisms such as the district health boards or committees and thus ensure a comprehensive care approach.

This chapter deals with the concept of a 'continuum of care', linking medical facilities and services with community-based and home care. It provides examples of how care and counselling can be organized, and of the problems to be addressed in implementation in Africa. Emphasis will be placed on various pre-requisites such as the need for pre- and post-test counselling, providing psychosocial care and networking among supporting agencies.

Rationale for comprehensive care

Care and support needs

To develop relevant, affordable and practical responses to meet the health care needs of people living with HIV/AIDS, we must first better understand what these needs are and why AIDS requires health care providers at various levels of the health care system – community level, district facility and referral level – to take approaches that differ from their routine ones.

In recent years several qualitative studies have been done to increase understanding of the needs of families living with HIV/AIDS, and how these differ from those of similar families which are not directly affected. In the context of a district programme, a participatory needs assessment including PLHAs, caretakers and families is the most appropriate method of collecting such information. Studies in Malawi, Uganda, Zimbabwe and Kenya reveal a similar picture of needs, mainly expressed in four areas: food, clothing, medicines and support for surviving children.

- Food: repeated illness of economically productive adult household members (women and/or men) results in a progressive decline in income and a complete lack of income when illness becomes terminal. In families where food is grown rather than bought, food production gradually falls, and when the PLHA is unable to work, no food may be available for the family;
- Clothing: skin lesions and repeated, prolonged episodes of diarrhoea make frequent changes of clothing and bedding, and the availability of soap, a necessity from the point of view of both hygiene and comfort;
- Medicines: common illnesses and opportunistic infections require treatment. Nearby dispensaries or clinics may lack supplies of essential drugs, forcing patients to go to private or more distant hospitals. Easy access to tuberculosis treatment is particularly needed, as patients' physical and financial capacity to obtain monthly supplies from a district hospital-based tuberculosis programme is severely limited;
- Support for surviving children: continued schooling is of great concern. Often when one or both parents are ill, a child is taken out of school due to dwindling income and need for help with household chores. Provision of school fees and uniforms is a commonly expressed need, since schooling is seen as the only hope for a brighter future. (See also Chapter 20.)

Most of these studies were conducted among families with a PLHA in a late stage of disease. The few studies focusing on healthy seropositive people as well as on non-infected surviving family members during the bereavement period show the additional need for emotional support to help in acceptance of the diagnosis, safeguard confidentiality and increase ability to cope with discrimination within the community, including among extended family members and health care workers.

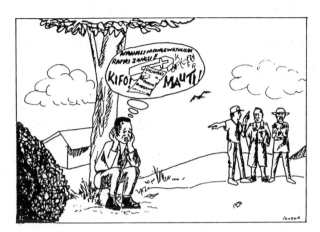

Stigma: men condemning and isolating a person with AIDS.

Psychosocial needs

In many respects, the psychosocial implications of AIDS are similar to those found in other chronic and fatal diseases (2). However, HIV/AIDS have certain distinctions that profoundly influences how psychosocial support is provided. First, HIV infection may be diagnosed many years before the first opportunistic infections occur; even then, a person may live a full and productive life for many months or years before full-blown AIDS develops. Second, as almost all HIV transmission occurs through sexual contact, the impact of AIDS is not limited to one individual. The sexual partner may already be infected, or be at risk of becoming infected. Because the majority of those infected are young adults, they are likely to have small children who are at risk of being orphaned and/or of having been infected perinatally. Third, the behaviours that lead to HIV infection frequently provoke social and moral judgements, and subsequent discrimination against the infected person. In addition, irrational fears of becoming infected through social contact, or through caring for the sick person, may also lead to ostracism and isolation of the infected person by family members or the surrounding community, including health care workers. Thus, HIV/AIDS is a condition laden with emotions of psychosocial distress, including denial, blaming others for the infection and feelings of hopelessness about the future.

The needs of PLHAs are only partially being met by formal government health and social services, but communities and NGOs have generated innovative responses to help patients cope and improve their quality to life. The introduction of cost-sharing in many countries means patients are asked to pay a part of their medical costs, adding an extra burden when illnesses are chronic. The result is that most cannot afford to pay for facility-based care plus the transport costs incurred. Therefore, they must be cared for in their homes, in the community and by traditional healers.

The burden on hospitals and the consequences

Many urban district or referral hospitals in the most heavily affected countries in east and central Africa now report that the majority of their adult beds in medical wards are occupied by persons with HIV-related conditions. For example, in a major hospital in Kampala, Uganda, 55% of patients admitted to medical wards were HIV-positive in 1992; in a major teaching hospital in Lusaka, Zambia the figure was 70%; in a referral hospital in Mwanza, Tanzania in 1994, 45%; and in a district hospital in West Kenya, 30%.

This is typical in most high-prevalence countries, where hospitals are bearing the brunt of the HIV/AIDS epidemic. One reason for this is that people who suspect they may be HIV-positive bypass local health care facilities, such as dispensaries and health centres, and seek help directly from higher health care levels within, or often outside, their district – even when their condition does not warrant care by a referral level hospital. Reasons given include the lack of drugs or trust, but more importantly, people's fear of their diagnosis being disclosed within their community. On the other hand, people admitted with AIDS or late stages of other diseases are often ignored by doctors and nurses, or may be discharged early or even rejected because 'there is nothing we can do'. These people stay home, without any support or palliative treatment, and often suffer a lack of food, clothing, blankets and simple nursing care and medicines.

Fear of disclosure is often mixed with denial of the medical diagnosis or the fact that no cure is available. This fear leads not only to bypassing nearby clinics, but also to a prolonged period of searching for care or cure at private hospitals or from traditional practitioners. People may also go directly to distant national referral hospitals where they presume sophisticated care is available from specialists. Disappointment is the usual result, combined with serious depletion of the family budget. Public health budgets are also affected, if the clinician orders repeated unnecessary diagnostic tests and prescriptions in response to patient demand and to avoid difficult discussions when HIV is diagnosed.

Experiences with district care approaches

Community responses

Case studies from eastern and southern Africa illustrate how communities, health care providers and people affected by HIV/AIDS have found better responses to the needs expressed above. Box 1 describes the cost and impact of home-based care in Zambia, where many home-based care programmes have been initiated since 1987. The AIDS Support Organization (TASO) in Uganda is perhaps one of the best-known responses to the increased need for HIV/AIDS patient care in Africa. A brief description of TASO is given in Box 2. Another initiative is the establishment of a residential hospice unit which provides palliative care to terminal patients. Here several PLHAS can receive care from members of other households in turn. Supplies and resources can be pooled and households are relieved of their caring duties when others take their turn. An example of a care facility in Zimbabwe is described in Box 3.

Box 1. Cost and impact of home-based care in Zambia

In Zambia, AIDS is already the most common cause of death for adults admitted to hospital. Total HIV infection projections for 1998 are as high as 1.8 million, or nearly 28% of the total population. The vast majority of those infected will seek health care at some point in their illness, causing demand for hospital beds to rise as much as 20% annually in the next decade. PLHAs are expected to occupy 90% of the country's 25,000 hospital beds by 2010.

Forty-seven home-based care programmes have been set up since 1987 to provide services for PLHAs in their communities. Further, the Zambian government has responded by formally endorsing home-based care as a part of its health strategy, urging district health boards to support home-based care and encouraging home-based care programmes to improve efficiency through increased integration with other community health care systems.

A study has been carried out to examine some home-based care programmes initiated by hospitals and communities. Broad comparisons were made between these two major types of infrastructure to explore their relative efficiency and success in integrating into existing health care services. Unit cost per home visit varied significantly, ranging from US$ 10 to $ 40 for the hospital-initiated programmes (due to the difference in structures, services and productivity of these programmes) to US$ 2 for a community-initiated programme. Major costs include transport, supplies, salaries and training. Hospital costs varied between US$ 3 and $ 8 per day, although neither costs incurred by visiting family members nor loss of opportunity costs could be calculated.

The key conclusion of the study is that although external financing is required, support for the home-based care movement in Zambia should be continued and increased. Home-based care programmes in Zambia have been exemplary and an inspiration to the rest of the world. They have clearly brought immeasurable comfort and service to thousands of PLHAs, their families and communities.

Nevertheless, there is an urgent need to improve the efficiency and lower the cost associated with current home care services as carried out in some countries. Increased use of home care could alleviate some of the pressure on tertiary care centres. Costs can be lowered by avoiding vertical programmes based on outreach activities which require vehicles, have low coverage and demand a great deal of senior staff time. The demand for hospital care could be diverted to community care: if the existing primary care facilities located closer to households were to be better utilized and supported, including the availability of comprehensive care. Communities would be able to organize and offer a broader spectrum of clinical, as well as emotional and spiritual support. To accomplish this, however, the capacity of communities and families to care for PLHAs will need to be increased and made more sustainable (3, 4). Often, as shown in the case studies, capacities are available but underutilized and not linked together, such as church groups, local health workers, traditional healers, caring by family members, etc.).

Box 2. TASO: an AIDS support organization in Uganda

The first cases of AIDS in Uganda were reported in Rakai District, west of Lake Victoria, in 1982. More than 40,000 cases have been reported since then, but this is only a fraction of the total. Moreover, these figures cannot convey the scale of human suffering and loss which the people of Uganda have faced for more than a decade.

TASO has its origins in a small group of people who began meeting in one another's homes in Kampala in 1986. All but one had HIV or AIDS, which meant rejection and isolation. They met to exchange information, to give each other support and encouragement, and to pray. They had no office, no transport and no funds. But they did have initiative, vision and a deep commitment to practical action on behalf of people with HIV and AIDS, people who were neglected by the health service and ostracized by the rest of society.

From these humble beginnings, by 1993 TASO had grown into an organization with 22,795 clients registered in counselling centres throughout Uganda. Using its first counselling centre as a model, TASO has supported the establishment of eight centres on district hospital premises throughout Uganda. At TASO centres clients receive counselling, AIDS education, medical care and material assistance. Hospital staff volunteers provide services at these clinics.

Since 1989, TASO has continued to develop its technical capacity to train various categories of people to provide a continuum of care, and support from home to hospital. Increasingly, attention has been focused on providing training for other organizations, both locally and internationally. This allows TASO's work to be replicated by trained counsellors and volunteers. There is no doubt that part of TASO's success is due to the inspired leadership and its staff's bond to AIDS. But its success is also due to the fact that providing comprehensive AIDS care does seem to make a difference, creating an atmosphere of hope and job satisfaction for volunteer health workers, as an addition to the often-demoralizing working conditions in the hospital wards.

Emphasis is now being placed on the integration of AIDS-related services into district government activities throughout Uganda. For example, TASO staff in the community, in collaboration with the tuberculosis control programme, supervise tuberculosis treatment follow-up and thus limit the risk of developing multi-drug resistance. TASO staff are also involved in counselling in the hospital wards and making referrals to sensitize staff in peripheral clinics and home care programmes. Most initiatives originate from NGOs. In future it will be necessary to involve formal district services, and successful projects initiated by NGOs may be used to expand coverage through joint efforts with district health services. TASO's experience suggests that coordination and planning for home-based care services work best when the district level is involved (5).

Box 3. Hospice care in Harare, Zimbabwe

Mashambanzou is an AIDS support NGO established in 1989 with three aims: to develop a drop-in centre and support groups for people with HIV/AIDS, to establish a home care service and to provide a residential hospice unit. Mashambanzou began by establishing a palliative care ward in a major hospital as a hospice to care for terminally ill, destitute patients with AIDS and other illnesses who could not be cared for at home. At first there was a negative response, as people felt stigmatized and shunned the ward. However, since the ward was accepted it has been fully utilized.

In addition, the organization has established a residential unit within its main premises in a high density suburb of Harare. Patients can be admitted for a few days, along with a family care giver who learns how best to look after the patient through 'on-the-job' training. Although it also draws people from a much wider area, one important characteristic of the centre is its location in the community. Early experience with this unit has been generally positive. The environment is homelike, and patients gain support from each other as well as from their relatives and the professional support staff. A doctor visits weekly, a nurse is always on duty and two pastors provide spiritual support. A wide range of books and magazines is available and there are radios in each room (6).

These examples and others show that with commitment and goodwill it is possible to create opportunities to deliver services which respond to the needs of people living with HIV and their families. Most of these initiatives are NGO-based, and religion often plays an important role. Other important factors in success include, first, leadership: a charismatic leader can motivate individuals and communities, and help the programme establish a solid base. TASO in Uganda and Chikankwata in Zambia are good examples of organizations with charismatic leadership. A second factor is community resources and involvement. These are absolute requirements to sustain home-based care programmes. The final essential requirement is a continuous link with a functioning health system for support, referral and supervision.

Home-based care programmes may be cheaper than in-patient care, but are not inexpensive. While external financial resources are usually needed to set up such an initiative, this may stand in the way of mobilizing local resources, thus limiting sustainability. Interestingly, however, when a programme is successful, community resources become easier to find. Churches, industrial service clubs in urban areas, local NGOs and other private organization and companies may contribute to the programme. The efficient use of available resources may also be a problem. Accountability is thus another important requirement.

The continuum of care
In the context of these and other examples and initiatives, the concept of 'comprehensive care across a continuum' has evolved (6). Comprehensive care means taking a more

integrated view, in response to the interrelated needs of a person and his/her environment as a whole. In this sense plans for comprehensive care should include:

- the types of needs addressed: these include medical, information, social, material and psychological needs;
- the persons whose needs are addressed: not only the patient and his/her family during the illness, but also surviving family members after the patient dies. The surrounding community's needs should also be addressed, with respect to issues of stigma and rejection;
- duration of care: care is needed not only in times of crisis but in all phases of HIV infection as well as during the bereavement process;
- prevention: this can be discussed with the patient and family in the process of providing care in hospital and at home. To avoid stigmatization, discussions of awareness raising and prevention can be carried out while emphasizing solidarity with those in need of care.

Comprehensive HIV/AIDS health care comprises four main types of responses to needs.

Clinical management. Early diagnosis of illnesses resulting from HIV infection (including opportunistic infections) and rational treatment are crucial to improving quality of life. Flow charts and handbooks have been produced to guide the care provider in appropriate clinical management at the district hospital level, the health centre level and at home (see 'Further reading and resources' at the end of this chapter). Box 4 provides a schematic way of looking at the flow from voluntary counselling and testing to home care.

Tuberculosis deserves special attention. Early suspicions by the care provider at any hospital, health centre, family care provider or visiting health worker at home should be followed up; patients who are confirmed should be treated, to minimize the spread of tuberculosis. Follow-up treatment for tuberculosis can also be provided at the health centre or community level. Returning to the district hospital for follow-up treatment is cumbersome, particularly for people with HIV/AIDS. Community-based health workers trained in direct observed treatment with a short-term regimen can improve adherence to tuberculosis treatment. In this way AIDS home care programmes and the district tuberculosis programme can be linked and strengthen each other's work (see Chapter 19).

If resources are available, clinical care should also be considered for those in the early stages of HIV, including preventive therapy for toxoplasmosis, recurrent candidiasis, tuberculosis or pneumonia. More emphasis should also be placed on the role of the clinician in referrals. For example, a patient might be referred to a counsellor for help in accepting the diagnosis, to the health centre for simple ailments and follow-up treatments, to a nearby home care programme or to social or religious groups in response to material and spiritual needs. (See also box 5.)

Nursing care. Promoting and maintaining hygiene and nutrition, both at the institutional level and at home, is another essential component of comprehensive care in responding to the patient's needs. Emotional support and taking opportunities to discuss and listen to family members, and so to facilitate STD/HIV preventive education, should take place

Box 4. The HIV/AIDS continuum of care

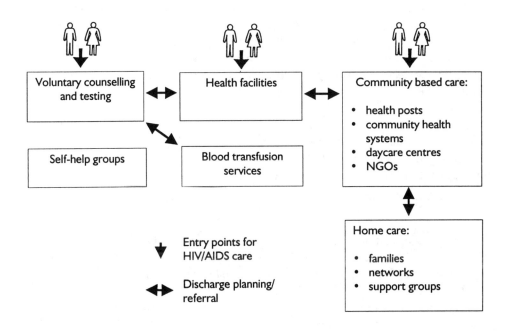

Source: See (7)

in clinical wards, clinics and at home. During the late stages of disease, when 'nothing can be done', the provision of palliative care in the ward or at home is vital. Pain management with simple treatments such as codeine phosphate, symptomatic treatments for cough, diarrhoea, skin and mouth lesions, and providing physical and mental comfort are important aspects of this care.

In addition, the prevention of blood-borne transmission should be emphasized by following the basic principals of universal precautions (see Box 5) in wards and clinics. Simple and effective disinfectants such as chlorine household bleach should be promoted for use at all levels, including at home, as a cheap and very effective way to nullify transmission risks. WHO's *Home care handbook* (see 'Further reading and resources') is an essential guide to learning more about comprehensive care at home.

Counselling. Counselling is defined as a confidential dialogue between a client/patient and a care provider, aimed at enabling the client to cope with stress and take personal decisions, such as those related to HIV/AIDS. Counselling enables a client/patient to open up and share his/her emotions, fears, guilt and anxiety as well as more practical issues with regard to the future, survival and planning for one's children.

Box 5. Who should be seen as 'infected'

HIV (and other bloodborne pathogens, e.g. Hepatitis B virus) may be transmitted in the health care setting from patient to patient, from patient to health care provider or, more rarely, from health care provider to patient. In each of these forms of transmission, the risk depends on the prevalence of infected individuals in the population, the frequency of exposure to contaminated medical instruments, the nature of such exposures, the relative infectivity of the virus, and the concentration of the virus in the blood.

Since it is not practical or desirable to identify everyone who is infected with HIV, the strategy for preventing HIV transmission in the health setting is to view everyone as having the potential to be infected. The only reason to focus on known infected individuals is to provide care, counselling, treatment and support.

Good counselling can only be done by those who are personally committed to care, and may involve nurses, social workers, doctors, paramedics, religious leaders or others. Training in counselling skills to improve communication and enable crisis handling is best done at the district level (see Chapter 12). Counsellors can play an important role as well as focal points before discharge from the hospital, to ensure follow-up by a committed person at community level (home care team or clinic staff) and to ensure admittance to the hospital in a confidential manner.

Anyone who is considering an HIV test for any reason should receive pre-test counselling. Explicit informed consent for HIV testing at the request of the client and for diagnostic purposes must be obtained as part of pre-test counselling. Pre-test counselling is defined as a dialogue between a client and a care provider about the HIV test, and the possible implications of knowing one's HIV sero-status, which in turn leads to an informed decision as to whether to take the test or not. The purpose of counselling is to help clients assess whether they are at risk, learn about the test and its implications, reflect on these, and decide whether or not to be tested. Counselling should also address post-risk behaviours and plans to reduce risks.

Post-test and follow-up counselling eases the provision of care and facilitates disclosure to a family member who may be willing to provide home care. One post-test counselling session is frequently not enough. A person may need ongoing support or the option to return for more sessions if they wish. Counselling after a positive test result thus involves breaking the bad news to the individual, assessing understanding and emotional acceptance of the result, and dealing with any immediate reactions. However, post-test counselling is not complete until the client has made plans to meet the challenges of living with HIV infection. The client should be helped to confront key questions such as: Who and how will I tell about my HIV status? How will I conduct my sexual life from now on? Who will I discuss my worries with? How will I make plans for members of my family? In other words, the client should be helped to find a balance between confidentiality and revealing his/her HIV status to a few significant people. Counselling will ensure the integration of prevention and care.

Social support. Material assistance such as food, school fees and exemption from cost-sharing can be provided by welfare offices or NGOs. Often PLHAs may be reluctant to seek help, fearing disclosure, or may not be aware of social services. This again stresses the need for counselling at the district level to provide referrals or discharge planning so that the client becomes aware of all available services.

Another useful social support is provided by PLHA support groups run by and for PLHAs and others affected by HIV. The main focus is usually on meeting material needs, but mutual moral support has proved useful, helping members to open up to each other and to foster a strong educational role in the community for PLHAs. PLHAs might for example present informative programmes that answer questions, allow for discussion and advocate prevention and solidarity for youth groups or factory workers. Mutual support in facing discrimination, obtaining legal assistance or making a will are other important activities of these support groups.

Comprehensive HIV/AIDS care should be accessible at several points along a continuum, ranging from district health and social facilities to community-based services and home care (see Box 6). This continuum should be linked by means of networking or coordination, so that at any point of contact with the PLHAs an active referral can be made to achieve more comprehensive care. It is helpful to have a list of potential service-providing organizations available to all care providers for use in advising and making referrals to the most suitable and convenient service.

The needs of a PLHAs and his/her family will change over time. For example, in the late stages of the disease, home care will become a more important option within the continuum; but at any stage various parts of each component of comprehensive care will need to be addressed. Care must be responsive to fluctuating needs. This approach requires coordination among the points on the continuum, including a referral mechanism operation among them which can be achieved for example through regular meetings at district or municipal level, involving all care organizations and by having a directory of care-providing organizations which can be consulted by the counsellor in the hospital before discharge of the patient.

The health facilities involved may include hospitals, health centres, clinics and dispensaries – whether operated by government, NGOs or privately. Community-based services include day-care centres, PLHA support groups, traditional health care, organizations providing welfare or income-generating activities, and various other services provided by NGOs and voluntary groups. Closely linked to community-based services is home care, which includes teaching family members to become care providers. This can give the family the information and support needed to manage common symptoms, establish links with community health workers, provide palliative care and moral support, maintain hygiene and nutrition with the help of social welfare programmes and obtain religious support.

Another essential service for PLHAs and their kin is legal support, including helping PLHAs to write a will, and helping survivors to enforce those wills or to obtain proper-

Box 6. Care along a continuum (7)

Home	Community	Health centre	District level
Person with HIV or other *chronic illness* *Family* *Friends and neighbours*	**Trained volunteers*** **Community health or** **TB workers*** *Traditional healers* *Red Cross groups* *Local leaders* *Teachers* *Youth groups*	**Nurse*** *Other staff*	*District hospital, e.g.* **doctors, nurses,** **counsellors*** *Welfare, e.g.* **social** **workers*** *Educational service* *Legal*

* Possible home care team members
Source: Living with AIDS in the Community/WHO/GPA

ties that should be theirs according to legislation instead of being bound by traditional customs alone. In Uganda projects such as FIDA and Concern have incorporated legal literacy (training families about legal issues) and supported community 'paralegals' (see Box 7).

Box 7. Legal support for communities in Uganda

Concern International has initiated a programme to reduce human rights violations against widows and orphans in Rakai, Uganda. Community-based paralegals are selected by their communities and trained by government lawyers in basic laws pertaining to sexual abuse, marriage, inheritance, divorce, domestic violence, children's rights and responsibilities, and the Ugandan legal system. They lead seminars in their communities using simplified booklets on legal issues developed by the Ministry of Gender and Development. Both magistrates and probation officers participate in the programme, which has promoted the development of a working relationship between them and the paralegals. There is also a referral structure for court cases, which helps people submit their claims to the appropriate courts of law without paying high fees to lawyers. The most common legal cases associated with HIV/AIDS relate to inheritance and marriage rights, and to sexual abuse, which are becoming much more commonly reported.

Box 8. Networking in Mwanza, Tanzania

An NGO-coordinating forum for networking among facility, home care and counselling was set up in Mwanza District. The forum includes three Protestant churches of different denominations, two Catholic parishes, one Islamic organization, the referral hospital, an NGO providing services for homeless children and various other NGOs. The support programmes of these organizations differ in emphasis, ranging from support for street children to home-based AIDS care. The municipal medical officer of health provided an office building, which was renovated and equipped by two NGOs.

The spectrum of networking collaboration activities includes counselling in hospitals, offices and at home; visits to the district hospital and to homes; AIDS education for communities, schools and special groups; assistance to clients (clothing, food, medicines, psychosocial help); and assistance to orphans (school fees, uniforms, clothing). No member of the network covers all activities, but by collaborating, the organizations involved can cover the whole range of HIV prevention and AIDS care activities.

Each member of the forum contributes at least US$ 6 monthly to meet the cost of keeping the forum functioning. The forum meets for several hours every three months to share problems and experiences. A walk-in HIV testing centre has been jointly established by four organizations. Counsellors from various NGOs meet every week at the hospital, and collaborate on providing services for patients about to be discharged. However, not all of these will contact the NGO after returning home. To avoid over-lapping services and potential conflicts, the town has been divided into geographically-defined areas, with each organization providing support in a specific area.

Box 9. Networking in South Africa

In Kwazulu, South Africa, a pilot home-based care programme developed a network involving a well-functioning community health worker programme and five mission and government hospitals, including their mobile and fixed clinics. Training and involving existing health staff responsible for tuberculosis, maternal, children's and primary health care, made earlier recognition of HIV-related illnesses and better services (including counselling and palliative care) possible at all levels. An additional advantage is improved patient compliance with tuberculosis treatment, since direct observation therapy could be decentralized: health centres and community members now handle much of this work. Steps for setting up such a programme are detailed in AIDS Action, Issue 28, 1995.

Networking for a continuum of care
Especially in urban areas, often several organizations are involved in providing home-based care within a district. The district has a key role to play in coordinating efforts to provide home-based care and linking it to government health and social services. Three examples of networking to provide a continuum of care coordinated by the district are shown in Boxes 8, 9 and 10.

Box 10. Nyakato AIDS outreach programme, Mwanza, Tanzania

In 1992–1993 19 counsellors/home care supervisors received training at the town's referral hospital which is equipped with training, HIV testing and referral facilities. They were from a ward six miles from the centre of Mwanza; while the programme was initiated by a parish, people of all denominations – Christians, Muslims and those who had no declared religion – were involved. Both community workers and health workers were included in the programme. To avoid the 'stigma' attached to AIDS as a sexually transmitted disease, these 19 counsellors/home care supervisors were asked to make visits to sufferers of all terminal illnesses, including cancer.

The counsellors/home care visitors have continued their involvement as volunteer workers throughout the last three years. The counsellor making home visits is not a stranger, but knows and lives in the area. An initial visit is used mainly to establish a relationship with the sick person, to become familiar with the home and individual's background, and to know when he/she may be needed. The counsellor is expected to stay in touch, also visiting the families of persons who have died and helping the orphans left behind.

A benefit of early diagnosis is that it allows patients to receive early treatment for opportunistic infections; thus they can continue to be productive and help their families for a longer period. Tuberculosis patients can receive effective treatment, so that the spread of the disease is stopped. The PLHAs can also help prevent the spread of AIDS by making a commitment to avoiding risk behaviour.

In 1994 the NGO decided to add a much-needed nurse to the programme, strengthening the quality of medical services. This has enabled quicker assessment of patients, and some help for very sick patients in assuring they get and take their medications. Valuable help has also come from the local government dispensary nurse, whose assistance is needed to accompany counsellors visiting a patient who is unable to walk to a facility. Spiritual help is provided by a parish priest.

The Nyakato project has also demonstrated the importance of using the community in which a person lives; that is friends of the family or others who have shown an interest in giving physical help or moral-spiritual assistance to the family of the sick person with his/her explicit consent. Counsellors meet each month to discuss problems they encounter and to exchange ideas on how to deal with problems that may arise. The counsellors have also had 'retreat days' – days set aside for prayer and meditation, and to become 'refreshed' for the daily work.

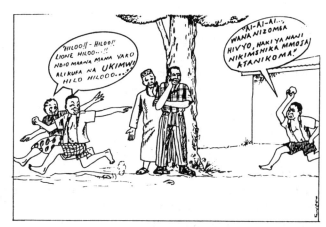

Stigma: children shouting at their friend whose mother is thought to have died of ukimwi (AIDS).

Challenges ahead

Community-based care and family home counselling programmes face several problems:

- Sustainability: NGO or church funds that cover running costs may be depleted; further, volunteer workers are indeed voluntary, and may end their involvement in the programme at any time.
- Obtaining supplies (drugs, food, clothing, dressings) often relies on charities or on donations from local businesses or organizations, and thus may be irregular.
- Many (or even the majority) of people in rural areas believe that sick people have been 'bewitched' and are likely to send them to a local traditional healer. This results in financial demands that may be substantial over time, in addition to emotional and symptomatic consequences.
- The tremendous stigma and fear attached to the disease may cause patients to be isolated by their families or even to be chased away by neighbours.
- If a husband dies without leaving a will, local customs may call for all family possessions to be distributed among the relatives, leaving nothing for the remaining members of the immediate family.
- Maintaining confidentiality and trust is difficult. Even when a husband has HIV/AIDS, wives may not be informed. Then they run the risk of becoming infected. Patients do not always consent to discussions between themselves, their partner and the counsellor.
- The extended family may not be able to accommodate and provide for the education of all orphans, especially when they have lost both parents (see Box 11). Some may become homeless street children in nearby urban centres.

Box 11. Muno Mu Kabi – supporting orphans

Muno Mu Kabi (which means 'a friend in need' in the local language) are informal groups of women operating on a voluntary basis, whose aim is to assist members in times of difficulties. These groups originated in Masaka, Uganda, in the 1960s. They were later introduced in Rakai District, Uganda – a district hard hit by AIDS – by visionary women who realized the importance of communal participation in problem solving.

When a member of this group loses a relative, or she is weak and needs assistance, the women typically intervene voluntarily, contributing labour or food, or drinks for mourners in case of a death. In 1993 one of the authors of this chapter visited Rakai and was taken to visit ten homes of 'orphan-breadwinners', children who received support so that they could continue to live in their parents' residences and farms, contrary to the African tradition of being scattered among relatives. Thus they managed to retain their parents' property, including the land and crops. The women of Muno Mu Kabi render needed services to the children and provide them with peace of mind. This type of arrangement could also be adapted to provide care for the sick, orphans and the elderly.

Conclusion

AIDS care and counselling is becoming an increasingly important issue in many African districts. Experiences with AIDS care programmes in areas affected early in the epidemic reveal the multiple obstacles to be overcome if an effective programme is to be achieved.

AIDS care and counselling is most effective when based on a continuum of care. In most districts, this will need to be established, or at the least, existing elements will need to be strengthened, to cope with the consequences of the epidemic. A set of linkages connecting home care to health facilities is needed, along with improved referral mechanisms, counselling and home care. A concerted effort will be required, including sharing available resources and mobilizing additional ones for AIDS care and counselling. To facilitate this and coordinate services, a network including all those involved in such activities will be essential. The long-term sustainability of care and counselling for people with HIV/AIDS in communities will depend on how well the continuum of care is established, operated and funded.

Further reading and resources
Evian C. *Primary AIDS care: a practical guide for primary health care personnel in the clinical and supportive care of people with HIV/AIDS,* second edition by C. Evian, Jacana, (Private Bag 2004, Houghton 2041, Johannesburg, South Africa) 1995.

WHO. *AIDS home care handbook.* Addressed to health care workers, the handbook sets out the essential information and advice needed to help individuals, families and communities manage AIDS-related problems and build confidence in their ability to provide AIDS care at home. WHO/GPA/AIDS/HCS/93.2. Geneva. 1993. Swahili version available from AMREF, Dar es Salaam, Tanzania. (Huduma kwa wenye Ukimwi majumbani).

WHO. *Source book for HIV/AIDS counselling/training.* WHO/GPA/TCO/HCS/94.9. Geneva, 1994.

WHO. *Counselling for HIV/AIDS: a key to caring.* WHO/GAT/TCO/HCS/95.15. Geneva, 1995.

WHO. *Manual of group techniques to assess the needs of people with AIDS.* WHO/GPA/TCO/HCS/95.2. Geneva, 1995.

WHO. *Provision of HIV/AIDS care in resource-constrained settings, report of a meeting, Geneva, 21–23 September 1994.* WHO/GPA/TCO/HCS/95.14.. Geneva, 1995.

AIDS Action issue no. 28 on 'Home and Hospital', London, AHRTAG, March–May 1995.

AIDS Action issue no. 29 on 'Keys to counselling', London, AHRTAG, March–May 1994.

Matomora MKS, The district health systems approach. *Contact* 143. Geneva, World Council of Churches, 1995.

WHO. *TASO Uganda – the inside story: participatory evaluation of HIV/AIDS counselling, medical and social services, 1993–1994.* WHO/GPA/TCO/HCS/95.1. Geneva, 1995.

Adolescent Health Programme. *Counselling skills training in adolescent sexuality and reproductive health: a facilitator's guide.* Guide to running a 5–day workshop. Geneva, WHO.

Strategies for Hope series. TALC, P.O. Box 49, St Albans, Hertfordshire AL1 4AX, United Kingdom or Strategies for Hope, 93 Divinity Road, Oxford OX4 1LN, United Kingdom. Organizations in Kenya should order them from: Health Education Network, AMREF, P.O. Box 30125, Nairobi, Kenya. Organizations in Tanzania should write to: AIDS Project, AMREF Tanzania, P.O. Box 2773, Dar es Salaam, Tanzania. Organizations in Uganda can order them from: AMREF Uganda, P.O. Box 51, Entebbe, Uganda. The titles of the booklets are:

1. From fear to hope: AIDS care and prevention at Chikankata Hospital, Zambia
2. Living positively with AIDS: the AIDS Support Organization (TASO), Uganda
3. AIDS Management: an integrated approach (Chikankata Hospital, Zambia)
4. Meeting AIDS with compassion: AIDS care and prevention in Agomanya, Ghana
5. AIDS Orphans: a community perspective from Tanzania
6. The caring community: coping with AIDS in urban Uganda
7. All against AIDS: the copperbelt health education project, Zambia
8. Work against AIDS: workplace-based initiatives in Zimbabwe
9. Candles of hope: the AIDS programme of the Thai Red Cross Society
10. Filling the gaps: care and support for people with HIV/AIDS in Côte d'Ivoire

Churches' action for AIDS, World Council of Churches. *Learning about AIDS, a manual for pastors and teachers,* and *A guide to HIV/AIDS pastoral counselling.* (150 route de Ferney, 1211 Geneva 2.)

AMREF Tanzania, (P.O. Box 1482, Mwanza/P.O. Box 2773, Dar es Salaam) have produced a booklet in English and Kiswahili in collaboration with the NGO Kuleana, entitled *Life first! A practical guide for people with HIV/AIDS and their families.*

FACT (Family AIDS Caring Trust). Their publications include *100 questions and answers on AIDS* and *Living through AIDS. Advice, health care and hope for people affected by the AIDS virus.* (FACT P.O. Box 970, Mutare, Zimbabwe.)

World Health Organization. Guidelines for nursing management of people infected with human immunodeficiency virus (HIV). *WHO AIDS Series,* no. 3. Geneva, WHO.

AIDS counselling: a manual for primary health care workers, AIDS Control Programme, Ministry of Health, Zimbabwe, 1990. (Printers: Cameo Business & Secretarial Services Ltd., P.O. Box A437, Avondale, Harare, Zimbabwe.)

Hospice Africa. *Pain and symptom control in the terminal cancer and AIDS patient.* Hospice Africa (Uganda), (P.O. Box 7757, Kampala, Uganda) 1995.

AIDS/STD Health Promotion Exchange issue no. 3 on 'People living with HIV/AIDS: promoting health through partnership'. Amsterdam, Royal Tropical Institute, 1994.

AIDS Health Promotion Exchange issue no. 1 on 'Maximizing the existing health potential of people with HIV/AIDS: have we succeeded?' Amsterdam, Royal Tropical Institute, 1991.

Lamont AC, Greiff M, Rosenberg D, Wiggin TR. AIDS in Africa: what drugs do the carers want or need? *Tropical Doctor* 1996, 26: 72–76.

References

1. WHO/GPA. The current global situation of the HIV/AIDS pandemic 1995. *Weekly Epidemiological Record* 1995, 70: 353–360.

2. Schopper D, Kalibala S, van Praag E. Psychosocial care for AIDS patients in developing countries. In: Carr SC and Schumaker JF (eds.). *Psychology and the Developing World.* Praager, Australia (in press).

3. Chela CM, Msiska R, Sichone M et al. Cost and impact of home-based care for people living with HIV/AIDS in Zambia, 1994. Ministry of Health, Zambia and WHO, Lusaka, Zambia, 1995.

4. William S. From fear to hope, AIDS care and prevention at Chikankata hospital, Zambia. *Strategies for Hope,* no. 1. Action AID, AMREF, 1990.

5. WHO. *TASO Uganda – the inside story: participatory evaluation of HIV/AIDS counselling, medical and social services, 1993–1994.* WHO/GPA/TCO/HCS/95.1. Geneva, 1995.

6. Jackson H, Kerkhoven N. *Developing community AIDS care in Zimbabwe.* Harare, SAfAIDS, 1995.

7. Van Praag E. The continuum of care: lessons from developing countries. *International AIDS Society Newsletter* 1995, 3: 11–13.

19 Tuberculosis control and AIDS

Samuel Kalluvya, Matheus Lefi and John Bennett

- What are the chances that an adult with TB is also HIV-infected?
- How can TB and AIDS control programmes be integrated at the district level?
- What can the community do to improve TB case detection?
- Which drugs should be used for patients with both TB and HIV?
- Can the TB coordinator become an HIV/AIDS counsellor?

The consistent association between tuberculosis (TB) and HIV infection is now recognized as one of the most serious public health, social and economic threats in developing countries (1). Among tuberculosis patients in Africa, very high seroprevalence rates – over 60% – have been reported (2), and since the HIV/AIDS epidemic began, the number of tuberculosis cases have tripled in some countries (3).The sexually active part of the population, and in particular groups that are apt to be more frequently exposed to HIV infection, is at high risk. This chapter presents a brief overview of existing tuberculosis control measures, followed by the changes since HIV/AIDS appeared, the current situation, cost implications and the monitoring of tuberculosis.

Tuberculosis control measures

Tuberculosis has been a known problem for longer than AIDS; thus, there is apt to be an existing programme and structures for prevention and control in most districts. A national TB policy will be in place (sometimes combined with leprosy control) and a TB programme will have been established within the regional and district health services. Such a programme typically operates with a trained member of staff who maintains a register of cases in the districts, and is also responsible for ensuring standardized diagnoses and case management. In line with WHO protocols, the aim is identification and effective treatment of all contagious, sputum-positive cases. Early diagnosis and prompt, effective treatment of other forms of tuberculosis (that is, smear negative and extrapulmonary tuberculosis) is also important in HIV-infected individuals. This will significantly reduce morbidity and mortality associated with TB in immuno-compromised patients. For children, BCG vaccination is already a part of immunization programmes and may possibly decrease morbidity and mortality. However, it is unlikely to change infection rates in adults.

The district hospital and some health centres within a district may have laboratories which can examine sputum for acid-fast bacilli. Beds are also often available for the initial treatment of cases in the hospital. Many health centres and clinics or dispensaries are able to undertake continued patient management and education.

Changes since the appearance of HIV/AIDS

The seroprevalence rates of over 60% in some tuberculosis patients in Africa and the unprecedented increase in the number of tuberculosis cases, as mentioned above, are among the changes that have occurred since the appearance of HIV/AIDS. For example, at a referral hospital in Tanzania tuberculosis cases have increased by 329% since 1984. In rural districts, the increase may be less dramatic but will almost certainly be of significance to public health (see Box 1). In studies in Zaire, Burundi, Uganda, Zimbabwe, Ethiopia, Central African Republic and Zambia, between 30–50% of patients with tuberculosis have been found to be HIV-positive (1). In Abidjan, Ivory Coast, a necropsy study (4) revealed disseminated tuberculosis as the dominant pathological finding in nearly half of HIV-positive adults dying of severe wasting ('Slim syndrome'). The situation has been summed up by Narain et al. (5) who stated that the association between tuberculosis and HIV is evident from the high incidence of tuberculosis, the high HIV seroprevalence among patients with tuberculosis, the high occurrence of tuberculosis among AIDS patients and the coincidence of increased recording of tuberculosis with the spread of the HIV epidemic in several African countries.

Box 1. Increase in tuberculosis cases

In Magu District, Tanzania, where HIV prevalence was about 5% in 1993, there was a twofold increase in pulmonary tuberculosis cases between 1984 (142 cases) and 1993 (295 cases), with incidence rising from 50 per 100,000 in 1988 to 110 per 100,000 in 1992. The rate of increase was highest in females. The number of new tuberculosis cases is about one-fourth as large as the estimated number of new HIV infections in the district each year (about 300 new tuberculosis cases and about 1,200 new HIV cases among adults).

Population-based data are also available for the whole region. In 1991, 29% of tuberculosis cases were attributed to HIV infection (9), in a population where overall HIV prevalence was about 5% among adults aged 15–54.

Mycobacterium Tuberculosis is a potent opportunistic infection in HIV-infected individuals, causing tuberculosis with emerging immunosuppression. HIV-associated tuberculosis is predominantly due to reactivation of latent *M. tuberculosis* infection. This may occur beginning in the very early stages of HIV disease. Both HIV/AIDS and tuberculosis are still on the increase. While in immunocompetent individuals the lifetime risk of developing active tuberculosis is about 10% (6), in those with both latent *M. tuberculosis* and HIV infection it is estimated at 5–10% per year, with a cumulative lifetime risk of 30% or more (7). In severely immunocompromised patients, primary acquisition of tuberculosis also may occur.

With the advent of HIV infection a number of problems in tuberculosis control have surfaced. An important problem is the masked appearance of *M. tuberculosis* in the case of co-infection with HIV. In the early stages of HIV infection, it presents in the classical form: a predominance of open pulmonary tuberculosis with cavity formation, as in immunocompetent individuals. In advanced HIV disease, tuberculosis is usually disseminated and, although often secondary, presents in an atypical form resembling primary tuberculosis. This poses diagnostic problems to the unwary practitioner taught about TB during the pre-HIV era, and to district and other health workers without X-ray facilities.

With HIV testing reserved for blood donors in many districts, data are unlikely to be available at either the district or regional level to determine the local interaction of the parallel and synergistic epidemics of TB and HIV/AIDS. There is a need to increase the number of HIV testing kits, so that TB patients can be regularly tested for HIV. Apart from helping in the study of HIV/TB interaction at these levels, knowing the HIV status of TB patients is important – their treatment may need to be modified to avoid potentially adverse drug reactions (see below). Further, an AIDS diagnosis based on the clinical case definition may be incorrect, if the profound wasting and prolonged fever observed are due to tuberculosis.

HIV/TB interaction

With two diseases acting synergistically (that is, reinforcing each other), there are possibilities for collaborative work between programmes related to the two diseases. At district level, coordinators for tuberculosis control could become involved in selected areas of AIDS interventions (10). These include patient management and counselling of AIDS patients, pre- and post-HIV test counselling, preventive counselling and condom promotion for people living with HIV and AIDS patients. Tuberculosis control coordinators can also contribute to surveillance of HIV/AIDS by reporting AIDS cases and providing data on district levels and trends in the incidence of tuberculosis. On the other hand, counsellors at health facilities and HIV screening centres, AIDS community carers during home visits, and AIDS programme coordinators should be actively involved in tuberculosis case finding. This can be done by inquiring about chronic cough, coughing of blood (hemoptysis), night sweats, lymph node enlargement and sudden or profound weight loss. If such symptoms are present the person should be investigated for tuberculosis by sputum microscopy at the health centre. In case of doubt, a chest

X-ray could be done at a district or regional hospital; lymphnode biopsy specimens or the patient should be sent to a referral hospital. AIDS programme coordinators could also focus on health education, to encourage early recognition and appropriate health-seeking behaviour for tuberculosis.

Several other aspects related to HIV–TB interactions are considered below. Many of these offer possibilities for cooperation among programmes.

Diagnosis/case detection

Health workers' knowledge of HIV/TB should be updated regularly through workshops/ seminars which include health workers from different levels of health delivery units. Supervisory, reappraisal visits by regional and district tuberculosis control coordinators should ensure that TB diagnostic guidelines and referral criteria are being followed by health workers under their supervision. Aspects of patient education, counselling and confidentiality related to tests/laboratory examinations should also be improved upon as needed.

Health workers should be taught how clinical and radiological manifestations of HIV-related tuberculosis differ from what they may have learned in the past. Localization of tuberculosis lesions in the mid- and lower-lung fields is quite common. Lesions include hilar adenopathy, localized infiltrates, or a miliary pattern. A lobar pneumonia-like pattern may be observed. HIV-related tuberculosis pleural effusions are now commonly observed. Apical localization with cavitary disease is common in the early stages of HIV infection. Although Kaposi's sarcoma may be associated with chest nodular infiltrations and hilar adenopathy, the associated skin manifestations are usually present. Pneumocystis carinii, which may also be associated with chest infiltrations resembling those of tuberculosis, is thought to be rare in East African AIDS patients (12).

A number of diagnostic problems arise when tuberculosis is associated with HIV infection. In advanced HIV disease, the rarity of cavitary disease make sputum microscopy a less-sensitive method for the diagnosis of pulmonary tuberculosis. The diagnostic yield can substantially be increased by using concentration methods (centrifugation of sputum before examination). At a referral hospital in Mwanza, of 307 AIDS patients with pulmonary tuberculosis only 147 (47.9%) had positive sputum smears, compared to 91.1% in a control group (11).

Patients should be instructed to bring adequate purulent morning sputum. In patients unable to cough, chest physiotherapy to induce coughing and bronchial drainage may be helpful. Sputum examination must take place in all suspect cases of TB (including extrapulmonary cases) irrespective of the type of disease. Three sputum smears must be made for every suspect case. Patients at HIV testing points should be questioned about symptoms suggestive of TB. Those with such symptoms should be screened for tuberculosis by sputum microscopy for acid fast bacilli and chest X-rays.

Although tuberculin skin reactions may be positive in the early stages of HIV infection, tuberculin testing is not diagnostically useful in most African adult populations with a prevalence of antecedent *M. tuberculosis* infection of more than 50%. Cutaneous anergy in advanced HIV infection and HIV wasting syndrome preclude its usefulness, even in diagnosing recently acquired *M. tuberculosis* infection.

Surveillance and reporting

District health management information systems and their links with the regional office typically need to be strengthened. Case definition must be standardized and circulated to all staff. The first level of analysis must be the institution where diagnosis is made, the second level is the district office and the third the regional office. Each level should draw conclusions and initiate the appropriate action. Basic analyses of number of persons, place and year can easily be done at district or regional levels. It is these which have helped to focus on the interrelationship of tuberculosis and declining immunity due to HIV infection.

In patients with both tuberculosis and HIV infection, the cause of morbidity and mortality may be difficult to identify: studies done where microbiological investigations are possible have shown other causes to be operating, such as infection with salmonella or streptococcus-pneumonia (13).

Patient management and counselling

While some HIV-positive patients develop tuberculosis from a dormant pre-existing infection, others may be exposed to the organism after becoming seropositive. While the first objective of a tuberculosis programme is to interrupt transmission by effectively treating infectious cases, prevention of nosocomial transmission within health units is also important. With respect to treatment regimes, there is typically a national policy which should be followed; this helps to avoid confusion across districts. Several countries in Africa now use short-course chemotherapy (eight months total; two months isoniazid (H) + rifampicin (R) + pyrazinamide (Z) + streptomycin (S) followed by six months isoniazid (H) + thiacetazone (T): 2HRZS/6HT) or another rifampicin-containing regimen should be followed for all smear-positive pulmonary tuberculosis, and for seriously ill smear-negative cases. The long-course standard regimen (two months streptomycin + isoniazid + thiacetazone followed by ten months of isoniazid + thiacetazone + 2HTS/10HT) is reserved for less-ill smear-negative cases and extra-pulmonary tuberculosis.

A study in Uganda, comparing thiacetazone and rifampicin-containing regimens for HIV-associated pulmonary tuberculosis, showed that the 2HTS/10HT regimen was associated with only 37% sputa sterilization, compared to 74% sterilization among patients on rifampicin-containing regimens (14). This observation emphasizes the need to use short-course, potent rifampicin-containing drug regimens for all forms of HIV-associated tuberculosis to improve compliance, cure and relapse rates to levels comparable to those of HIV-negative patients (15).

A regimen without rifampicin is suboptimal in terms of efficacy when used for disseminated tuberculosis associated with advanced HIV infection, namely, extra-pulmonary and smear-negative tuberculosis. However, such a regimen is much less expensive. When it is not possible to use rifampicin for all cases, national policy may specify using e.g. the long course standard regimen as a cost-effective alternative for treating patients who are neither infectious nor seriously ill.

Treatment compliance is the key to successful control of tuberculosis. Short courses are more likely to be successful, but even there a concerted effort will be needed to obtain maximum user compliance during the course of drug treatment.

The occurrence of tuberculosis in HIV-infected patients poses four additional problems to tuberculosis treatment:

- *Streptomycin injections*: The dire shortage of syringes and kerosene for sterilization in district and rural health facilities increases the risk of HIV transmission through injections. This calls for serious consideration of adopting an all-oral drug regimen. A two-month intensive phase of isoniazid, rifampicin, pyrazinamide and ethambutol and six months of intermittent or daily administration of ethambutol and isoniazid is a safe, effective and reasonably-priced regimen: 2HRZE/6E3 (three times per week) H3 or 6HE.

- *Adverse drug reactions*: The likelihood of exacerbated reaction to drugs must be taken into account, especially for thiacetazone (see Box 2). Patients placed on thiacetazone + isoniazid (called thiazina) should receive an initial supply sufficient for one week only, with thorough information on possible adverse reactions and the instruction to report immediately after observing any adverse dermatological reactions. Patients suspected of being HIV-infected who are prescribed thiacetazone should be monitored closely for itching or any allergic skin manifestations within the first four weeks of treatment, as most reactions occur during this period. Those with documented HIV infection preferably should not be given thiacetazone – if possible this should be replaced by ethambutol in the treatment schedule. Thiazina should be withheld from (8):
  - HIV seropositive individuals;
  - patients with herpes zoster;
  - patients with Kaposi's sarcoma;
  - patients with chronic diarrhoea.

Box 2. Adverse drug reactions

At a referral hospital in Tanzania it was observed that treatment of AIDS-related TB with the national TB control programme schedule, with 2SRHZ/6TH, although effective, is associated with higher rates of adverse skin reaction (43.4%), and a significantly higher relapse rate of 14.3%, compared to 2.9% among TB patients who are not HIV-infected. The mortality rate associated with Stevens-Johnson Syndrome may be high: at this hospital it accounted for 40% of TB deaths (16).

- *Drug resistance*: The number of TB cases escalates pari-pasu with the prevalence of HIV. As for any disease, an increase in the number of cases also increases the need for information about the incidence of multi-drug resistant organisms. Ideally, this incidence would be continually monitored. However, few districts have their own surveillance programmes. Although the district is very limited in its ability to deviate from national and regional protocols for treatment, it does have a responsibility to advocate for change. Carefully maintained records will be needed to support arguments for change.

- *Isoniazid chemoprophylaxis*: The number of dually infected individuals with a very high risk of developing active TB continues to increase in sub-Saharan Africa. In Western countries infected individuals are given isoniazid chemoprophylaxis to prevent reactivation of latent *M. tuberculosis*. It has yet to be proven that the cost of treating all HIV-reactivated excess TB cases with multiple drugs is cheaper than using isoniazid chemoprophylaxis to prevent these cases. However, there are several arguments against such a policy in resource-deprived sub-Saharan Africa. The first is cost, and the amount of organization that would be required. In addition, there are other limitations to isoniazid preventive therapy, including hepatotoxicity, failure to adher to the treatment regime, and the fact that treatment is only effective if there is no isoniazid resistance. Operational problems can also be evident; for example it may also be difficult to exclude active tuberculosis before beginning the treatment. Furthermore, the efficacy, safety and optimal duration of isoniazid chemoprophylaxis when given to HIV-infected individuals still needs to be established by research.

There may be a lack of HIV testing at district level, but since filter paper specimens can be easily transmitted to larger laboratories, this can be overcome. When HIV status is known, it is easier to make good decisions on the choice of TB treatment schedules.

Follow-up
Chronic diseases such as HIV/AIDS and TB require continued follow-up for individuals and families, sometimes over many months or years. This, however, may be rather difficult in communities with high mobility, such as communities of herdsmen, where health services experience frequent staff shortages or transfers. The TB register is an invaluable tool for assisting in follow-up and monitoring of patients. There is also a need to have an HIV/AIDS register of counselled patients, which should be kept by the district/regional AIDS coordinator (with all the safeguards of confidentiality).

Home-based care
Home-based care is common for both TB and AIDS. For TB, it may be combined with direct supervision of drug compliance; AIDS care provided by relatives may be carried out with some support from clinic staff.

Health care staff follow-up combined with home-based care may also be used for patients with various HIV-related diseases such as tuberculosis or pneumonia, as well as surveillance to spot occurrence of these diseases: prompt treatment can then be instituted. Such follow-up also makes it possible to record reliable data on patients' morbidity and mortality; the 'verbal autopsy' technique can be used to obtain information about a patient who has died.

Although there is some evidence in favour of the conclusion that, because of lower bacillary load, HIV-positive patients with pulmonary tuberculosis may be less infectious than those who are HIV-negative (17), it is still necessary to assume that home-based care of HIV-infected patients with untreated tuberculosis can pose a threat to vulnerable contacts, especially to children and HIV-infected contacts. This underscores the need for early detection and prompt treatment of active tuberculosis cases. Once effective treatment is started, the sputum becomes sterile within a few weeks and thus, the threat of spreading tuberculosis within the community becomes insignificant.

Home-based care by clinic/hospital staff often falls outside national protocols but nevertheless requires proper training and logistic support – transport (a bicycle or other vehicle), drugs and other supplies such as food supplements. Even though patients' main problems may be social ones, social worker support may not be available unless there are cooperative NGOs with such staff in the district, or active social services committees.

Training and education
The additional stigma of not one, but two feared diseases will have social repercussions that call for counselling and support, so that patients can begin to accept their illness and deal with it in a realistic way. Workers who previously concentrated on tuberculosis need to be trained in HIV/AIDS counselling; this presents a good opportunity for joint training sessions (see Box 3).

Box 3. Integrating AIDS and tuberculosis training

In Mwanza Region a one-week course on HIV/AIDS, organized by the Ministry of Health, was organized for health workers to improve their skills in assisting patients and communities with the consequences of HIV/AIDS. The course included a special session on tuberculosis, presented by the regional tuberculosis and leprosy coordinator. This session aimed at refreshing health workers' knowledge of tuberculosis and discussing the interface between HIV infection and tuberculosis. In addition, the district tuberculosis control coordinator attended a training course for counsellors.

In the past basic and on-the-job continuing education were often compartmentalized, making it easy to overlook interrelationships between conditions. Suitable health learning materials which bring together information about HIV/AIDS/STD/TB/malnutrition/poverty and their interrelationships, and make it accessible for staff, patients and the public – may not currently exist. These should be developed for the three target groups and pretested to ensure suitability and effectiveness.

BCG immunization of newborns
BCG immunization of newborns is widely used to prevent tuberculosis. There has been some concern about adverse effects of BCG vaccination, such as the possibility of disseminated BCG infection among HIV-infected infants. However, in countries with a

high risk of tuberculosis, the WHO recommends BCG vaccination of all infants at high risk, except those with AIDS symptoms (18).

Cost implications of TB and AIDS control

The district budget has been hit hard by the increasing incidence of two serious conditions, each making the other more difficult and costly to manage. With respect to TB, areas in which costs are apt to increase include:

- TB drugs and new regimes that cost more than the previous ones, e.g. ethambutol instead of thiacetazone. This increase may be partly offset by a decrease in costs if injectable streptomycin is omitted from the regimen. As HIV seroprevalence rises the incidence of TB also rises, and more drugs are needed. The costs of a short course with thiacetazone is US$ 46 (2HRZS $ 44 + 6HT $ 2) and with ethambutol US$ 55 (2HRSZS $ 44 + 6HE $ 11).
- more counsellors;
- more laboratory work;
- more TB and AIDS cases admitted to hospitals.

New costs will include:
- health learning materials;
- training workshops;
- more staff for home-based care and follow-up.

To keep costs under control, it is useful to review expenditures twice a year, to make sure they are in line with the budget.

Monitoring, evaluation and research

Monitoring
A set of simple indicators (Chapter 6) is needed to monitor the control of tuberculosis and AIDS. From the many possibilities, a few should be selected that can be routinely acquired and a few that require survey methods. Reference should always be made to the national tuberculosis programme to assure alignment with respect to indicators. Indicators such as the following can be monitored:

Input
- number of training sessions;
- drug availability;
- vehicles;
- health learning methods.

Process
- registration, reported cases;
- community involvement;
- coordination;
- people trained and type of training.

Output
- TB treatments completed;
- HIV tests;
- sputa examined for acid fast bacilli;
- number of trained staff;
- number of community members trained.

Outcome/ impact
- sputum-positive cases rendered sputum-negative;
- deaths TB + HIV;
- trends in number of cases;
- TB incidence.

Evaluation

Participation of all districts of a region in the evaluation process is important. All districts should collect adequate baseline information on the suggested monitoring indicators; comparisons between districts can then be made on a regular basis, such as every two years. This activity provides an opportunity to bring in impartial and critical people from the national and regional offices. It is useful to include a wide spectrum of disciplines on the evaluation team, such as nursing, pharmacy, education, a social worker, a sociologist, an epidemiologist and a manager; and to discuss methods and findings with communities.

Research

Research at district level is usually of a simple health systems/operational type. It is used to determine what is working well, what is not, and how improvements can be made. Introducing health management information systems in districts should make it possible to do simple analyses of district data, such as the prevalence, incidence and mortality pattern of tuberculosis, tuberculosis cure rates, relapses, reaction and defaulter rates. Examples of research questions include:

- Why is compliance poor and how can we improve it?
- How long are the delays between first symptoms of TB and sputum examination and treatment?
- Have our training workshops changed staff performance?
- How much do our HIV-positive patients know about tuberculosis?
- Are we targeting the right groups for TB/HIV education?

If donor funds and extra research workers are available, the district level is also an ideal setting for epidemiological and community studies. These could include placebo-controlled randomized clinical trials to demonstrate efficiency (e.g. of isoniazid preventive chemotherapy). A list of critically needed research has developed by the WHO (19), which can provide additional ideas.

Conclusion

In a sub-Saharan population with an HIV prevalence of 10%, about 30 to 40% of all tuberculosis cases are apt to be attributable to HIV infection (20). As a result of synergistic interaction of HIV and *M. tuberculosis* infections, there is no greater problem facing many districts in such a country than the raging tuberculosis and HIV/AIDS epidemics. For example, much of the increase in TB cases detected in Tanzania after 1982 can be attributed to HIV infection. Funds and staff are needed to provide good planning and management for control programmes. It is our belief that, to make the most of resources, it would be advisable to merge national tuberculosis and AIDS care programmes; alternatively, these programmes should integrate as many activities as possible, and work closely together.

Further reading

World Health Organization. *Treatment of tuberculosis: guidelines for national programmes.* Geneva, 1993.

World Health Organization. *Tuberculosis/HIV Research. Report of WHOReview.* Tuberculosis unit, GPA Geneva, 1992.

World Health Organization/Global Programme on AIDS. *Proposed recommendations for intensified collaboration between National Tuberculosis and AIDS programmes.* GPA/ACA/(2)/93.2. Geneva, Nov 1993.

AIDS Action, Issue on 'Tackling TB and HIV', no. 31, London, AHRTAG, December 1995–February 1996.

Crofton J. et al. *Clinical Tuberculosis.* London, TALC, 1992.

References

1. Harries AD. Tuberculosis and Human Immunodeficiency Virus infection in developing communities. *Lancet* 1990, 335: 387–390.

2. Pitchenik AE. Tuberculosis and the AIDS epidemic in developing countries. *Annals of Internal Medicine* 1990, 113: 89–91.

3. Raviglione MC, Snider DE, Kochi A. Global epidemiology of tuberculosis: morbidity and mortality of a world wide epidemic. *Journal of the American Medical Association* 1995, 273: 220–225.

4. Lucas SB, De Cock KM, Hounson A et al. Contribution of tuberculosis to slim disease in Africa. *British Medical Journal* 1994, 308: 1531–1533.

5. Navain JP, Raviglione MC, Kochi A. HIV-associated tuberculosis in developing countries: epidemiology and strategies for prevention. *Tubercle and Lung Diseases* 1993, 73: 311–321.

6. Sutherland I. Recent studies in the epidemiology of tuberculosis based on the risk of tuberculosis disease. *Advances in Tuberculosis Research* 1976, 19: 1–63.

7. WHO/Global Programme on AIDS. *Proposed recommendations for intensified collaboration between National Tuberculosis and AIDS programmes.* GPA/ACA/(2)/93.2. Geneva, 1993.

8. Nunn P, Kibuga D, Gathua S et al. Cutaneous hypersensitivity reactions due to thiacetazone in HIV-1 seropositive patients treated for tuberculosis. *Lancet* 1991, 377: 627–630.

9. Van den Broek J, Borgdorff MW, Pakker N et al. HIV-1 infection as a risk factor for the development of tuberculosis: a case-control study in Tanzania. *International Journal of Epidemiology* 1994, 22: 1159–1165.

10. Van Asten H. The Tanzania experience. In: WHO. *Potential for intensified collaboration between national AIDS and tuberculosis programme.* GPA/ACA(2)/93.5 rev., Geneva, 1993.

11. Kalluvya S, Mkumbo EN. *AIDS and tuberculosis at Bugando Medical Centre N.W. Tanzania.* Paper presented at 2nd National Seminar on AIDS Research in Tanzania, Dar es Salaam. September 26–28, 1994. (Abstract.)

12. Serwadda D, Goodgame H, Lucas S et al. Absence of pneumocystosis in Uganda AIDS patients. *AIDS* 1989, 3: 478.

13. Brindle BJ, Nunn PP, Batchela BIF et al. Infection and morbidity in patients will tuberculosis in Nairobi Kenya. *AIDS* 1993, 7: 1469–1474.

14. Okwera A et al. Randomised trial of thiacetazone and rifampicin containing regimen for pulmonary tuberculosis in HIV infected Ugandans. *Lancet* 1995, 344: 1323–1328.

15. Ackal A, Coulibaly D, Digben H et al. Response to therapy, mortality and CD4 + Lymphocyte counts in HIV-infected persons with tuberculosis in Abidjan, Cote d'Ivoire. *Lancet* 1995, 345: 603–610.

16. Kalluvya S, Mkumbo EN. *Treatment of tuberculosis with the national tuberculosis programme regimen of patients with advanced HIV infection: response to therapy and prognosis.* Paper presented at 2nd National Seminar on AIDS Research in Tanzania, Dar es Salaam. September 26–28, 1994. (Abstract.)

17. Elliott AM, Hayes RJ, Halwiindi B et al. The impact of HIV on infectiousness of pulmonary tuberculosis: a community study in Zambia. *AIDS* 1993, 7: 981–987.

18. Quinn TC. Interactions of the Human Immunodeficiency virus and tuberculosis and the implications for BCG vaccination. *Reviews of Infectious Diseases* 1989, 2: 5379–5383.

19. WHO. *Tuberculosis/HIV research. Report of WHO Review.* Tuberculosis unit, GPA, Geneva, 1992.

20. Van Cleeff MRA, Chum HJ. The proportion of tuberculosis cases in Tanzania attributable to human immunodeficiency virus. *International Journal of Epidemiology* 1995, 42: 637–641.

20 Consequences of the AIDS epidemic for children

Marc Urassa, Gijs Walraven and Ties Boerma

- Can the risk of mother-to-child transmission be reduced?
- Will child mortality in a district increase because of AIDS?
- How many more orphans will there be because of AIDS?
- Are more orphanages needed?
- Should breastfeeding be discouraged in HIV-infected mothers?

HIV/AIDS among children is a consequence of the adult epidemic. Most HIV transmission and AIDS occurs among adults, as the main mode of transmission is sexual contact. The principal forces driving the HIV epidemic in children in sub-Saharan Africa are the maturation of the heterosexual epidemic in the adult population, the large number of infected women in their child-bearing years, high fertility, substantial transmission from mother to child and the almost universal practice of breast-feeding. An additional factor is the frequent administration of blood transfusions to young children and the difficulties involved in securing a safe blood supply. In many children, the disease develops rapidly and severely; they die in early childhood. This chapter examines the magnitude of the impact of HIV/AIDS on children at the district level. Interventions are described which may help to reduce mother-to-child transmission. Children are also affected by severe HIV disease in adult family members, which adds to child morbidity, and when parents die children become orphans. The extent of the orphan problem and options to cope with it are discussed.

Mother-to-child transmission

HIV can be passed from an HIV-infected mother to an infant during pregnancy, childbirth or breastfeeding. The risk of transmission from mother to child has been estimated at 20% to 45% in Africa (1), though more recent estimates from studies with good controls are around 25% (2, 3). Transmission rates in developing countries are higher than in undeveloped countries. It appears that most transmission occurs during birth. The risk of transmission resulting from breastfeeding is estimated at about 14%, with a range from 7 to 22% (4).

The risk of transmission from mother to child is thought to be higher when the mother is in an advanced stage of HIV or has AIDS, when complications occur during delivery (e.g. premature rupture of membranes, prolonged labour, prematurity – see reference 3), or when the mother has a vitamin A deficiency (5). The relationship found in a Malawian study between low serum levels of vitamin A in the second and third trimester of pregnancy and increased mother-to-child transmission (6) is important, because it suggests that improving vitamin A intake during pregnancy may lower transmission. The risk of transmission may be higher for vaginal delivery than for delivery by Caesarian section (about twice as high according to a European study (7)). An American trial also found that the antiviral drug zidovudine reduces transmission if given to pregnant mothers and their newborns. A recent study from Malawi suggests that maternal malaria may also contribute to increased mother-to-child transmission rates in Africa (8).

Considerable research is now focusing on reducing mother-to-child transmission, because it is believed that affordable medical interventions have a good chance of being effective. Box 1 lists interventions currently being considered (5, 8). The most attractive interventions, because of their affordability, are vitamin A supplementation and malaria chemoprophylaxis during pregnancy. However, even if these interventions are proven to be efficacious (that is, shown to have substantial impact in controlled settings), problems of coverage, cost and user compliance remain.

Box 1. Interventions to reduce mother-to-child HIV transmission

Intervention	Prospects
Vaginal disinfection with virucide before delivery	Easy to apply if delivery is in health facility (but more than 50% of births take place at home); efficacy not clear
Caesarean section	Not feasible as a large scale intervention
Vitamin A supplementation	Perhaps feasible, since costs are low, but depends on whether multiple doses are needed during pregnancy and at the time of delivery
Avoid breastfeeding	Benefits likely to be offset by health problems that accompany use of breast milk substitutes in African settings
Malaria chemoprophylaxis	Efficacy not clear; even if efficacy is high, coverage, cost and user compliance will remain a problem
Antiviral drugs (zidovudine)	Efficacy of zidovudine proven (single trial) but too expensive for large scale application; whether short or prolonged course is needed is unclear

Breastfeeding

If possible, all infants should be breastfed; this is one of the most important ways to improve a baby's survival chances during the first year of life. However, breastmilk can also transmit HIV from an HIV-infected mother to her infant. This has generated debate on whether breastfeeding should be discouraged among HIV-positive mothers. In resource-poor settings, where infections and malnutrition are the primary causes of infant death, WHO/UNICEF recommendations encourage all mothers to breastfeed (9). In these circumstances, the benefits of breastfeeding outweigh the risk of HIV transmission (4). In addition, the costs of alternative feeding methods, such as artificial feeding, are too high for the budget of many households and, even if available, products are sometimes over-diluted or prepared with contaminated water. A policy of screening women for HIV and advising those found positive to use breastmilk substitutes can only be considered if resources are adequate to establish a sound system of voluntary testing and counselling (during the antenatal period) and if there is no stigma associated with having HIV/AIDS (4). In most districts HIV prevalence among adults is less than 10%. Here only a small number of HIV infections would be prevented by discouraging breastfeeding, at the cost of many child deaths. Where the mother is known to be infected, the risk of infection must be weighed against other risks: for example, whether money is available to provide alternative nutrition. Ideally, parents should be given information by the health worker, so they can make their own informed choice.

Box 2. Sexual abuse

Sexual abuse of children is little discussed. The evidence, however, increasingly shows that such practices are common, although the extent is difficult to establish. In a study of street children in Mwanza town, 89% of children cited violence at home as one of their reasons for choosing to live on the streets; virtually all children reported being physically or sexually abused (10). Also, street children who had been remanded or imprisoned reported sexual abuse by gang leaders among adult prisoners.

HIV or AIDS and STDs in young children, especially girls, may point to sexual abuse, such as in a case in Tanzania: an 11-year-old rural girl had been living with her blind grandmother and a male farm labourer who had AIDS. A year after the labourer died of the disease, she came to town with AIDS symptoms, and died within a few weeks. There was no history of blood transfusion or injections in the past ten years – sexual abuse was thought to be the most likely cause of her disease and death.

Other routes of infection

As mentioned, there are also other ways a child can become HIV-infected; of these, the most significant is blood transfusion (see Chapter 16). Improper use of needles and syringes (see Chapter 17), sexual abuse of children by an infected adult (see Box 2) and ritual scarification and other practices (such as circumcision using improperly sterilized equipment) also contribute to the number of infections. However, children do not (not a single case is known) become infected with HIV from ordinary physical contact with HIV-infected adults or other children.

Children with HIV/AIDS

HIV infection in children is fairly common, but it is a hidden and often unrecognized problem. Diagnosis and management of sick children in Africa have become more difficult because of HIV (11). Most HIV-infected children become ill during their first year of life, but symptoms may resemble many other childhood diseases. Furthermore, a positive HIV antibody test is only reliable in a child older than 18 months; before that HIV antibody tests may be false positive due to the mother's antibodies, which may remain in the child's body for prolonged periods. More sophisticated tests (such as the polymerase chain reaction, or PCR) can detect HIV in infants, but at present such tests are neither feasible nor affordable for African district hospitals.

In the absence of HIV testing, diagnosing HIV infection or AIDS must be made on the basis of clinical signs and symptoms. The case definition developed by WHO is not very useful for either surveillance or clinical use (11), and should not be used. Instead, districts should refer to guidelines for management of sick children in areas where HIV infection is prevalent and laboratory facilities limited, such as the guidelines recently been developed by WHO in consultation with other authorities (see 'Further reading').

A common symptom of HIV infection in children is failure to grow. However, many children suffer from growth faltering, most of whom are not HIV-infected. Bacterial infections, pneumonia, septicaemia, diarrhoeal diseases and measles may seem more severe in immunosuppressed HIV-1 infected children. They may respond more slowly and require a longer course of antibiotics as treatment for bacterial infections. Furthermore, HIV-infected children often fail to respond to nutritional rehabilitation efforts. Because it is difficult to distinguish between HIV and tuberculosis, a trial using tuberculosis treatment plus fortified feeding may be justified. When chronic or repeated bouts of diarrhoea occur, a course of co-trimoxazol (which cures the most common HIV-associated gastrointestinal bacterial infections) is worth trying if a laboratory diagnosis cannot be obtained. If the response to treatment is not satisfactory, a short course of metronidazole (to treat other common microbial infections) may be useful. Fungal infections of the throat or oesophagus (candidiasis) may improve if nystatin or ketoconazole is available, allowing the child to swallow food again. (However, these are expensive and rarely obtainable.) The implication of all these conditions among infected and possibly-infected children is an increasing need for medications. Yet expensive anti-viral treatments are inappropriate for African countries, treatment for many other opportunistic infections is lacking and nervous system conditions and malignancies defy any treatment.

In child health care and clinical management of malnutrition and infectious diseases, it is important to take HIV/AIDS in young children into account: hospitals and health centres are seeing more sick and dying children with HIV-associated disease. However, this may not be a priority public health problem in a district. For example, in a district with a population of 300,000, 5% HIV prevalence and a fairly high level of fertility, every year about 200 children can be expected to be born with HIV infection. This may have relatively few consequences for outpatient services. For example, in a district with these characteristics and 40 health facilities, each facility can expect about five such patients per year. The increasing burden on inpatient care and hospitals, however, may be substantial.

There seems to be no substantial risk in giving routine immunization (BCG at birth, tuberculosis, diphtheria, pertussis, tetanus, and oral polio) to HIV-infected children, although the immunological response in those infected with HIV may be diminished (12). The international policy of the WHO is to continue vaccinating HIV-infected children.

Child mortality

Although the exact increase in mortality risk in Africa is unknown, the mortality of children infected with HIV is higher than the mortality of children who are not. It is assumed that about 50% of children with HIV acquired through vertical transmission from their mother die before they reach their third birthday, and 75% before the age of five.

How does HIV/AIDS affect child mortality at district level? The extent depends on how common HIV infection is among pregnant women. The increase in child mortality also depends on pre-existing child mortality levels, that is, prior to the AIDS epidemic. Box 3 shows four situations with respect to changes in under-five mortality (number of children dying before the age of five years per 1,000 live births) in a district with 300,000 inhabitants. Vertical transmission from mother to child is assumed to be 25%. The estimated increases in child mortality in these situations range from 3–26%.

Much of the responsibility for child care falls on mothers and other female caretakers. When the mother is ill, poorer preventive health care (immunizations, home hygiene, etc.) and lowered ability to seek treatment are often the result. Older siblings or the extended family may not always be able to help. Delays in seeking care are increasingly explained by telling about a sick mother. This also has direct consequences for hospitals. In the past African hospitals often relied on parents and families to provide general and nursing care to children on the wards. With more and more illnesses among parents, such arrangements are no longer possible. HIV/AIDS in parents also affects children in another way, as prolonged illnesses affect a household's economy: family income decreases and at the same time much is spent on treatment for AIDS patients.

Box 3. Child mortality due to AIDS

In a district where HIV prevalence is 3%:
- where under-five mortality was high before HIV/AIDS (184 per 1,000 live births), child mortality will increase by 3% (to 189 per 1,000), and the number of child deaths will increase from 2,554 to 2,628 per year;
- where under-five mortality was fairly low before HIV/AIDS (85 per 1,000 live births), child mortality will increase by 6%, to 90 per 1,000. The number of child deaths will increase from 1,032 to 1,109 per year.

In a district where HIV prevalence is 10%:
- where under-five mortality was high before HIV/AIDS (156 per 1,000 live births), child mortality will increase by 9% (to 174 per 1,000). The number of child deaths will increase from 2,330 to 2,610 per year;
- where under-five mortality was fairly low before HIV/AIDS (76 per 1,000 live births), child mortality will increase by 26% (to 96 per 1,000). The number of child deaths will increase from 870 to 1,116 per year.

Source: Nicoll et al. (13)

Orphans

An orphan is defined here as a child under 15–18 years of age who has lost one or both parents. Since HIV/AIDS increases mortality in adults aged 25–49 years, many more children are likely to become orphans in the near future. Prior to the AIDS epidemic adult mortality rates (15–49 years) were typically about 0.5% per year in much of Africa. While adult mortality levels and HIV prevalence vary considerably across districts or countries, a two to three-fold increase due to HIV/AIDS is likely to occur. When both parents die, AIDS is more often the cause than any other reason for adult death; it therefore generates more two-parent orphans. How can a district best cope with the burden of this increasing number of children who have lost one or both parents?

The first issue is how many orphans there will be, or more important, how many more than prior to the AIDS epidemic. In the past, fairly high levels of adult mortality meant that orphans were common: as many as 5% of children under 15 had lost at least one parent. In Tanzania, 5.3% of children 0–14 years were estimated to be orphans (14). Of these, about 1 in 10 had lost both parents (0.5% of all children). More recent data from the Kagera Region in Tanzania showed an orphan rate of 7.5%, including 1.3% who had lost both parents. About 22% of these are estimated to have become orphans because their parent(s) died of AIDS. For two-thirds of children who have lost both parents, AIDS is believed to be the cause. Moreover, this is only the beginning of an increase in numbers of orphans. Statistical models of the impact of the AIDS epidemic suggest the number of orphans is likely to increase dramatically during the next decade (15).

Data from studies of two communities with high and medium HIV prevalence are shown in Box 4. These studies suggest that in a district with 300,000 people one can expect 7,000 to 20,000 orphans, including 1,000 to 4,000 who have lost both parents.

Box 4. Orphans in districts

A survey in Manicaland, Zimbabwe, where adult HIV prevalence is well above 10%, found that 12.8% of children under 15 were orphans (16). A community study in rural Mwanza, Tanzania, where adult HIV prevalence is 6%, showed 7.6% of children 0–14 to be orphans (17). The figure classifies the orphans into types: the majority are paternal orphans, having only a mother.

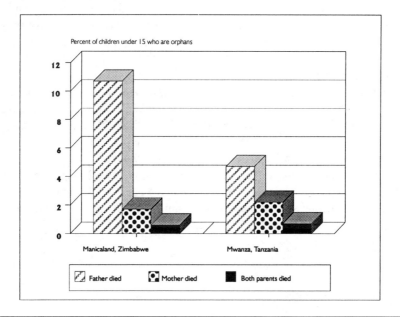

What can a district do to cope with the increasing numbers of AIDS orphans? The options include orphanages, direct support and feeding programmes (14).

- *Orphanages*: these are costly and can only cover a small group of orphans for which no other solution can be found. The cost per orphan in rural Tanzania has been estimated at US$ 160 per year. Orphanage may also not be conducive to the social development of children.
- *Direct support for basic needs*: this could include transfers of food, clothing, other basic commodities and/or cash. Such programmes may help poor families through acute crises, but are neither feasible nor sustainable in the long run.
- *Direct support for education*: such support may focus on subsidizing school fees

and uniforms. High cost, difficulties in determining targeting criteria (who is included), unknown effectiveness and low sustainability indicate that caution is warranted in using this intervention.

- *Feeding posts and child care centres*: these centres are mainly supported by the community, with limited outside assistance (10–20% of total costs), and focus on children under seven years (mostly under two years). Such centres are relatively successful in parts of Tanzania. In addition to the advantage of nutritional supplementation for the children, the intervention frees up adult labour time, which can be used to increase income.

It is essential to consider the orphan problem in the local context. Child fostering is very common in many parts of Africa. For example, a large study in rural Mwanza, Tanzania, found that only 58% of children under 15 lived with both parents (17). Seven percent of children lived with their father only, 22% with their mother only and 13% did not live with either parent. Death of a parent was given as the reason for only one-fourth of these children becoming a 'foster child'. Prior to the AIDS epidemic, orphans were already common, and in the past satisfactory solutions appear to have been found for the majority of children.

The capacity of traditional coping systems is unknown. In Zimbabwe, where 18% of households include orphans and 13% of children have been orphaned, the majority of children receive satisfactory care within extended families or through adaptations of community coping mechanisms (16). It should therefore not be assumed that the life and health experiences of orphans are inevitably poor. Most of African society remains rurally based and in many places people have always coped well with such children. Supporting these existing coping mechanisms may be the best way to care for orphans. The need for establishing special support programmes may be limited to poorer children and households in urban and peri-urban areas (see Box 5).

Box 5. Orphan assistance

In Kagera Region, Tanzania, 12 community-based and international NGOs assist about 47% of all orphans. External aid seems to create some degree of dependency: people or communities are likely to wait for external NGOs to come to their aid. The UKIMWI Orphan Assistance project provides limited assistance to communities to help in solving their own orphan problems. Family and community resources are mobilized, primarily to increase food production, including cultivation of plots and keeping two cows for local consumption, and banana/coffee cash crop farming. Other activities include community support to carry out housing repairs for orphans, providing school fees for a number of orphans, medical assistance for orphans, and income-generating activities for women's groups (tailoring, needle work, baskets and so forth) or female orphans (restaurant) (18).

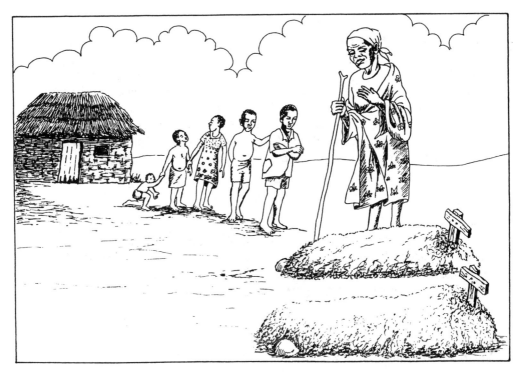

Young children with their grandmother, burying their parents.

In Zimbabwe, where HIV prevalence is high in many districts, changes in traditional child care practices have been observed, especially in peri-urban areas. Such changes were already taking place before the AIDS epidemic, but AIDS mortality has accelerated these changes. Foster et al. (19) describe these changes as follows:

- in traditional marriages, inheritance of widows is no longer practised;
- paternal orphans are cared for by the widow rather than the paternal relatives;
- orphans are cared for by maternal rather than paternal relatives;
- grandparents increasingly care for orphans;
- orphans are cared for by older sisters and brothers;
- relatives are refusing to accept responsibility for supporting orphan households;
- orphans from the same family are being cared for by different caregivers.

Street children

The AIDS epidemic may also contribute to increasing numbers of street children in urban areas. Street children are also at higher risk of HIV infection and other STDs because of the financial need to be involved in prostitution, the lack of adult protection and socialization, the inherent dangers of street life and greater freedom to experiment with sex (20). In several cities and towns NGOs provide support to street children (see Box 6).

Box 6. Protection for street children

In Mwanza town, an NGO (kuleana) provides an integrated programme for approximately 140 street children at any one time. The programme covers health, education, advocacy (through the Center for Children's Rights), counselling, business support and community awareness. About 100 children also receive shelter and food. One very successful project is the establishment of a bakery and pizzeria. These sell to town residents, providing full-time employment for eight street children.

Community care
An increasing number of villages have now established care committees to help households cope with AIDS. Such committees identify and organize assistance for orphans or families who care for orphans. An example of such a committee, which relies on some external support, is given in Box 7.

Box 7. Community care for orphans

In Katete District in Zambia, community AIDS care committees support about 1,500 orphaned children. This programme was established in 1994, initiated by the district hospital AIDS team after it carried out a survey to assess the magnitude of the orphan problem. Committees made household visits to assess orphans' and caretakers' situations. Standard forms were used to record data on children's clothing, nutritional status, school attendance and the household's socioeconomic circumstances. The community committees selected children to be admitted to the programme: criteria included the loss of both parents, or identification by community members as having serious problems.

A major problem was keeping children in school when they lacked the money to buy school uniforms and other needed items. The committees purchased sewing machines and materials, and community members sew uniforms for the children. Children are also given exercise books, pencils and pens, soap, a cup for school use and other items. The committees visit school headmasters to obtain their cooperation in keeping the children in school. Furthermore, committees provide agricultural support to some families and assist grandmothers who need help in repairing or building houses (20).

Conclusion

The AIDS epidemic affects children in many ways. Although ways are being sought to reduce mother-to-child transmission, children may become HIV-infected by their HIV-infected mothers. HIV infection in children may be expressed in a wide variety of forms, making treatment problematic: it is often impossible to distinguish HIV infection from other illnesses that afflict children. When adult family members suffer from HIV/AIDS, child morbidity and mortality increase. Furthermore, orphans are becoming much more common in HIV-affected populations, especially orphans who have lost both parents. Supporting traditional coping mechanisms and taking special measures only for those not covered by those mechanisms appears to be the most appropriate and feasible way to cope with increasing numbers of orphans. Communities are also beginning to develop new mechanisms, as suggested by a number of examples.

Acknowledgement

The authors would like to thank Dr Angus Nicoll for his helpful comments.

Further reading
World Health Organization. *Guidelines for the clinical management of HIV infection in children.* WHO/GPA/AID/SHC/93.3. Geneva, Global Programme on AIDS, 1993.

WHO. *Consensus statement from the WHO/UNICEF consultation on HIV transmission and breastfeeding.* WHO/GPA/INF/92.1. Geneva, Global Programme on AIDS, 1992.

Strategies for Hope Series, no. 5. AIDS Orphans: a community perspective from Tanzania. TALC, P.O. Box 49, St Albans, Hertfordshire AL1 4AX, United Kingdom or Strategies for Hope, 93 Divinity Road, Oxford OX4 1LN, United Kingdom. Organizations in Kenya should order them from: Health Education Network, AMREF, P.O. Box 30125, Nairobi, Kenya. Organizations in Tanzania should write to: AIDS Project, AMREF Tanzania, P.O. Box 2773, Dar es Salaam, Tanzania. Organizations in Uganda can order them from: AMREF Uganda, P.O. Box 51, Entebbe, Uganda.

The orphan generation (Part 1: 10 minutes; part 2: 40 minutes, VHS PAL. A video about community-based care and support for children orphaned by AIDS. Standard price: GBP 45; available for GBP 25 for charitable and educational organizations in sub-Saharan Africa. Charitable and educational organizations in sub-Saharan Africa who cannot pay may request a free copy. Available in English and French: TALC, P.O. Box 49, St. Albans, Herts AL1 4AX, United Kingdom.

World Health Organization/UNICEF. *Action for children affected by AIDS. Programme profiles and lessons learned.* Geneva, 1994.

References
1. Lallemant M, Le Coeur S, Samba L et al. Mother-to-child transmission of HIV-1 in Congo, central Africa. *AIDS* 1994, 8: 1451–1458.

2. Lepage P, Van der Perre P, Mesllati P et al. Mother-to-child transmission of HIV-1 and its determinants: a cohort study in Kigali, Rwanda. *American Journal of Epidemiology* 1993, 137: 589–599.

3. St Louis ME, Kamenga M, Brown C et al. Risk for perinatal HIV-1 transmission according to maternal immunologic, virologic, and placental factors. *Journal of the American Medical Association* 1993, 269: 2853–2859.

4. Nicoll A, Newell ML, Van Praag E et al. Infant feeding policy and practice in the presence of HIV-1 infection. *AIDS* 1995, 9: 107–119.

5. Van de Perre P, Meda N. Interventions to reduce mother to child transmission of HIV. *AIDS* 1995, 9(suppl A): S59–S66.

6. Semba RD, Miotti PG, Chiphangwi JD et al. Maternal vitamin A deficiency and mother-to-child transmission of HIV-1. *Lancet* 1994, 343: 1593–1597.

7. European Collaborative Study Group. Caesarean section and risk of vertical transmission of HIV-1 infection. *Lancet* 1994, 343: 1464–1467.

8. Bloland PB, Wirima JJ, Steketee RW et al. Maternal HIV infection and infant mortality in Malawi: evidence for increased mortality due to placental malaria infection. *AIDS* 1995, 9: 721–726.

9. WHO. *Consensus statement from the WHO/UNICEF consultation on HIV transmission and breastfeeding.* WHO/GPA/INF/92.1. Geneva, Global Programme on AIDS 1992.

10. Rajani R, Kudrati M. The varieties of sexual experience of the street children in Mwanza, Tanzania. In: Zeidenstein S, Moore K (eds.). *Learning about sexuality: a practical beginning.* New York, The Population Council/International Women's Health Coalition, 1996. pp. 301–323.

11. Nicoll A, Walraven G, Kigadye RM et al. Difficulties in the diagnosis of HIV-1 infection and disease in children in Africa. *Medical Virology* 1995, 5: 87–96.

12. Ryder RW, Oxtoby MJ, Mvula M et al. Safety and immunogenicity of Bacille Calmette-Guerin, diphtheria-tetanus-pertussis, and oral polio vaccines in newborn children in Zaire infected with human immuno-deficiency virus type 1. *Journal of Pediatrics* 1993, 122: 687–702.

13. Nicoll A, Timaeus I, Kigadye RM et al. The impact of HIV-1 infection on mortality in children under 5 years of age in sub-Saharan Africa: a demographic and epidemiologic analysis. *AIDS* 1994, 8: 995–1005.

14. Ainsworth M, Rwegarulira AA. Coping with the AIDS epidemic in Tanzania: survivor assistance. *Technical Working Paper,* no. 6. Washington DC, Population, Health and Nutrition Division, Africa Technical Department, World Bank, 1992.

15. Gregson S, Garnett GP, Anderson RM. Assessing the potential impact of the HIV-1 epidemic on orphanhood and the demographic structure of populations in sub-Saharan Africa. *Population Studies* 1994, 48: 435–458.

16. Foster G, Shakespeare R, Chinemana F et al. Orphan prevalence and extended family care in a peri-urban community in Zimbabwe. *AIDS Care* 1995, 7: 3–17.

17. Urassa, M, Ng'weshemi JZL, Isingo R et al. *Orphanhood, child fostering, and the AIDS epidemic in rural Tanzania.* Paper presented at the IUSSE conference on sociodemographic impact of AIDS in Africa, Durban, 3–6 February 1997 and forthcoming in *Health Transition Review.*

18. Rutayuga JBK, Muta CF, Kidza M. *Families and communities manage the orphan problem, a Tanzania/Uganda example.* Paper presented at the IXth International Conference on AIDS and STD in Africa. Kampala, December 1995. (Abstract MoD062.)

19. Foster G, Drew R, Makufa C. Am I my brother's keeper? Orphans, AIDS and the extended family's choice of caregiver. *Sociétés d'Afrique and SIDA* 1995, 10: 14–16.

20. AIDS Coordination Bureau. *Support to children orphaned due to HIV/AIDS.* Discussion paper. Amsterdam, Royal Tropical Institute, February 1996.

Part six
Financing and
sustainability

21 Costs of district AIDS programmes

Ties Boerma and John Bennett

- How can a district best use limited resources?
- How much does a safe blood supply cost?
- When should a district focus mainly on high-transmission areas?
- What are the costs and effectiveness of STD control?
- Given one US dollar per capita, what can be done to reduce HIV transmission?

HIV prevention and AIDS care programmes address priority problems, with significant economic and development repercussions for individuals, communities and health care systems. Prevention and care programmes need to be implemented urgently and efficiently, yet districts have to fit AIDS care into their already limited budgets. This makes it essential to compare the costs and benefits of possible interventions, and to set priorities based on the resources available.

This chapter outlines the economic priority of AIDS versus other conditions. The costs and effectiveness of specific interventions and AIDS care are estimated, mainly based on the experience in Tanzania. These costs will vary among countries, due to large differences in salaries or types of constraints faced in different countries. What matters here is comparing the relative costs of HIV/AIDS interventions, in relation to their effectiveness. In the final section, examples are given of how district AIDS programmes can develop intervention packages for different levels of resources.

AIDS as a priority problem

The World Bank has estimated that in sub-Saharan Africa STDs and HIV are among the top illnesses in terms of loss of disability-adjusted life years (DALY) (1). STD/AIDS comes in fifth place, with 8.8% of all DALYs lost, after malaria (10.8%), respiratory infections (10.8%), diarrhoea (10.4%) and vaccine-preventable diseases (9.6%). Of course, the relative importance of STD/AIDS will increase in the coming decade, as the AIDS epidemic is still in its early stages.

By 1993 AIDS expenditures were already absorbing an estimated 20–60% of government health expenditures in some eastern and southern African countries. Treatment costs are expected to soar even higher in the next few years. The economic impact of adult illnesses has many facets; health costs comprise only one of these. HIV infection and AIDS produce costs to the patient, as well as to a variety of sectors such as education, agriculture and social welfare. The illness may affect production and earnings, consumption and investment, household health and composition, and may also have psychological costs (2).

Considering the consequences of AIDS and the coping mechanisms required bring out the human aspect of the epidemic. In making a case for deep consideration of the wisest ways to spend the limited financing allocated to prevention and care, and how to use data to support advocacy to obtain more funds, it is really only in such human terms that the full consequences of the epidemic can be brought home. However, a case cannot be made for increasing the funding of activities if there is no information about how cost-effective they are. Unfortunately, for many interventions aimed at changing behaviour (not only sexual behaviour but other types as well) our knowledge of cost-effectiveness is lacking.

In the following sections, we make an attempt to estimate the costs and effectiveness of interventions that can be implemented at the district level. Cost estimates are based partly on the literature from Africa, and partly on local experience in Mwanza Region during 1993–1995.

Estimating the costs of HIV prevention and AIDS care

Calculation of costs is a difficult process. In principle, both costs of the providing agencies and costs of clients (such as time, transport, burial and so forth) should be included. In practice, only the former are usually covered. Costs also need to be discounted – that is, spread out over the budget years for which they are relevant (capital expenditure on premises, 20 years; computers, 3–4 years and training, 3–4 years). In the following section, we will outline the costs and effectiveness of selected interventions. However, our estimates of costs are only meant to give an idea of provider costs, particularly in relation to the estimated costs of other HIV/AIDS interventions. The calculations are based on a district that is assumed to have a population of 300,000, including 125,000 adults/adolescents and an estimated 100,000 sexually active individuals, and unless otherwise stated are based on our experience in Mwanza Region. We will consider the following interventions:

1   promotion of safer sexual behaviours: general population
2   promotion of safer sexual behaviours: youth
3   promotion of safer sexual behaviours: high-transmission areas
4   STD control: general population
5   STD control: core groups
6   condom promotion and distribution
7   reduction of HIV transmission through blood transfusions
8   reduction of HIV transmission through injections
9   AIDS care: training of health workers

10   counselling
11   care for AIDS patients
12   survivor assistance.

The first eight interventions are entirely preventive, the next two are both preventive and curative, and the last two are curative interventions.

1. Promotion of safer sexual behaviours: general population

In promoting safer sexual behaviour to prevent HIV, one possible strategy is to target the general population. Such an intervention entails working with government staff, NGOs and communities throughout the district. It may include AIDS awareness campaigns in villages or small towns, and establishment of and support for community AIDS action committees. Provision and promotion of condoms may or may not be part of this strategy.

Costs: If a whole district is to be covered, its community leaders must be mobilized to promote safer sexual behaviour. Transport availability is essential to set up the programme and to supervise it. If we assume that our district of 300,000 people has an average community size of 5,000, it then consists of 60 communities. The costs of this intervention per community can be roughly estimated:

Mobilization and initial training for community leaders	$ 250
Three-day AIDS awareness campaign in the community	$ 1,500
Follow-up activities	$ 750
Total	$ 2,500

For the 60 communities in the district the total would then be US$ 150,000. This includes only the time, transport, training materials and allowances used during health education activities, not condoms or capital costs (such as vehicles), and takes the necessary government/NGO staff preparation time into account.

Effectiveness: The effectiveness of an intervention within the general population, in terms of preventing HIV infections, depends on the level of HIV transmission in the area. For example, in the majority of communities (which are typically rural) in most districts, HIV incidence is likely to be low. Therefore, using a strategy that targets the general population will prevent only a few new HIV infections, even if interventions are successful.

2. Promotion of safer sexual behaviours: youth

Another strategy is to target youth aged 12–19 years, an important group for HIV prevention activities. The majority of youth can easily be reached through school programmes. However, the proportion of youth not in school increases rapidly with age: AIDS programmes will also need to target these out-of-school youth.

A school youth programme may simply introduce a national AIDS curriculum in primary and secondary schools. It could also involve a peer educator programme, plus establish a parent-teacher committee to address issues such as sexual behaviour and AIDS. Such a programme also involves and educates the community. Out-of-school youth can be reached by extending the school programme or planning special activites for them (e.g. clubs).

Costs: A district with a population of 300,000 may have 150 primary schools and 3–10 secondary schools, with as many as 15,000 students in the higher levels of primary education. Teachers from each school will need to be trained to introduce the new curriculum, and continued supervision and support will be needed following the training. Training and supervision of three teachers per school is estimated at US$ 200 per year. Health education materials could add another US$ 100 per year. This minimal version of a school youth programme would thus cost US$ 300 per school (or US$ 3 per pupil); for 150 schools, costs would amount to US$ 45,000.

A more extensive school programme, as outlined in Chapter 10, would involve more training (school committees, trainers of peer educators, peer educators), more supervision, and more health learning materials. Costs of the programme per pupil could easily double (US$ 6 per pupil), so that coverage of the whole district would amount to US$ 90,000.

Out-of-school youth are more difficult to reach and programmes for them are therefore likely to be more costly. It is also more difficult to estimate their cost, since much depends on the approach chosen. Efforts can be part of general community efforts or special programmes, whether in liaison with the school programme or not.

Effectiveness: Youth programmes have the potential to prevent a large number of HIV infections, especially in adolescent girls. Perhaps not so much on the short run – for example, HIV incidence among boys under 20 years is very low, even without inter- ventions – but long-term benefits are potentially high. However, estimates of effective- ness are hard to find. Most evaluations of school programmes have shown improvements in knowledge and attitudes, but very few have documented changes in sexual behaviour. A possible spillover effect of school programmes is that knowledge is taken home and shared with other family members.

Promotion of safer sexual behaviours: high-transmission areas
Instead of focusing on the population as a whole, a more intensive set of activities could be specifically targeted to all of the populatiion in selected high-transmission areas. A district can identify five to ten priority areas to promote safer sex, offer condoms and STD control in an attempt to limit the spread of HIV throughout the whole district. Examples of safer sex promotion programmes that focus on condoms are also given in the section on STD control in high-transmission areas in this chapter.

Costs: These are similar to those outlined above for the general population, but since the intervention is intensified, costs will also be higher. We also include a peer educator programme (for the community in general or for vulnerable groups such as bar workers), intended to sustain the effort after AIDS awareness campaigns are completed, and to stimulate behavioural change. Communities with high-transmission areas are

Table 1. Annual costs of promoting safer sex in a high-transmission area

Type	Number	Price per unit ($)	Total costs ($)
Mobilization	Community leaders' meetings (3)	250	750
Peer educator training	Workshop (1)	750	750
Peer educator support	Monthly supervision, allowances	–	1,000
Health education	Books, leaflets, videos, etc.	500	500
Campaign	One week	2,500	2,500
Monitoring and evaluation	Ongoing	2,500	2,500
Total			6,000

often larger (10,000 or more population). Estimated costs for the initial year (summarized in Table 1) amount to US$ 6,000 per high-transmission area, excluding the STD component (which is covered in point 4).

Effectiveness: The potential effectiveness of such interventions is high, since they target areas where HIV transmission is high. There are, however, very few studies which examine the impact promoting safer sex has on actual sexual practices and subsequent HIV/STD transmission. Combining condom provision and STD control appears to be the best option. Recent evidence from Mwanza has shown that reducing the number of sexual partners is also possible and can be achieved with limited inputs (3).

4. STD control – general population

Treating STDs has two benefits. First, it reduces the burden of STDs among the adult population and (through transmission at birth) young children. Second, controlling STDs reduces the risk of HIV transmission. Recent studies in Mwanza Region have shown that strengthening STD management in government health facilities can reduce HIV transmission by as much as 40% (4) (see Chapter 14). Treatment in the district programme is now based on a syndromic approach, but serology is still used as a screening technique for syphilis in women, and may also be carried out for selected STD cases.

Costs: Costs include the following:
- Drugs (mostly antibiotics): in Tanzania in 1996 costs for drug treatment ranged from $ 1.04 per case for chancroid to $ 1.60 for gonorrhoea and $ 1.40 for syphilis (5). In Kenya, average costs were $ 1.93 per STD. Much higher costs have been reported in other settings, most likely due to higher salaries, use of laboratory tests and more expensive treatment schedules ($ 9.46 in Maputo versus $ 10.16 in Johannesburg per STD episode) (6).
- Laboratory tests (RPR and possibly TPHA for syphilis, Gram stain and culture for gonorrhoea, wet prep for trichomonas, etc.): the cost of RPR and TPHA tests for syphilis is about US$ 1.50 (including drawing blood), and for RPR alone about

Table 2. Annual costs of a district STD treatment programme

Type	Number	Price per unit ($)	Total cost ($)
Drugs	5,000 patients	2.00	10,000
Lab tests and equipment	1,500 tests	2.50	3,750
Training	2 courses/every 3 yr	6,000	4,000
Supervision	6 times, yr (including vehicle)	2,000	12,000
Condoms	50,000 (10 per patient)	0.025	1,250
Total			31,000

US$ 1.00. Gram stain testing for gonorrhoea is cheap, but cultures for Neisseria gonorrhoea and tests for chlamydia infection tend to be expensive.
- Training health workers in the syndromic approach and new treatment schedules, and supervision: a health worker needs training every three years to keep up-to-date with new treatment schedules and the like. Supervisory visits covering the health staff need to be carried out every two months.
- Condoms (e.g. ten) are usually supplied to each STD patient to prevent further transmission.

The annual costs of providing STD treatment services in a district with 300,000 people and 100,000 sexually active persons are roughly estimated in Table 2. Total costs are US$ 31,000 per year. This may double if opportunity costs for health workers are included (see Chapter 14).

Effectiveness: STD control is considered one of the most effective ways to reduce HIV transmission. Treatment costs per STD case may seem high (more than $ 4 in the example), but direct (STDs treated) and indirect (HIV infection prevented) benefits are considerable.

If district resources are insufficient to improve STD management services in the whole district, a cost-effective approach is to focus on areas with suspected or established high-transmission of HIV/STD (e.g. truck stops, small towns, marketplaces). This is likely to increase cost-effectiveness, since the focus is on a population in which the transmission of HIV is high and STDs are more common than among the rural population of a district. Interventions in high-transmission areas may also have a beneficial effect on areas with lower transmission.

5 STD Control – core groups
STD control among specific populations with high levels of sexual activity (also called core groups) is generally considered a cost-effective way to control STDs and prevent HIV transmission. Such interventions focus on commercial sex workers (prostitutes, bar workers) and often include their clients as well.

Table 3. Annual costs of target group interventions: examples from two projects (in US$)

Type	Nairobi, Kenya[1]	Mwanza, Tanzania[2]
Salaries	17,100	9,000
Training	10,000	2,000
Rental premises	7,300	1,000
Drugs	17,400	3,000
Condoms	13,000	free
Transport	2,200	500
Lab tests	10,000	500
Total	77,000	16,000

[1] Clinic for 500+ prostitutes
[2] Reproductive health programme for 100 bar workers

Costs: Variations in cost are related to the type of project, the specific characteristics of the target population and the country of implementation:

- In Nairobi, Kenya, a health clinic was established to provide comprehensive health services, focusing on STDs, for 500 resident prostitutes in Pumwani (7). The annual costs of this project were US$ 77,000 (see Table 3).
- In Yaounde, Cameroon, a peer education project among 7,000 prostitutes included social marketing of condoms (sold by the 40 peer educators, who completely recovered purchase costs) (6). The project costs were about US$ 200,000, of which 96% was for salaries. More than half a million condoms were distributed ($0.34 per condom).
- In Bulawayo, Zimbabwe, peer educators, who got a small honorarium, focused their attention on sex workers and their clients, people in bars and bar workers, and those attending STD clinics (6). Annual costs were US$ 72,000, of which 30% were salaries and 27% were condom costs. About 700,000 condoms were distributed ($0.10 per condom).
- A mobile STD service provided outreach services to bar workers in Mwanza, Tanzania, at an estimated cost of $ 25,000 per year, reaching about 100 bar workers. However, the mobile services were considered too costly and centres for bar workers were established in fixed locations in 1994.
- In Mwanza, Tanzania, a women's centre initially provided STD services and health education to 60 female bar workers in the area. This was later expanded to include other reproductive health services and another 40 bar workers. Peer educators were at the heart of the project (ten in the first phase). The total costs of this project, which was provided with free condoms, were US$ 16,000 per year.

Effectiveness: Treatment of STDs is highly cost-effective if targeted at high STD prevalence groups. A comparison of core versus non-core groups has shown that an STD treatment strategy which targets highly sexually active groups such as prostitutes may be ten times more cost-effective than one which targets less-sexually active groups (5).

For example, prostitutes in Nairobi tend to have a high number of sexual partners (usually more than 4–5 per night), making it easy to understand why STD control measures among prostitutes there may be cost-effective. Many districts, however, do not have the same type of prostitutes as in Nairobi. In such districts, commercial sex workers can be identified, but the number of partners is lower and consequently, also the cost-effectiveness of core group interventions. A broader approach focusing on high-transmission areas rather than on core groups may be more cost-effective, but so far no evidence is available.

6. Condom promotion and distribution

When used as prescribed, condoms prevent both HIV infection and STDs (which, as noted, facilitate HIV transmission and infection). This intervention involves increasing condom availability and, by promoting condoms, also increasing use.

Costs: Condom costs are associated with the condom itself, plus its distribution and promotion. WHO-promoted condoms cost $ 0.024, USAID condoms cost US$ 0.045. In addition, storage and distribution costs are incurred: from the central to the regional and district levels, and from the district to health facilities, bars, and other points of distribution. Distribution costs can be reduced by sharing transport, for example, with the immunization programme (EM) vehicles. Condom promotion activities include printing health education materials, using peer educators and advertising – perhaps with posters, newspapers, radio or TV.

Social marketing (see Chapter 11) of condoms has become increasingly popular. Social marketing involves the private sector in selling donated condoms at a subsidized price. Costs per condom sold (after subtracting the purchase price) vary from US$ 0.07 in Ghana to US$ 0.18 in Zimbabwe. The costs per condom distributed by programmes that promote safer sexual behaviour in Zimbabwe, Uganda and Cameroon were found to be US$ 0.10, US$ 0.21 and US$ 0.34 respectively (8).

At the district level, donated condoms are often supplied free of charge. District costs are thus limited to distribution and promotion costs, which for this calculation we assume to be US$ 0.15 per condom distributed. In a district of 300,000, with 100,000 sexually active persons, the number of condoms needed depends on a number of factors. Therefore, to calculate the number required, we must make a few assumptions: condoms are used only for casual contacts and sometimes with regular extra-marital partners; on average, the number of sexual encounters for which condoms are wanted is six per year (or three condoms per couple). Thus, 300,000 condoms will be needed, which will cost US$ 45,000 per year.

Effectiveness: The proper and regular use of condoms during sexual intercourse reduces the risk of HIV and STD transmission to negligible levels. Inconsistent and inappropriate use are thought to be common, which lowers effectiveness. For example, the interaction of casual sex and alcohol abuse is likely to have an adverse effect. The limited negotiation power of women in sexual transactions may also affect consistent use.

Effectiveness is increased by targeting vulnerable groups – both for promotion and for condom distribution. In a simulation exercise Robinson et al. have demonstrated the value of condom use, even when used only with less-regular partners (9). If condoms are used consistently and effectively by 50% of men in their contacts with one-off sexual partners (such as female bar workers and commercial sex workers) 39% of all adult HIV infections can be prevented.

7. Reduction of HIV transmission through blood transfusions

Blood transfusions are an important health intervention, which can, however, also transmit HIV (see Chapter 17). Transmission of HIV to transfusion recipients has become a public health problem; thus HIV screening of blood and blood products is now a prerequisite for transfusion in all donor centres and hospitals.

Costs: The costs of providing safe blood for transfusion depend on the prevalence of HIV among blood donors (HIV-positive donors must be deferred and HIV-positive blood must be destroyed), whether counselling of donors is carried out (this is not done in most countries), whether blood is collected by individual hospitals or by a centralized blood transfusion service, and the number of safe units to be transfused (6). Costs per unit produced may vary from US$ 21 to $ 52.

In Zimbabwe, with a donor seroprevalence of almost 4%, the costs of HIV safety per unit of blood produced were US$ 3.90 (in addition to the regular costs). This included HIV screening (testing and associated costs) ($ 2.10), replacement of infected blood ($ 1.30), confirmatory HIV testing ($ 0.23) and counselling ($ 0.21) (6). In a hospital in Zambia, where HIV prevalence among donors was 16%, HIV tests accounted for one-third of blood collection costs (10). The total cost of HIV safety per blood unit was US$ 9.10.

Medical and laboratory staff need to be trained to follow guidelines or criteria for blood transfusion. Such training sessions can eventually decrease costs, since strict adherence to guidelines can reduce the number of blood transfusions. Continued supervision, however, is necessary for success (11).

The number of discarded blood units can be reduced by selecting low-risk donors and by using a deferral strategy. Selecting low-risk donors also incurs costs: donor recruiters must be employed, health education materials need to be developed and incentives may be necessary to retain donors (see Chapter 17). Donor deferral, based on the use of a set of screening questions, may also save costs (ref. 12; see also Chapter 17).

The total cost of HIV screening of all blood units also depends on the number of units produced per capita, which may vary from 70 to 600 per 100,000 per year (6). If we assume 400 transfusions per 100,000 population, then a district with a population of 300,000 can expect about 1,200 blood transfusions in a year. The cost of HIV safety is then only $ 6,000 per year (assuming $ 5.00 per unit), mainly for HIV tests. Additional costs, including donor recruitment, may add another $ 4,000–$ 6,000. Training medical staff and subsequent supervision may cost another $ 2,000.

Effectiveness: Blood screening cannot prevent all transfusion-associated HIV transmission. The test may fail to detect HIV (due to a sensitivity lower than 100% or an inappropriately conducted test), or the donor may be in the window period (see Chapter 16). The effectiveness of blood screening, however, is high. In a study in Zambia, it was estimated that financial benefits exceed costs by a factor of three (10). The cost per case of HIV infection prevented was $ 31.62, while the cost of this protection for the total population was only $ 0.03 per person.

8. Reducing HIV transmission through injections and other blood contact

HIV transmission can take place via the re-use of needles and syringes, although the proportion of HIV infection attributable to re-used syringes and needles in southern Tanzania has been estimated at only 0.4% (13). HIV risk for health workers is also low, although some professions such as surgeons are at increased risk. A study of traditional birth attendants in Rwanda showed a high frequency of blood–skin contact but the risk of HIV was only marginally increased compared to that of the overall population (ref. 14; see also Chapter 16).

Costs: The main components needed are supplies, training and supervision. Supplies may involve needles and syringes, sterilizing equipment, and protective gear including gloves for high-risk groups such as surgeons and midwives.

Training focuses on persuading health staff to improve injection and sterilization practices and to use protective gear regularly. Supervision is needed to ascertain that guidelines are properly followed. Workshops may also be needed for traditional healers and other non-medical staff who provide health care, including injections.

In a district with 300,000 people, the costs of providing needles and syringes for injections that are safe for both patients and health workers are estimated at US$ 45,000 (based on data from Mwanza Region: 2.5 injections per person per year and $ 0.06 per needle and syringe, including distribution costs). These calculations assume the use of disposable needles and syringes, which, contrary to common practice in most of Africa, are actually disposed of after use. In addition, sterilizing equipment that will last three years costs about US$ 2,000 (one pressure cooker at $ 50 for each of 40 health facilities). Training and supervision may add another US$ 3,000. Since the costs associated with improving injection and sterilization practices will also benefit many other programmes, we have arbitrarily decided that one-fourth of these costs should be allocated to general HIV prevention, which corresponds to a reduction of US$ 11,667 per year. Supplies of gloves for medical staff in high-risk professions cost about US$ 3,750, assuming 50 such staff each use about 300 pairs of gloves per year ($ 0.25 per pair). Table 4 sums up these costs.

Effectiveness: The number of HIV infections attributed to injections is estimated to be low. Therefore, the effectiveness (including that with respect to cost) of this intervention is also likely to be low.

Table 4. Annual costs of providing safe injections for both patients and health workers

Item	Cost per year ($)
Needles/syringes	45,000
Sterilizing equipment ($ 2/3 years)	667
Training and supervision ($ 3/3 years)	1,000
Subtotal	46,667
Minus 1/4 (costs attributed to HIV prevention in general)	- 11,667
Subtotal costs	35,000
Gloves	3,750
Total costs	38,750

9. AIDS Care – training health workers

Training health workers to deal with HIV/AIDS and its consequences has many aspects. Training is needed to bring health workers' knowledge of HIV/AIDS up to date and allow them to provide better care to HIV/AIDS patients. It should also improve their skills in diagnosing tuberculosis and other related illnesses and undertaking appropriate action. Counselling skills should also be included, and the ability to support community home-based care initiatives should be strengthened. In addition to the care component, training courses for health workers can enhance their ability to educate the public about HIV/AIDS, and thus contribute to reducing HIV transmission. STD control can also be integrated into this course, or a separate course on STDs may be given (budgeted under STD control).

An independent learning programme described in the Chapter 12 is a way of training a broader group of health workers. While courses on HIV/AIDS usually are given for staff in charge of health facilities, an independent learning programme can include all staff of facilities (nurse attendants, cleaners and others).

Costs: A one-week training course, such as proposed in Chapter 12, will cost in the range of US$ 1,500–5,000 depending on the availability of training facilities, the level of allowances paid to trainers and the cost of facilitators. Training materials, including written and audiovisual materials, may add another $ 500 per course. Two to three such workshops of about 25 participants each will be required to cover all health facilities in a district.

A district in Tanzania with 40 health facilities required about US$ 15,000 to cover all health facilities and all staff working in those facilities via an independent learning programme. This included a set of five books for 525 health workers (US$ 2,000), allowances for trainers (US$ 2,000), and facilitators' workshops for follow-up training (US$ 9,000). This programme involves health unit-based training, and should be repeated every three to four years to keep skills up-to-date (see Chapter 12).

Table 5. Estimated annual costs of voluntary testing centre

Item	Lower salaries (US$)	Higher salaries (US$)
Renting premises	500	500
IEC	2,000	2,000
Counsellor salary (1)	2,000	10,000
Transport	200	200
Lab staff salaries	500	2,500
HIV tests (1)	1,100	1,100
TOTAL	6,300	16,300
Cost per test	6.30	16.30

Effectiveness: The effectiveness of training is difficult to estimate, but common sense indicates it is necessary to provide health workers with training on HIV/AIDS, as they are likely to be the main source of care for HIV/AIDS patients. Medical care-associated transmission through needles and injections will be reduced somewhat and the quality of care should improve. The role of health workers as catalysts for change in sexual behaviour in the community may be less visible, but can be important.

10. Counselling for HIV prevention

Counselling can be seen as both an HIV prevention activity and a component of AIDS care. The aim of HIV-prevention counselling is to encourage people to change their sexual behaviour, irrespective of their HIV status. Counselling is also part of proper medical and psychological care for HIV-infected patients. In this case the process involves multiple contacts between counsellor and patient. This form of counselling is discussed below, under Care for AIDS patients.

Costs: The costs of running a voluntary HIV testing and counselling centre may include renting premises, IEC to increase public awareness about the existence of the testing centre and the importance of knowing one's HIV status, salary for a counsellor (usually a trained health worker), equipment to draw and collect blood (filter paper is the cheapest method), a reliable HIV laboratory (which does HIV testing in accord with well-established procedures) and transport to the laboratory.

Follow-up counselling of HIV-positive and HIV-negative individuals or groups may also be included. The number of counsellors needed depends on the number of individuals coming for counselling. If we assume an attendance of five persons per day (including pre- and post-test counselling), then the running costs of a small voluntary testing unit would be US$ 6,300 yearly if salaries are low, and about three times that if salaries are higher (see Table 5). Some costs can be recovered by charging for HIV testing (e.g $ 1–2 per test). It is likely that people will be willing to pay for this important service, so that a small fee will not affect utilization.

Effectiveness: The effectiveness of counselling in bringing about behavioural change in general populations is unknown. Some studies have found favourable changes in discordant couples after HIV testing or in other situations, but the evidence is not conclusive. In societies where AIDS is associated with considerable stigma, many clients – even with counselling – are likely to refuse to accept that their HIV-test results were positive: then no behavioural changes will take place. Many more people will not even bother to take an HIV test. Others, however, will change their sexual behaviour even if their test result is negative.

11. Care for AIDS patients

The number of AIDS patients who need terminal care in districts is increasing. The increase in adult morbidity during HIV infection may be fairly limited (about 25% increased morbidity and health services utilization by HIV-infected adults compared to HIV-negative adults) (14), but medical expenditures increase sharply in the terminal phase of the illness. AIDS in children is less common than in adults, but may also affect health services, notably in-patient care. This increase is of particular concern to district hospitals, where the heaviest burden of AIDS care may fall. As part of a continuum of care, home-based care programmes may also be an option (see Chapter 18).

Cost: Costs per AIDS patient in Tanzania have been estimated at US$ 290 per adult case and $ 195 per pediatric case, assuming that drugs are available. Three-quarters of these costs are attributable to nursing and institutional care, while drugs account for one-fourth of the total. It was assumed that 25% of these adults would develop tuberculosis, and estimated that the average cost of tuberculosis care for each of these HIV-infected adults would be $ 59 (5).

In a district with a population of 300,000 and a stable HIV situation (that is, where incidence has been 1% for at least ten years) about 1,000 adults develop AIDS each year. The cost of providing medical services for these patients for one year will be about US$ 200,000. Children with AIDS may add another US$ 50,000 to this amount. Since not all patients seek care, and available treatment may be limited (more likely in particularly resource-poor countries like Tanzania than in more affluent countries such as Zimbabwe), actual expenditures may be lower.

Decentralizing AIDS care – that is, using home-based care – may reduce district costs by 25–28% (5), even when the cost of support from the necessary peripheral health workers is taken into account. Both morbidity and concomitant use of outpatient treatment services might be expected to increase by 25% for HIV-infected persons compared to HIV-negative persons, that is, averaged over the whole duration of HIV infection. In a population with an HIV prevalence of 10%, increases in outpatient costs during HIV infection are thus moderate: in this case the overall increase in outpatient care utilization is about 2.5% (15).

The effectiveness of AIDS care in terms of preventing new HIV infections is very low, and therefore it cannot be considered an intervention to reduce transmission. The main objective is humanitarian, although community-based care does increase AIDS awareness, and institutional care enhances health worker and media awareness.

12. Survivor assistance

Widows and children may need assistance in terms of adequate food, shelter and funds for school fees (16). Even prior to the AIDS epidemic, adult mortality (15–49) was about 0.5% per year, so the problems of orphans and widows are not new. Extended families were generally able to cope with this in the past. In the current situation there will be more two-parent orphans than before, since AIDS often affects both parents, and the number of orphans may become too high for the traditional coping system to handle. Finally, AIDS expenditures may be higher than those of other illnesses that lead to death, since the final stages may be prolonged.

Costs: If adult mortality due to AIDS is about 1% in a district with a population of 300,000 (suggesting close to 1,000 annual adult deaths), and we assume each adult has three children on average, almost 3,000 children may be newly orphaned each year. In a district with lower HIV incidence and prevalence (about 0.5% and 5% respectively), this is about 1,500 children. The number of two-parent orphans is assumed to be 300 and 150 respectively, at 10% and 5% HIV prevalence levels (at age 15 a child ceases to be classified as an orphan by our definition).

Orphanages are considered to be rather expensive (16). They may be budgeted at US$ 500 per child per year in rural areas. If the majority of two-parent orphans were to be put in orphanages, costs would easily exceed $ 200,000–$ 300,000 per year. If orphans are to be helped outside of orphanages, and if substantial coverage is to be achieved in a district – that is, if families taking in children are to receive meaningful help – costs are likely to reach US$ 20,000 or more per year. Direct transfers (food, clothing, basic commodities) may be useful to help poor families through the initial crises following the death of an AIDS patient. Costs may vary, from $ 5 to $ 15 per month per child, and may continue for a period of 6–12 months. Costs of a community child care centre and feeding post are US$ 20–40 per day. Subsidies for school fees and uniforms range from US$ 10–20 for primary school children and US$ 70–100 for secondary school children.

Where community help is not sufficient, small orphanages costing less than $ 50,000 per year, with heavy external support for children who are not caught by the community safety net, plus a district fund of US$ 20,000–50,000 for temporary assistance in the more difficult initial period, may be a feasible solution.

Effectiveness: It is not clear which approach is the most effective in alleviating the difficult circumstances of orphans and widows. Among the concerns is how to avoid undermining traditional coping mechanisms and creating dependency. Moreover, apart from any other considerations, relying on orphanages on a large scale is very costly.

Comparing interventions

A comparison of the costs and effectiveness of the interventions described above suggests that reducing HIV in high-transmission areas (promotion of safer sex), condom distribution, STD control, safer sex promotion for youth and ensuring a safe blood supply are high-priority interventions. Priorities may change as the epidemic progresses. Initially, it may be necessary to use all resources to provide interventions aimed at reducing HIV transmission. Later on, care and survivor assistance may become relatively more important.

In our example of a district with 300,000 people and an HIV prevalence of 5% to 10%, a comprehensive HIV prevention programme covering the whole district population with STD control, intensive health education, youth activities, condom promotion and distribution, training of health workers, and a safe blood supply could easily cost $ 350,000, or $ 1.16 per person ($ 3.50 per sexually active adult). This does not include capital costs or most government or other staff salaries. The additional costs associated with AIDS care depend on the proportion of adults in a community who develop AIDS, how many of them seek care, and the level and cost of the care available. We estimate, based on the discussion in points 11–12 that a further US$ 200,000–300,000 per year may be needed in our example for basic care of AIDS patients, including a home-based care programme and a fund for survivor assistance. This comes to US$ 1 per capita per year, or US$ 3 per adult.

Examples of district approaches

Many factors affect the ultimate choice of an AIDS programme in a district. What is beyond doubt is that informed choices must be made and priorities set. In the following analysis we focus on economic resources as a major factor in making these choices. In making these decisions, it is important to remember that the amount of money available to a district is not static: if the government budget is low, efforts should be made to attract additional donor funding, to generate local resources and/or to invite NGOs to team up with the district to make a more comprehensive programme possible.

Table 6 shows options for district AIDS programmes at different funding levels, all in a district with a population of 300,000 and adult HIV prevalence between 5% and 10%. In this example safe blood supply and interventions in high-transmission areas (STD control, AIDS education, peer educator programmes) have been given the highest priority, followed by district-wide STD control and youth.
    Within a total budget of US$ 25,000 per year only a limited programme is possible in high-transmission areas, but a safe blood supply can be assured. With a budget of US$ 50,000, high-transmission area interventions can be expanded and a youth programme can be initiated there. Alternatively, if treatable STDs are a major public health problem, the focus could be on ensuring improved STD services with district-wide coverage. Within the US$ 50,000 budget, very little money is available to improve AIDS care: the funding in Table 6 provides for one training course, for health workers in high-transmission areas.
    With a US$ 100,000 budget, more than one-third of funds can go into comprehensive programmes for high-transmission areas, and a larger proportion of youth can be covered by AIDS and sex education. District-wide coverage with improved STD services via

Table 6. District AIDS programmes in relation to funding levels

Resources available	General population	HTA/ target groups incl. STD control	Youth	Blood & medical	Coun- selling	AIDS care	Survivor assistance
Very limited ($25,000)	–	15,000	–	10,000			
Limited ($ 50,000)	25,000 (STD control)	15,000	–	10,000			
Limited ($ 50,000)	–	25,000	15,000	10,000			
Moderate ($ 100,000)	30,000 (STD control)	30,000	25,000	10,000		5,000	
High ($ 200,000)	30,000 (STD control)	60,000	60,000	10,000		20,000	20,000
$1 per capita ($ 300,000)	30,000 (STD control)	80,000	110,000	10,000	10,000	40,000	20,000

health facilities can also be achieved.

If $ 200,000 is available, money can be set aside for AIDS care, and possibly also for a district survivor fund to help orphans and widows through the most difficult period. With $ 1.00 per capita ($ 300,000 total) a fairly extensive district HIV prevention programme can be set up, although district-wide coverage is not included. Funds available for AIDS patient care are still limited, but some AIDS care can be offered within existing health facilities.

Conclusion

There is no doubt that prevention of HIV and STDs ranks among the most cost-effective of health interventions. At district level, the choices made need to assure that the limited resources available are used in ways that will have the highest possible effect on HIV prevention. A careful analysis of the social dynamics and the distribution of sexually transmitted diseases in a district makes it possible to identify high-trans-mission areas. Resources, can then be targeted to increase their impact. Even when budgets are relatively limited, comprehensive HIV prevention activities directed specifically to high-transmission areas appear to be feasible and have considerably higher cost-effectiveness than diffuse low-intensity interventions aiming to cover the whole district population.

Further reading

WHO. *The costs of HIV/AIDS prevention strategies in developing countries.* WHO/GPA/DIR/ 93.2. Geneva, 1993.

Directory of European funders of HIV/AIDS projects in developing countries and *Guide to technical support available to HIV/AIDS projects in developing countries.* UK NGO AIDS Consortium, (Fenner Brockway House, 37–39 Great Guildford Street) London SE1 0ES.

WHO. *Provision of HIV/AIDS care in resource-constrained settings.* Geneva.

The hidden cost of AIDS: the challenge of HIV to development. The Panos Institute, (9 White Lion Street) London N1 9PD, United Kingdom, 1992.

References

1. World Bank. *World Development Report 1993. Investing in health.* New York, Oxford University Press, 1993.

2. Hanson K. AIDS: what does economics have to offer. *Health Policy and Planning* 1992, 7: 315–328.

3. Ng'weshemi JZL, Boerma JT, Barongo L et al. Changes in male sexual behaviour in response to the AIDS epidemic: 1. Quantitative evidence from a cohort study in urban Tanzania. *TANESA Working Paper,* no. 6. Mwanza, 1995.

4. Grosskurth H, Mosha F, Todd J et al. The impact of comprehensive management of sexually transmitted diseases on the incidence of HIV infection. *Lancet* 1995, 346: 530–536.

5. World Bank. *AIDS Assessment at planning study.* Washington DC, 1992.

6. WHO. *The costs of HIV/AIDS prevention strategies in developing countries.* WHO/GPA/DIR/93.2. Geneva, 1993.

7. Moses S, Plummer FA, Ngugi EN et al. Controlling HIV in Africa. Effectiveness and cost of an intervention in a high frequency STD transmitter care groups. *AIDS* 1991, 5: 407–411.

8. Soderlund N, Lavis J, Broomberg J et al. The costs of HIV prevention strategies in developing countries. *Bulletin of the WHO* 1993, 71: 595–604.

9. Robinson NJ, Mulder DW, Anvert B et al. Modelling the impact of alternate HIV interventions and strategies in rural Uganda. *AIDS* 1995, 9: 1263–1270.

10. Foster S, Buve A. Benefits of HIV screening of blood transfusions in Zambia. *Lancet* 1995, 346: 225–227.

11. Vos J, Gumodoka B, Van Asten HA et al. Changes in blood transfusion practices after the introduction of consensus guidelines in Mwanza Region, Tanzania. *AIDS* 1994, 8: 1135–1140.

12. McFarland W, Kahn JG, Katzenstein DA, Mvere D, Shamu R. Deferral of blood donors with risk factors for HIV infection saves lives and money in Zimbabwe. *Journal of AIDS and Human Retrovirology* 1995: 183–192.

13. Hoelscher M, Riedner G, Hemed Y et al. Estimating the number of HIV transmissions through reused syringes and needles in the Mbeya Region Tanzania. *AIDS* 1994, 8: 1609–1615.

14. Habimana P, Bulterys M, Usabuwera P et al. A survey of occupational blood contact among traditional birth attendants in Rwanda. *AIDS* 1994, 8: 701–704.

15. Kikumbi SN, Isingo R, Boerma JT. Consequences of adult HIV infection for outpatient morbidity and treatment costs: a prospective study in Tanzania. *TANESA Working Paper,* no. 10. Mwanza, 1996. (Forthcoming in *Health, Policy and Planning.*)

16. Ainsworth M, Rwegarulira AA. Coping with the AIDS epidemic in Tanzania: survivor assistance. *Technical Working Paper,* no. 6. Washington DC, Population, Health and Nutrition Division, Africa Technical Department, World Bank, 1992.

22 Integration and sustainability

Gijs Walraven and Japheth Ng'weshemi

- What are the advantages and disadvantages of vertical programmes for HIV/AIDS and for STDs?
- How do AIDS programmes relate to reproductive health in general?
- Does health sector reform affect AIDS programmes?
- How can NGOs, communities and districts join in programmes?
- What can be done to increase sustainability?

Introduction

The rapid spread of the AIDS epidemic in its first decade justified special efforts and increased funding directed toward assessing the magnitude and consequences of the epidemic. Such efforts have also been needed to single out the most useful approaches to reducing its spread and impact. However, it is now evident that the AIDS epidemic cannot easily be contained: for the coming decades, this will remain one of the health problems districts need to address. Even if HIV incidence were to decline rapidly in the near future, the associated health problems would last for decades.

This chapter examines the prospects for integrating an HIV prevention and AIDS care programme in a district health system, and the effects this can be expected to have on its sustainability. Before considering either integration or sustainability, though, it is necessary to outline the realities of the financial, organizational, and management problems that face the resource-constrained countries of Africa. Since integration is seen as essential to sustainability, this aspect is explored first. The chapter then turns to the more specific aspect of the sustainability of an HIV prevention and AIDS control programme.

Background

After achieving independence in the 1960s, many African countries undertook ambitious programmes, including an expansion of health care services: building referral and district hospitals, health centres, dispensaries and health posts; establishing basic health care and training large numbers of health workers. The district was regarded in many countries as the basic organizational unit for health care services, especially after the Alma Ata conference on primary health care (PHC) in 1978. Ministries of health were determined to strengthen district health systems, as a means of implementing PHC. Basic indices of health improved considerably during the 1970s, with substantial reductions in infant and under-five mortality and an increasing life expectancy (1). The role of health services in these improvements is controversial, but most authorities agree that advances in primary health care have made substantial contributions (2, 3).

Financial and technical support for primary health care programmes have often come via 'pump-priming' financing from international agencies, such as UNICEF and WHO, bilateral arrangements with donor countries, and international NGOs. The usual expectation has been that, with time, in-country resources would develop to the point of being able to pick up most or all of the costs of the programmes.

During the 1980s and 1990s progress faltered. Support for health services has been diminishing. Most African economies have been in recession for a number of years, resulting in a reduction of the internal resources available for health care expenditures. This problem has been compounded by competing internal priorities and imposed structural adjustment programmes, a number of which are considered to have been directly related to diminished government spending on health care in sub-Saharan African countries (4–7). Worldwide, per capita expenditures on health are estimated to average US$ 24 per annum in low income countries (range $ 4 to $ 158) and $ 1860 (range $ 383 to $ 2673) in countries with established market economies (1). External support – intended to be short term – has become essential to sustain programmes in the long term. Nevertheless, the priorities of international organizations and donor governments are moving elsewhere, and they are reducing their inputs to Africa. At the same time, it has been impossible for most African countries to pick up the cost of programmes that were initially funded externally, while individuals are also unable to pay a significant portion. Although families often incur considerable indirect costs in receiving health care, personal income has not increased sufficiently to allow health insurance schemes or full charges to individuals to pay health care costs (8).

Meanwhile, in many African countries government staff have experienced reductions in real wages, lowering their morale and often forcing them to look for additional sources of income. Even where the health pyramid has broadened its base, health planning has mainly followed a 'top–down' approach. At national level, PHC systems have been saved from total collapse only by vertical programmes, which have continued to receive external funding.

Decentralization has been seen as a way to improve management structures, and has been encouraged by organizations such as the World Bank. As decentralization has begun, it has changed the role of ministries of health in coordinating services and resources. There have been many changes, but in many countries no clear organizational structure has emerged. The critical preliminary analysis – including that of the political realities – was insufficient to understand the complexities of decentralization. Often there has been a failure to understand that for decentralization to work, not only responsibility but also authority (including authority over use of funds) would also have to be devolved. In addition, the tropical climate in much of sub-Saharan Africa makes for high maintenance costs, thereby increasing the burden of recurrent costs on health budgets. There are increasing difficulties, as the buildings and equipment purchased by the major investments of the 1960s and 1970s are now often in poor condition. HIV/AIDS thus add to the difficulties of health services that are already under considerable stress. The examples in Box 1 illustrate the nature of some district health care management problems that may affect AIDS programmes.

Box 1. Examples of management problems in district health care

- The district AIDS coordinator and the district tuberculosis/leprosy coordinator work in isolation from each other. The two programmes are funded by different donors and have separate information and reporting systems, separate accounts and separate supply systems.
- The district medical officer has just attended an STD control workshop in the regional capital. When she returns to the district, she finds it impossible to hold a workshop: all available funds have been earmarked for specific programmes, and district workers refuse to participate in the workshop if they do not receive allowances.
- The AIDS programme falls under the multisectoral district PHC committee. Its budget depends entirely on resource allocations from national level – but no resources to implement plans have been received for more than one year. The committee rarely meets.
- The district AIDS programme coordinator reports directly to the regional AIDS coordinator in the office of the regional medical officer, and a similar procedure exists for most other district officers. This undermines the district medical officer 's potential role as a team leader.
- AIDS has spread unevenly throughout the district, so that allocations of staff and drug supplies for health facilities need to be adjusted, but no decisions are taken.

Various approaches have been used in attempts to strengthen the management of health services. A district study in Tanzania has concluded that without changes to the system as a whole, the three main interventions used until recently (management training, development of information systems, use of planning and evaluation methodologies) will make only marginal improvements to health services management. Changes are needed, for example, to provide managers and health professionals with both incentives for improving efficiency and quality of care and the authority that will be required to improve the situation (9).

Integration

At present, lack of resources is not the only problem; also, the resources that are available may not be used effectively. In particular, the resources of vertical programmes may duplicate each other and their separate management may be wasteful. NGOs and programmes of the district government may include different elements. If these were to be integrated, they could form the basis for a more comprehensive approach, in which programmes would reinforce and strengthen each other. Integration of vertical programmes is thus a major point of interest. However, integration may be complex: for example, staff may have incompatible job descriptions and salary scales. Integration implies bringing different partners and components together in one system; their varied objectives and resources will need to be harmonized. Further, the potential for integration is affected by many factors outside the district. In planning to fund programmes, donors from other countries who want to ensure sustainability need to bear these points in mind during planning phases: the more integrated a programme is, the more sustainable it is apt to be.

An integrated health system comprises not only government and non-government health services; it involves communities, other government sectors (such as education, water, community development), private practitioners and the traditional health care system as well.

Vertical programmes

Many districts have vertical programmes with specific trained staff who have their own supplies and possibly transport. Their supervision is often carried out by a higher level of administration. Common vertical programmes include tuberculosis and leprosy control, an expanded programme on immunization (EPI), control of diarrhoeal disease (CDD), maternal and child health, family planning and in wealthier urban areas, even school health. And now AIDS programmes and STD control programmes have been added to this list. These programmes are often heavily funded by donors. At district level, integration of such programmes is advantageous on many levels, from the possibility to plan a coordinated approach, involving a broader spectrum of staff and providing supervision with a more local focus, to daily questions of cost efficiency such as sharing transport among workers. These possibilities for encouraging linkages and making more efficient use of scarce resources lie behind the assertion that integrating programmes and organizations can increase sustainability.

While some are more easily integrated than others, integration could involve a broad variety of vertical programmes. However, the benefits of integration are greater when programmes overlap with respect to contents and operational aspects. The most obvious partner for an AIDS programme is one for control of STDs; in many countries this integration is already taking place. Tuberculosis control also needs to be integrated with HIV/AIDS programmes, although its link with AIDS care is easier to demonstrate than that with HIV prevention (see Chapter 19).

Many arguments can be put forward in favour of integrating AIDS programmes with other aspects of reproductive health, such as family planning, prevention of infertility and unsafe abortion, and even child survival. Integration of HIV prevention activities into more general reproductive health programmes makes sense not only because of overlap in programme contents; HIV prevention may be more effective when addressed in a broader context. This points up the error in a common assumption of vertical programmes, that 'their' health problem is perceived as a priority by the community. HIV/AIDS provides an example in which this is often not the case: other health problems may provide a much better entry point for prevention than a programme focused on HIV/AIDS alone (see Box 2).

Box 2. Should HIV prevention activities be integrated into reproductive health? Examples from the field

After the first decade of the AIDS epidemic the disease appears to have become endemic in many areas of Africa, including Mwanza Region, Tanzania: HIV prevalence (based on surveillance of antenatal clinic attenders) has been stable since 1991. Efforts to contain the AIDS epidemic need to continue relentlessly, but there is a particular need to expand AIDS control efforts and address the issues related to reproductive health. Further, integration of the two programmes is likely to increase the effectiveness of AIDS education efforts.

During the implementation of the TANESA programme multiple linkages between AIDS prevention and control and reproductive health issues have been encountered.

schoolgirls: role plays in rural schools make clear that for sexually active schoolgirls the primary concern is pregnancy, not AIDS;
fishermen: fishermen include a large group of young unmarried and mobile males, who are accustomed to risk-taking behaviour. The main health concern is STDs, which are rampant, not AIDS;
bar workers: many claim that abortion, prevention of pregnancy, infertility and STDs are more immediate and greater problems for them than AIDS;
infertility: after controlling for other factors, a rural survey and a hospital-based case control study both showed HIV prevalence to be considerably higher among infertile women than for others. Infertility was also associated with marital instability and with a greater number of sexual partners over a lifetime;
gender issues: members of women's groups complain about their limited ability to insist that men, including their spouses, use condoms. This is also clear from in-depth interviews with female office workers. In those interviews women tend to picture their spouses as an important health threat (AIDS and STDs), while the mere suggestion of condom use is out of the question.
antenatal care: STDs are all highly prevalent among antenatal women in Mwanza Region, affecting both mother and child and putting women at increased risk of HIV/AIDS.

These practical experiences of the TANESA project not only demonstrate the many natural linkages between AIDS control activities and reproductive health, but also suggest that AIDS activities may benefit considerably from broadening the scope of 'reproductive health' to encompass AIDS issues as well.

Intersectoral linkage and coordination

Health is an integral part of the socioeconomic development of a community. Thus it is preferable to coordinate health activities with those of other sectors. Cooperation among sector specialists – needed to help villages and larger communities prepare operational plans, supervise, monitor and evaluate health-related activities – is better at district level than at central level. Working together facilitates information sharing and generation of new ideas, and can both increase political support and lead to more efficient utilization of resources. In the absence of cooperation, duplication and fragmentation are likely; the resulting failures stand in the way of the goal of improving physical, mental and social well-being.

The district level could also provide an opportunity to bring government administrators together with NGOs and the private sector. This could happen in a far more informal and less threatening environment than would have been possible at national or regional level. However, at all levels there has been a lack of dialogue between the government and NGOs and among NGOs themselves. This interferes with the establishment of a partnership and coordination of efforts. Full NGO involvement in the formulation and implementation of health policies is a vital step in districts.

Training. Integrating opportunities and facilitating cross-programme and cross-sector training of staff in a district with respect to AIDS are important steps. An integrated training programme can be prepared, based on a training needs assessment (see also Chapter 12). Here too, the possibility of making use of the strong points of the varied organizations involved is a valuable part of programme integration. For example, training for counselling and community involvement is often done very effectively by NGOs, while training for treatment can be well-organized by government agencies. Trainers can thus be drawn from the district, region, and from NGOs. Such training should cross programme boundaries, involving government workers from multiple sectors, NGOs, private sectors and traditional medical practitioners. This is also a chance to begin real integration: for example, in courses on HIV/AIDS, tuberculosis and STD control need to be included, 'modern' counsellors and traditional medical practioners can discuss counselling approaches to patients with HIV/AIDS, and the health and education sector can jointly conduct training for school HIV/AIDS programmes.

Community involvement

The primary goal of an integrated programme is to develop community-based interventions that will increase the knowledge and ability of the community to facilitate behavioural changes – changes that hopefully will lead to better reproductive health. In integrating comprehensive reproductive health programmes, it is important to plan for capacity building, both at community and health facility levels, and for ways to forge strong links between the newly-joined programme elements. Even a mobilized community, fully aware of the meaning of safe motherhood, fertility issues and safe sex, can make a significant impact (on e.g. maternal mortality, birth rates or HIV incidence) only if the health personnel at local level are trained, have proper equipment and supplies and know how to work with the community. Similarly, the best equipped and supplied district hospital, health centre or dispensary, with a staff of well trained workers can achieve the desired objectives only if the community is aware of the importance of interventions available to promote safe motherhood, control fertility and prevent HIV and STDs. Working simultaneously towards community involvement and staff development is also essential because as the community begins to understand more – and to feel ownership for programmes – they are apt to place increased demands on health workers to deliver more adequate services.

Community health development refers to activities that help individuals, families and communities deal with problems of living, in particular in relation to health problems. Communities are often seen in a simplified way, as homogeneous, harmonious, relatively autonomous, and well-bounded entities (10). The local leaders who are often accepted as spokespersons are frequently relatively better-off people, generally older men, whose interests can be quite different from others in the community.

Involvement of a broad spectrum of the community does not generally arise spontaneously. Initial stimulation is needed (see also the chapter on community involvement). This may even be more so given a topic like AIDS which, especially in the beginning of the epidemic, is a less obvious health problem. Community development workers who have been trained to take an egalitarian and 'participatory' approach to their work are apt to be better equipped to guide community involvement and empowerment than health workers. For the more 'technocratic' health workers who may feel that the quickest way to change behaviour is to tell people what to do and how to do it, it is a meaningful and challenging learning experience to work together with community development workers and staff of the other sectors present at local level. This gives them a chance to begin to realize that the initially slower, more difficult approach of community involvement is, in the long term, the way to achieve real and lasting change.

Integration of prevention and care. Relief from personal suffering is clearly the top health priority of every individual. It follows that curative care, backed by a good, regular input of drugs and other supplies, is felt as a major need by many individuals and communities. Part of the process of increasing community awareness is to help the community to begin to understand the benefits to individuals and families of comprehensive services, which should include health promotion, specific prevention, treatment and rehabilitation and cover all aspects (including social and emotional) of care. The need for comprehensive services also pertains to AIDS programmes, although the link is less obvious because there is no cure for AIDS. As suggested earlier, however, building an AIDS care component into an HIV prevention programme may help to make the latter more effective.

Integration of traditional medicine with PHC can also be an asset in working toward community involvement. Traditional healers retain their popularity because they are a part of community life – they offer a more or less integrated system of social measures and curative procedures, with important individual and community health effects. Further, they have often been cited as being accessible, available, acceptable and adaptable. They survive because they represent a culturally understood approach to managing many physical and psychosocial illnesses. Integration with traditional medicine requires 'modern' district health workers to acquire more knowledge of the possibilities of local traditional medicine. It can also be a way for them to learn more about the needs of individuals and communities. Dialogue, which assumes two-way communication and cooperation between modern and traditional medicine, is a necessary element in the development of an integrated district health system. Particularly with regard to AIDS, traditional healers can play an important role, because they are able to provide the spiritual and psychological care that is one of the greatest needs of AIDS patients. Further, training for traditional healers may encourage them to avoid inappropriate use of drugs and perhaps to refer patients who can be best helped within the modern district health system.

Non-discrimination against AIDS. Vulnerable groups – those who are seen as being at high risk – are often marginalized within the community, and may not have access to current health programmes. If for example female bar workers are targeted, it is necessary to first check if this group can be reached by the regular health services (Box 3). If targeted groups are not reached, integration of HIV/AIDS programmes with others will be more difficult.

Box 3. Special services for vulnerable groups

In an urban ward in Mwanza, female bar workers did not make much use of existing health services. Health authorities felt these women needed extra services to control STDs and to provide an entry point for on-going HIV prevention activities (health education, condom distribution). Therefore, special services were set up for these women, run by government staff seconded to a donor-aided project. This service was only open to female bar workers.
At a later stage, services were expanded to include other reproductive health issues. This was used as an opportunity to enhance integration of health services for female bar workers into the regular health system. A nurse-midwife from the local government clinic became responsible for family planning and maternal and child health services among the bar workers and their children. In addition, STD services at the local government and private clinics were also strengthened, to treat the STDs of the bar workers' clients as well as others.

In the longer term, integration of information, education and legislation are needed to create a societal environment that protects the individual rights of people with AIDS. Often people with AIDS do not make their disease public because they fear discrimination. AIDS was and is still often perceived as the problem of others – marginalized people. This makes their integration and participation in programmes difficult. Yet this participation is needed to assist in attaining sustainability and prevent the spread of the disease. Where organizations of people with AIDS exist, they should be given a prominent place, encouraged and stimulated.

Facilitating and ensuring integration

The management problems in district health management shown in Box 1 are related to factors including lack of resources, lack of information, lack of coordination, lack of skills, unclear procedures, and poorly motivated staff. An integrated district health system with good management and organization is well-positioned to initiate integration and begin to solve some of the related problems. However, as noted above, for such a system to fulfil its potential, it needs to be situated within a clear organizational structure and line of authority. Among other points, the role, responsibilities and authority of the district medical officer and the district health management team within the system must be made emphatically clear. When vertical programmes such as tuberculosis, family planning or STD/HIV control are decentralized and are to be integrated with general health care programmes in a district, this should be facilitated by placing not just responsibility but also full financial and administrative authority at district level.

Decentralization of authority is particularly important because the district level can be more sensitive than a distant central administration to the needs of local people, and is better able to encourage their participation in the planning and management of their health services. This level should also be the best equipped to encourage intersectoral cooperation to promote health at the level where motivation can be greatest. It is in the district that 'top–down and bottom–up meet, if they meet at all' (11). To be able to 'meet', the district should be a large enough unit to have supporting technical and managerial staff available. Policies can then be adapted, thus making them more responsive and relevant to local needs and circumstances; flexibility can be fostered; community participation can be enhanced; innovation and creativity can be initiated and tried out without having to be enacted for the whole country. Admittedly this is textbook language; the realities are still somewhat different.

Integration does not just happen. It requires organization, as well as educated and discerning staff and communities. The organizational structures most commonly involved are district development committees, PHC committees, district health management teams, and NGO coordinating networks. When advocacy for the integration and sustainability of an AIDS programme is effective, local government structure and organization can also be a strong force for integration. Some of the several factors that are needed to shape an integrated district health system are summarized in Box 4.

Sustainabily

The idea that investments in health and social programmes involve heavy expenditures without providing a significant return is a misconception. Proper access to health care, is an economically productive life- and money-saving force (12). As the number of people affected by HIV/AIDS rises, the direct and indirect impacts and costs are becoming more clear. We are combatting a severe epidemic, and yet will have to answer difficult questions about the future of the programmes being set up: how many of the activities related to prevention and care are sustainable? Should all elements of an HIV/AIDS control programme be established with the idea that they will become sustainable?

Box 4. Important factors in an integrated district health system

- responsible decentralization
- clear organizational structure, with appropriate authority for health care delegated to the district level
- community involvement
- intersectoral cooperation
- partnership and coordination with NGOs and organizations of people who have AIDS
- dialogue and cooperation between modern and traditional medicine
- involvement and protection of marginalized groups
- a health information system based on two-way communication
- effective education for health and other areas
- joint training
- human resource development
- curative and preventive care
- integration of vertical programmes: such as AIDS, STD, tuberculosis, maternal and child health, family planning

---

Or is it warranted to have some components that are unsustainable, which will pay off later because they are expected to have an important pay off.

No matter which components are seen as essential, to maintain programme continuity several aspects of an AIDS programme will need to be sustained, including resource inputs (e.g. skilled personnel, equipment, funds for allowances, maintenance for buildings and transport). There are also processes that have to be kept going to maintain the volume and quality of work (supervision, organization, training and continuing education, community involvement and empowerment).

Previously the assumption was that after initial help from donors in creating a system and facilities, recipient organizations would manage the systems that had been established, and take care of future needs. This belief has lost its credibility. Health care can never, if equity is taken into account, become an investment that pays for itself in terms of cash, as might be expected in industry (13). At present, the burden of unpayable recurrent costs is reaching a point of crisis.

This crisis with respect to funding for recurrent costs suggests that if sustainability is only about economic aspects, it cannot be achieved. Health care in low income, resource poor areas requires financing from outside. Recently the World Bank proposed a minimum package of essential public health and clinical services based on the cost-effectiveness of the interventions, the size and distribution of health problems, and the resources available (1). The most cost-effective package contains all elements of primary reproductive health care (see Box 5). However, the total cost of even this 'sub'package already exceeds the estimated total amount presently available for health in countries such as Tanzania, Malawi and Zaire.

Box 5. Per capita costs of primary reproductive health care

Antenatal and delivery care	US$ 3.8
Family planning	US$ 0.9
AIDS prevention	US$ 2.0
STD treatment	US$ 0.2
Total	**US$ 6.9**

Source: World Bank. World Development Report 1993

Where is the necessary funding to come from? At a time when enormous savings should be possible in many countries, for example by decreasing military expenditures, pressure must be put on politicians and government representatives to re-examine the priority they accord the health and social sectors. At district level, local leaders need to be made aware of the situation and mobilized to help in obtaining resources.

Apart from additional funds, a more efficient and effective use of available resources will be required. This makes substantial health system reform and reallocation of public spending, based on national level policy changes, important. This would mean, for example, spending far less on cost-*in*effective interventions like tertiary hospital care. Decentralization, combined with more consistent and coordinated support to district health systems and reinforcement of management capacity at this level, will be needed.

Increasing efficiency and effectiveness will demand the conceptualization of a practical approach to 'minimum district health care': a way to realize maximum benefits from the minimum resources available. This approach has to do with developing flexibility and creativity and learning to weigh competing needs in a variety of situations. It will require real community involvement and concerted attention to other issues discussed in this chapter. The cost of AIDS care can also be reduced and the well-being of people with AIDS enhanced by improving services in a cost-effective way. While such programmes are not inexpensive, there are several examples of alternative approaches to inpatient care, which focus on home and community ambulatory care. These can improve quality of life for people with AIDS and still reduce costs, in comparison to inpatient care (see Chapter 18).

Policy changes and implementation of concepts such as minimum district health care are essential; however, major improvements in financial support to the system will still be needed (14). Supplementation of domestic resources with considerable long-term, external donor assistance will remain vital to filling the resource gap in many countries.

Fees for services
In the search for funding sources, cost recovery is clearly one of the options that must be evaluated. Charging fees can contribute to better care, for example by encouraging

quality-based competition among providers and giving patients a feeling that they have a right to expect adequate services. However, fees raise diverse issues. For example, they generate revenue from those patients who judge services to be worthwhile at the going price; and they divert those patients who either cannot pay, or judge services to be less desirable than some alternative, to other sources of care. Experiences with cost recovery have been quite varied (15); communities in Africa have demonstrated a willingness and ability to pay for services they feel to be important. One factor that must be taken into account in establishing cost recovery programmes is that when the community makes a financial contribution, the system should be open for them to audit, thereby reassuring everyone that their money is being used for the intended purposes.

The question of how to provide health care for the poor is of great importance. Financial contribution systems must be designed in ways that do not increase poverty and poor health, but the exemption of the poor is difficult to handle. To leave the determination of who cannot afford to pay to the discretion of health workers would not be very satisfactory; it would be bound to result in decisions that were arbitrary and/or inconsistent from one centre to another, and possibilities for favouritism, if not outright corruption. One option might be a system in which proposals for exemption are made by village committees, based on their local knowledge of household circumstances. Since traditional healers seem to use a system of exemptions and price scales related to wealth, their participation in these village committees has been advocated (16).

In the context of HIV prevention and AIDS care, fees for services may not be feasible. Generally, people are not keen on paying for preventive activities, although sometimes local initiatives may be used to raise money. For example, in Magu District, Tanzania, the village AIDS action committees raised money for HIV prevention activities by having spectators pay to see videoshows on AIDS during campaigns. Terminal AIDS patients are also very willing to pay for any type of treatment. Such payments are however often funded by selling off property, which has a disproportionate effect on the survivors in the family (see Chapter 18).

Condoms are a somewhat separate issue. Within social marketing programmes, payments cover some of the costs associated with purchase and distribution. Yet, as shown in Chapter 21 the costs of such programmes are still considerable, so that it remains necessary to rely on donor assistance. Perhaps at a later stage when condoms have been sufficiently popularized condom programmes will be able to recover their costs.

Other aspects of sustainability
Sustainability is more than a matter of sustainable financing. Sustainability refers to the ability of activities to remain functional after the parent project or programme, often funded and stimulated from outside, has ended. Thus sustainability depends on how well the knowledge, attitudes and practices and technology that have been introduced take root in the district and its communities, and the extent to which a programme encourages and facilitates community involvement. Communities may participate at different levels. At first they participate only in *programme benefits* (using a service),

followed by participation in *activities* (e.g. participatory in a health education session) and later in *implementation* (e.g. helping the health worker to organize a health education session planned by the health worker). Those who are more involved and committed may eventually participate in *monitoring and evaluation*, and perhaps go on to take part in *planning* (17). The term 'stages' may be preferable to 'steps', because this is a continuing process from minimal to full social participation. In AIDS health education programmes the participation of a broadly representative group from the community is desirable. Including infected people is very important. Their participation may lead to a strong emotional reaction within the target group; HIV/AIDS becomes visible in a person from the same community. The target group then becomes aware that HIV is not only a problem of 'others'.

In addressing the issue of sustainability of health services, another important aspect is human resource development (18). Health workers often operate under difficult circumstances. To prevent further 'burn out' or drop outs among health workers from the district health services several issues will have to be addressed. This includes the conditions under which they work, the need for proper management strategies that increase motivation (for example, an emphasis on feedback that is positive rather than negative, plus incentives and career possibilities), encouraging teamwork and support among peer groups, provision of continuing education and regular supportive supervision, and skilled management of non-performance (using a compassionate approach but with realistic possibilities for disciplinary action). Decentralization of responsibilities to the district level will need to be gradual, and accompanied by training to increase capabilities. This will need to be relevant to the district and to include ongoing support: there has been a tendency to provide training or seminars in national or regional capitals, without providing for continuity and on-the-spot support, and without a realistic consideration of factors that inhibit implementation. Further, much training is still conducted with material prepared for industrialized countries. This implies a risk of irrelevance and of placing too high a value on technology that is inappropriate for the local situation. The concept of appropriate technology – which emphasizes that the most sophisticated technology is not always the best – also applies to learning materials. The local production of or adaptation of these materials is important (19). Materials need to be reviewed and possibly produced that are relevant to the situation, take local conditions and traditions into account, and teach technologies that are appropriate.

Box 6 presents a list of issues that need to be considered by a project or programme that wants to maximize the chances of sustainability for its activities.

Box 6. Checklist: sustainability issues in projects/programmes

- consider sustainability from the beginning
- consider links between vertical programmes and aim to integrate programmes: for example, establish a reproductive health care programme, rather than separate programmes for safe motherhood, family planning, AIDS and STDs
- use appropriate technology; standardized equipment with locally available spare parts, local purchasing and maintenance
- pay close attention to organization and administration; work toward having a well trained and cost-conscious staff
- seek a close working relationship among all partners and programmes at both district and more central levels
- involve key local leaders, politicians, businessmen and church leaders
- do not pay higher salaries and allowances than government guidelines
- use a participative approach, encouraging community involvement and contribution
- carry out fundraising in the community and seek contributions in kind e.g. drinks, food and venues
- involve local cultural groups
- apply flexibility and creativity in management
- implement cost recovery, with exemption of the poor

Conclusion

HIV/AIDS programmes began as vertical programmes, which made an attempt to rapidly control a serious epidemic. It is now evident that rapid control is not possible, but that instead a concerted, long-term effort will be required to prevent as many new HIV infections as possible and to contain the multiple consequences of the epidemic.

The integration of HIV/AIDS programmes with one or more other vertical programmes has multiple advantages. In particular, HIV/AIDS programmes need to work together with those concerned with other elements of reproductive health. HIV/AIDS programmes also need to be integrated in overall district health plans. What is needed is an integrated plan involving government, NGOs and the private sector as well as traditional medical practitioners in the joint, cooperative delivery of comprehensive health services.

The general context, in many countries in sub-Saharan Africa, of declining government resources and declining budgets – especially for health and social services – limits the sustainability of AIDS programmes funded by governments. Nevertheless, communities are a long way from being able to pay the total costs of their health care. It is essential to seek ways to help them. Integrated district level programmes that are more efficient and effective can provide a part of the answer. Current reforms in the health sector in many countries are an important way of strengthening district management. These, however, cannot realize their potential without a national context conducive to well-functioning decentralization. Moreover, increased commitment to health at national level is vital, and continued external funding will be needed to sustain efforts and achieve high levels of coverage. Equally important is the need to involve local communities and mobilize their resources to help in sustaining programmes. Strengthening local capacity to plan, implement and evaluate HIV prevention and AIDS care programmes should be at the core of all HIV/AIDS programmes.

Further reading

World Health Organization. *The challenge of implementation; district health systems for primary health care.* Geneva, 1988.

AIDS Management: an integrated approach (Chikankata Hospital, Zambia). *Strategies for Hope Series, no. 3.* TALC, P.O. Box 49, St Albans, Hertfordshire AL1 4AX, United Kingdom or Strategies for Hope, 93 Divinity Road, Oxford OX4 1LN, United Kingdom. Organizations in Kenya should order them from: Health Education Network, AMREF, P.O. Box 30125, Nairobi, Kenya. Organizations in Tanzania should write to: AIDS Project, AMREF Tanzania, P.O. Box 2773, Dar es Salaam, Tanzania. Organizations in Uganda can order them from: AMREF Uganda, P.O. Box 51, Entebbe, Uganda.

WHO. *AIDS prevention: guidelines for MCH/FP programme managers. I. AIDS and family planning* and *II. AIDS and maternal and child health.* Geneva, 1990.

AIDS/STD Health Promotion Exchange issue no. 4 on 'Reorienting health and social services', Amsterdam, Royal Tropical Institute, 1995.

References

1. World Bank. *World Development Report 1993. Investing in health.* New York, Oxford University Press, 1993.

2. Grant J. *The State of the World's Children 1992.* Oxford, Oxford University Press, 1992.

3. King, M. Health is a sustainable state. *Lancet* 1990, 336: 664–667.

4. Editorial. Structural adjustment and health in Africa. *Lancet* 1990, 335; 885–887.

5. Editorial. Structural adjustment too painful. *Lancet* 1994, 344: 1377–1378.

6. Cornia GA. Adjustment policies 1980–85: effects on child welfare. In: Cornia GA (ed.). *Adjustment with a human face.* Oxford, Oxford University Press, 1987.

7 Chabot J, Harnmeijer JW, Streefland PH (eds.). *African Primary Health Care in times of economic turbulence.* Amsterdam, Royal Tropical Institute, 1995.

8. Abel-Smith B. Rawal P. Can the poor afford 'free' health services? A case study of Tanzania. *Health Policy Planning* 1992, 7: 329–341.

9. World Health Organization. *The challenge of implementation; district health systems for primary health care.* Geneva, 1988.

10. Sandiford P, Kanga GJ, Ahmed AM. The management of health services in Tanzania: a plea for health sector reform. *International Journal of Health Planning and Management* 1994, 9: 295–308.

11. Serkkola A. Primary health care in pluralistic settings. In: Lankinen KS, Bergstrom S, Makela PH et al. (eds.). *Health and disease in developing countries.* London, Macmillan, 1994.

12. Bargzar M, Kore I. A solid base for health. *World Health Forum* 1991, 12: 156–160.

13. Valtonen H. Health systems financing. In: Lankinen KS, Bergstrom S, Makela PH et al. (eds.), *Health and disease in developing countries.* London, Macmillan, 1994.

14. LaFond AK. Sustaining health care in poor countries. *Tropical Doctor* 1994, 24: 145–148.

15. McPake B, Hanson K, Mills A. Community financing of health care in Africa: an evaluation of the Bamako initiative. *Social Science and Medicine* 1993, 36: 1383–1395.

16. Walraven G. Health insurance in rural Africa (Letter). *Lancet* 1995, 345: 521.

17. Rifkin SB. Lessons from community participation in health programmes. *Health Policy Planning* 1986, 1: 240–249.

18. Van Bergen J. District health care between quality assurance and crisis management. *Tropical and Geographical Medicine* 1995, 47: 23–29.

19. Folmer H et al. *Testing and evaluating manuals: making health learning materials more useful.* Amsterdam, Royal Tropical Institute, 1992.

Appendix: Additional resources

Free publications

AIDS Action, quarterly in English, French, Spanish and Portuguese, includes information on IEC, care and STD treatment. Target audience: health workers, teachers, media workers, community groups, international and local non-governmental organizations. Subscription address: AHRTAG, Farringdon Point, 29–35 Farringdon Road, London EC1M 3JB, United Kingdom.

AIDS & mobility: materials for HIV/AIDS education aimed at travellers, ethnic minorities, and migrant communities. This catalogue lists brochures, posters, videos and other educational materials developed in European countries. Materials in a wide variety of languages are listed (e.g., Arabic, Bengali, Chinese, Gujerati, Hindi, Kiswahili, Lingala, Luganda, Punjabi, Somali, Trigina, Urdu).
   Order from: AIDS & Mobility Project, NIGZ, P.O. Box 500, 3440 AM Woerden, The Netherlands.

AIDSCAP Information Mailing, periodic mailings of selected articles in English, French and Spanish; contains articles on topics such as transmission, testing, clinical and social aspects, education, etc. *AIDScaptions* (published three times yearly in English, once annually in French and Spanish) and *Network* (quarterly in English) contain articles on AIDS and other health-care issues.
   Subscription address: Family Health International, P.O. Box 13950, Research Triangle Park, NC 27709, USA.

AIDS/STD Health Promotion Exchange, quarterly in English published by the Royal Tropical Institute (Amsterdam, The Netherlands) and Southern Africa AIDS Information Dissemination Service (SAfAIDS, Harare, Zimbabwe). Theme issues focus on the development, implementation and evaluation of HIV/AIDS- and STD-related health promotion activities by governmental and non-governmental groups. Themes cover target audiences and/or methodologies. Past themes have included: use of theatre, mobility and HIV/AIDS, sensitization and training for health promotion, health promotion for people living with HIV/AIDS, programmes targeting learning-disabled persons, incorporating a gender perspective into sexual health education, networking, and monitoring and evaluation. A subject index is available.
   Subscription address: Royal Tropical Institute, P.O. Box 95001, 1090 HA Amsterdam, The Netherlands.

All about STDs: information on sexually transmitted diseases, English and Dutch.
   Order from: STD Foundation, P.O. Box 9074, 3506 GB Utrecht, The Netherlands.

Counselling skills training in adolescent sexuality and reproductive health: a facilitator's guide, English, French and Spanish; guide to running a 5-day workshop.
   Order from: WHO, Adolescent Health Programme, 1211 Geneva 27, Switzerland.

Directory of European funders of HIV/AIDS projects in developing countries and *Guide to technical support available to HIV/AIDS projects in developing countries*. UK NGO AIDS Consortium, Fenner Brockway House, 37–39 Great Guildford Street, London SE1 0ES, United Kingdom.

Essential AIDS information resources (resource list), *HIV/AIDS and sexual health: key resources for development workers*, *Youth and sexual health* all provide information on books, training materials, teaching tools, videos, newsletters and journals. Other publications that are free for organizations in developing countries include *Let's teach about AIDS* (six pamphlets describing participatory learning exercises) and *Practical guidelines for preventing infections transmitted by blood or air in health-care settings*.
   Order from: AHRTAG, Farringdon Point, 29–35 Farringdon Road, London EC1M 3JB, United Kingdom and WHO/GPA, Documentation Centre, 1211 Geneva 27, Switzerland.

Facing the challenges of HIV/AIDS/STDs: a gender-based response: a resource pack containing a book and set of activity cards to show how a gender-based approach can be integrated into HIV/AIDS/STD programmes. Produced by the Royal Tropical Institute and Southern Africa AIDS Information Dissemination Service on behalf of WHO/GPA. It will also be available in French and Spanish sometime in 1996.
   Order from: WHO Documentation and Sales, 1211 Geneva 27, Switzerland.

IPPF Open File, monthly news digest in English, gives short descriptions of articles appearing in the press concerning family planning, HIV/AIDS and STDs.
   Subscription address: IPPF International Office, Regent's College, Inner Circle, Regent's Park, London NW1 4NS, United Kingdom.

HIV/AIDS project planning manual for NGOs in English.
   Available from: Regional Bureau for Asia and the Pacific, UNDP, 55 Lodi Estate, New Delhi 110 003, India.

Methods in AIDS education: a training manual for teachers, gives information on methods and implementation/evaluation of school-based programmes.
   Order from: UNICEF, P.O. Box 1250, Harare, Zimbabwe.

Pacific AIDS Alert Bulletin, quarterly newsletter in English and French.
   Subscription: South Pacific Commission, B.P. D5, Noumea Cedex, New Caledonia.

Population Reports, five times yearly in English, French, Spanish and Portuguese; includes information on family planning, HIV/AIDS and STDs.

Subscription address: Johns Hopkins University, Population Communication Services, 527 St. Paul Place, Baltimore, MD 21202, USA.

Resource pack on sexual health and AIDS prevention for socially apart youth. This manual contains information for youth workers and educators working with young people who may be homeless and living on the streets or in refugee camps. It contains lists of resources and contacts and offers ideas about how to develop activities. It is free of charge to organizations working in developing countries and can be ordered from AHRTAG (see address for newsletter *AIDS Action*).

Strategies for Hope Series, booklets on various AIDS-related programs in English, French and Portuguese. NGOs in developing countries may request a limited number of those booklets pertaining to their region free of charge; others must pay.
   Addresses: TALC, P.O. Box 49, St Albans, Hertfordshire AL1 4AX, United Kingdom or Strategies for Hope, 93 Divinity Road, Oxford OX4 1LN, United Kingdom. Organizations in Kenya should order them from: Health Education Network, AMREF, P.O. Box 30125, Nairobi, Kenya. Organizations in Tanzania should write to: AIDS Project, AMREF Tanzania, P.O. Box 2773, Dar es Salaam, Tanzania. Organizations in Uganda can order them from: AMREF Uganda, P.O. Box 51, Entebbe, Uganda.
   The titles of the booklets are:
1. From Fear to Hope: AIDS Care and Prevention at Chikankata Hospital, Zambia (GBP 2)
2. Living Positively with AIDS: The AIDS Support Organization (TASO), Uganda (GBP 2)
3. AIDS Management: an Integrated Approach (Chikankata Hospital, Zambia) (GBP 2)
4. Meeting AIDS with Compassion: AIDS Care and Prevention in Agomanya, Ghana (GBP 2)
5. AIDS Orphans: A Community Perspective from Tanzania (GBP 2)
6. The Caring Community: Coping with AIDS in Urban Uganda (GBP 2)
7. All Against AIDS: the Copperbelt Health Education Project, Zambia (GBP 2)
8. Work against AIDS: workplace-based initiatives in Zimbabwe (GBP 2.75)
9. Candles of Hope: the AIDS Programme of the Thai Red Cross Society (GBP 2)
10. Filling the gaps: care and support for people with HIV/AIDS in Côte d'Ivoire (GBP 2.75).
11. Broadening the front: NGO responses to HIV and AIDS in India (GBP 2.75)

What is AIDS? Manual for health workers in English, French, Spanish, Portuguese, Swahili; address: Churches' Action for AIDS, World Council of Churches, 150 route de Ferney, 1211 Geneva 2, Switzerland.
   Also available are *Learning about AIDS, a manual for pastors and teachers, A guide to HIV/AIDS pastoral counselling* and the pamphlet *Youth: AIDS, why we care.*

Organizations with materials and resources available at low cost

ABIA (Associação Brasileira Interdisciplinar de AIDS), Rua Sete de Setembro 48, 12o andar, 20.050–000 Rio de Janeiro, RJ, Brazil.
   ABIA has several informational pamphlets on various topics as well as a guide for

AIDS education in school (*A AIDS e a escola: nem indiferenca nem discriminação*) in Portuguese.

African Research and Educational Puppetry Programme (AREPP), P.O. Box 51022, Raedene 2124, South Africa.

AREPP will send an AIDS-related puppet show on tour upon request; the organization also offers workshops to train people in providing AIDS education and information via puppetry and other methods. People can also train with AREPP in Johannesburg for several months and during this period can earn a wage as staff members. Though AREPP cannot offer the plays and workshops for free on tour, they can assist organizations in requesting financing for the tours and workshops.

AHRTAG (Appropriate Health Resources and Technologies Action Group), Farringdon Point, 29–35 Farringdon Road, London EC1M 3JB, United Kingdom.

AHRTAG provides an information and enquiry service to health workers in developing countries and publishes practical manuals and free newsletters on various health-related problems (e.g., AIDS, diarrhoeal diseases, respiratory infections). They have also published a free directory of HIV/AIDS-related newsletters.

AMREF Tanzania, P.O. Box 1482, Mwanza, Tanzania and P.O. Box 2773, Dar es Salaam, Tanzania.

In collaboration with the NGO Kuleana, AMREF has produced a booklet in English and Kiswahili entitled *Life first! A practical guide for people with HIV/AIDS and their families*.

Copperbelt Health Education Project, P.O. Box 23567, Kitwe, Zambia.

This organization has produced brochures and programmes targeting various community groups.

FACT (Family AIDS Caring Trust), P.O. Box 970, Mutare, Zimbabwe.

Their publications include flashcard series for use in transmitting information on AIDS via story-telling (thus far stories have been prepared concerning schoolchildren, young women and working men), *100 questions and answers on AIDS* and *Living through A.I.D.S. (advice, health care and hope for people affected by the AIDS virus)*.

Family Planning Association Education Unit, 27–35 Mortimer Street, London W1N 7RJ, United Kingdom.

Publishes *Working with uncertainty; a handbook for those involved in training on HIV and AIDS* (H. Dixon and P. Gordon).

IPPF (International Planned Parenthood Federation), Sexual Health Department, P.O. Box 759, Inner Circle, Regent's Park, London NW1 4LQ, United Kingdom.

IPPF has produced numerous printed materials available free of charge or at a low cost; included among these is the booklet *Talking AIDS; a guide for community work*.

International Federation of Red Cross and Red Crescent Societies, P.O. Box 372, 1211 Geneva 19, Switzerland.

The Red Cross/Red Crescent Societies in many countries are involved in AIDS education and information programs and have produced various free materials in this respect. Two useful resources: *Action for youth – AIDS training manual*, which is available in English, French and Spanish and *AIDS, health and human rights: an explanatory manual* (ISBN 92-9139-014-3; 1995).

Rural Center for the Study and Promotion of HIV/STD Prevention, Indiana University, Poplars 617, 400 E. 7th Street, Bloomington, IN 47405-3085, USA

The Center produces 2-page fact sheets on various topics. Up to 25 copies of each can be ordered free of charge; the first four titles are: *Behaviour change models for reducing HIV/STD risk, Evaluating HIV/STD education programs, HIV infection and women* and *Preventing HIV/STD among adolescents.*

SAfAIDS (Southern Africa AIDS Information Dissemination Service), 17 Beveridge Road, P.O. Box A509, Avondale, Harare, Zimbabwe.

SAfAIDS produces a newsletter entitled *SAfAIDS News* and also has a resource centre which provides documentation especially related to the socio-economic impact of HIV/AIDS.

TALC (Teaching Aids at Low Cost), P.O. Box 49, St Albans, Hertfordshire AL1 4AX, United Kingdom.

Among the materials produced by TALC are three slide sets on HIV infection for medical and other experienced health workers, a slide series on HIV prevention and counselling, videos on counselling and care of children orphaned due to AIDS, and a flannelgraph on family planning, STDs and AIDS.

WHO, Distribution and Sales, World Health Organization, 1211 Geneva 27, Switzerland.

GPA, WHO's disbanded Global Programme on AIDS, produced the *WHO/AIDS Series* which includes the following titles in English, French and Spanish. The prices (in Swiss francs) listed are those for developing countries.

1. Guidelines for the development of a national AIDS prevention and control programme, 27 pp., Sw. fr. 5.60
2. Guidelines on sterilization and disinfection methods effective against human immunodeficiency virus (HIV), 2nd edition, 11 pp., Sw. fr. 2.80
3. Guidelines for nursing management of people infected with human immunodeficiency virus (HIV), 42 pp., Sw. fr. 6.30
4. Monitoring of national AIDS prevention and control programmes: guiding principles, 27 pp., Sw. fr. 5.60
5. Guide to planning health promotion for AIDS prevention and control, 71 pp., Sw. fr. 9.80
6. Prevention of sexual transmission of human immunodeficiency virus, 28 pp., Sw. fr. 5.60
7. Guidelines on AIDS and first aid in the workplace, 12 pp., Sw. fr. 2.80

8. Guidelines for counselling about HIV infection and disease, 48 pp., Sw. fr. 7.70
9. Biosafety guidelines for diagnostic and research laboratories working with HIV, 28 pp., Sw. fr. 5.60
10. School health education to prevent AIDS and sexually transmitted diseases, 79 pp., Sw. fr. 12.60
11. The Global AIDS Strategy, 23 pp., Sw. fr. 6,30

Other publications available from WHO include:
- *AIDS: images of the epidemic* (1994, Sw. fr. 22.40)
- *AIDS prevention through health promotion: facing sensitive issues* (1991, English, French, Spanish, Japanese, Indonesian, Sw. fr. 11.20)
- *School health education to prevent AIDS and STD: handbook for curriculum planners* (1994, free)
- *School health education to prevent AIDS and STD: teacher's guide* (1994, free)
- *School health education to prevent AIDS and STD: student activities* (1994, free)
- *AIDS prevention: guidelines for MCH/FP programme managers. I. AIDS and family planning* and *II. AIDS and maternal and child health* (May 1990, free)
- *Living with AIDS in the community* (1992, English, French, Portuguese, Amharic, Efik, Kiswahili, Thai, Sw. fr. 6/US$ 5.40)
- *Source book for HIV/AIDS counselling training* (free)
- *Counselling for HIV/AIDS: a key to caring* (free)
- *Provision of HIV/AIDS care in resource-constrained settings* (free)
- *AIDS home care handbook* (1993, English, French, Portuguese and Arabic, US$ 16.20)
- *Manual of group interview techniques to assess the needs of people with AIDS* (1995, free)
- *HIV prevention and care: teaching modules for nurses and midwives* (1993, English, French, Portuguese, free)
- *AIDS in Africa – handbook for physicians* (English, French, Portuguese, US$ 14.40)
- *Guidelines for the clinical management of HIV infection in adults* (1991, English, French, Sw. fr. 13/US$11.70)
- *Guidelines for the clinical management of HIV infection in children* (1993, Sw. fr. 13/US$ 11.70)
- *Evaluation of a National AIDS Programme: a methods package. 1. Prevention of HIV infection* (1994, free)
- *Guidelines for blood donor counselling on HIV* (1994, free)
- *TASO – the inside story. Participatory evaluation of HIV/AIDS counselling, medical and social services 1993–1994* (1995, free)

Useful books (some of these are expensive)

The AIDS handbook: a guide to the understanding of AIDS and HIV . This fully revised second edition by John Hubley now takes into account not only programmes in Africa but also Asia, the Pacific region and South America. Increased attention is given to control of STDs and drug injection as well as educational programmes in the workplace and prisons. Order from: Macmillan Education Limited, Houndmills, Basingstoke, Hampshire RG21 2X1S, United Kingdom.

Facing the challenges of HIV/AIDS/STDs: a gender-based response (free of charge), M. de Bruyn et al., Royal Tropical Institute, Mauritskade 63, 1092 AD Amsterdam, The Netherlands. Also available from SAfAIDS, 17 Beveridge Road, P.O. Box A509, Avondale, Harare, Zimbabwe and from WHO, ASD Office, 1211 Geneva 27, Switzerland.

Women and AIDS: an international resource book, M. Berer & S. Ray, 1993, AHRTAG, 1 London Bridge Street, London SE1 9SG, United Kingdom.

A resource manual for AIDS educators, 1991, Canadian Public Health Association, AIDS Education and Awareness Program, 400-1565 Carling Avenue, Ottawa, Ontario K1Z 8R1, Canada. ISBN 0-919245-50-1.

STD/AIDS peer educator training manual, 1992. Can be ordered from three addresses:
- AIDSCAP, Family Health International, P.O. Box 13950, Research Triangle Park, NC 27709, USA;
- National AIDS Control Programme, United Republic of Tanzania, Ministry of Health, P.O. Box 9083, Dar es Salaam, Tanzania;
- AMREF, P.O. Box 2773, Dar es Salaam, Tanzania.

Talking AIDS: a guide for community workers, G. Gordon and T. Klouda, 1988, AIDS Prevention Unit, IPPF, Regent's College, Inner Circle, Regent's Park, London NW1 4NS, United Kingdom & Macmillan Publishers, Houndmills, Basingstoke, Hampshire RG21 2XS, United Kingdom. ISBN 0-333-49781-3.

AIDS: working with young people, P. Aggleton et al., 1990, Avert, P.O. Box 91, Horsham, West Sussex, RH13 7YR, United Kingdom. ISBN 0-9515351-0-2.

The handbook for AIDS prevention in Africa, P. Lamptey and P. Piot, eds., Family Health International, AIDSCAP, P.O. Box 13950, Research Triangle Park, Durham, NC 27709, USA. ISBN 0-939704-06-4.

Puppets for better health: a manual for community workers and teachers, G. Gordon, 1986, Macmillan Publishers, Houndmills, Basingstoke, Hampshire RG21 2XS, United Kingdom. ISBN 0-333-39138-1.

Tools for project evaluation: a guide for evaluating AIDS prevention interventions, 1992, AIDSCAP, Family Health International, P.O. Box 13950, Research Triangle Park, NC 27709, USA.

Preventing a crisis: AIDS and family planning work, 1989, G. Gordon and T. Klouda, AIDS Prevention Unit, IPPF, Regent's College, Inner Circle, Regent's Park, London NW1

4NS, United Kingdom & Macmillan Publishers, Houndmills, Basingstoke, Hampshire RG21 2XS, United Kingdom. ISBN 0-333-51721-0.

Developing health and family planning print materials for low-literate audiences: a guide, M. Zimmerman et al., Program for Appropriate Technology in Health (PATH), Communication Department, 1990 M Street, N.W., Suite 700, Washington, D.C. 20036, USA.

AIDS and primary health care: the role of non-governmental organizations, 1992, c/o I. Wolffers, Dept. of Social Medicine, Van der Boechorststraat 1, 1081 BT Amsterdam, The Netherlands.

Altering the image of AIDS, M. de Bruyn (ed.), 1994, Bailey Distribution, Learoyd Road, Mountfield Industrial Estate, New Romney, Kent TN28 8XU, United Kingdom. (This book focuses on how images and reporting on HIV/AIDS can be influenced by governments, the media and NGOs.)

Primary AIDS care: a practical guide for primary health care personnel in the clinical and supportive care of people with HIV/AIDS, second edition by C. Evian, Jacana, Private Bag 2004, Houghton 2041, Johannesburg, South Africa (1995.; about US$ 20).

A colour atlas of AIDS in the tropics, M.A. Ansary et al., Wolfe Medical Publications Ltd, Brook House, 2-16 Torrington Place, London WC1E 7LT, United Kingdom. ISBN 0-7234-1629-X.

AIDS in the world II, 1996, Oxford University Press, 198 Madison Avenue, New York, NY 10016, USA. ISBN 0-19-509097-7.

AIDS and the Third World, 1988, ISBN 1-870670-04-3.
Triple jeopardy: women and AIDS, 1990, ISBN 1-870670-20-5.
The 3rd epidemic: repercussions of the fear of AIDS, 1990, ISBN 1-870670-12-4.
The hidden cost of AIDS: the challenge of HIV to development, 1992, ISBN 1-870670-29-9.
All can be ordered from The Panos Institute, 9 White Lion Street, London N1 9PD, United Kingdom.

We miss you all; AIDS in the family, N. Kaleeba, Women and AIDS Support Network, P.O. Box 1554, Harare, Zimbabwe.

Testing and evaluating manuals: making health learning materials more useful, H.R. Folmer et al., Royal Tropical Institute, Mauritskade 63, 1092 AD Amsterdam, The Netherlands. ISBN 90-6832-046-7.
E-mail: acb@support.nl

About the authors

Dorica Balyagati holds an advanced diploma in community development from the Community Development Training Institute in Arusha, Tanzania. She has worked as a community development officer, first in Dar es Salaam and later in Bukoba district, focusing on women's programmes. In 1993 she joined TANESA as a coordinator for women and gender activities.

Longin Barongo has an MMed in Community Medicine from the University of Dar es Salaam and received an MSc in Epidemiology from the London School of Hygiene and Tropical Medicine in 1995. He has worked with the National Institute for Medical Research in Mwanza since 1988 and joined the TANESA project in 1990.

John Bennett has a medical degree and specializes in community health. He taught on faculties of medicine in East Africa for 20 years, first as professor of Preventive Medicine at Makerere University, Kampala, Uganda, subsequently as professor of community medicine at Dar es Salaam University, Tanzania, and later as professor of community health at Nairobi University, Kenya. He then was appointed regional adviser in Primary Health Care for UNICEF/WHO in Eastern, Central and Southern Africa, and remained in that position for nine years. In the following four years he worked as director of publications at AMREF, Nairobi, and as UNICEF consultant in Namibia, before moving to the republic of South Africa in 1994. He is presently based at the Institute of Social and Economic Research, Rhodes University, Grahamstown. In recent years he has served as consultant to the TANESA project and as adviser on several HIV/AIDS/STD committees in the Eastern Cape Province of South Africa.

Zacharia Berege obtained an MD in 1976 and an MMed (obstetrics and gynaecology) in 1984, both at the University of Dar es Salaam. He has worked as a clinician, and district and regional medical officer for many years. Since 1991 he has been the director of Bugando Medical Centre, a consultant referral and teaching hospital in Lake Zone, Mwanza, Tanzania.

Ties Boerma received a medical degree in 1981, a MSc (demography) at the University of Groningen, the Netherlands, in 1983 and a PhD in medical demography at the University of Amsterdam in 1996. He has worked as PHC adviser for UNICEF/WHO in eastern and southern Africa for five years, and as coordinator for health analysis for the USAID-sponsored Demographic and Health Survey (DHS) programme for four years. In 1993 he joined the Royal Tropical Institute, Amsterdam, to work on the TANESA project in Mwanza.

Maria de Bruyn is a medical anthropologist who works on health projects for the Royal Tropical Institute in Amsterdam, the Netherlands. Her current HIV/AIDS-related work includes management of the AIDS Coordination Bureau (the secretariat and resource centre of the AIDS Coordination Group in the Netherlands, an informal consortium of Dutch NGOs that support HIV/AIDS programmes in developing countries) and editing of the international quarterly newsletter *AIDS/STD Health Promotion Exchange*.

Wil Dolmans is associate professor of Tropical Medicine and head of the Nijmegen Institute for International Health at Nijmegen University in the Netherlands. He was trained as a medical doctor, completed a PhD in 1978, and has worked intermittently in Mwanza Region and other places in Tanzania since 1969.

Isabelle Favot graduated as a medical doctor in France in 1987. She earned degrees in Tropical Medicine and Epidemiology, and has worked in Guyana and the West Indies. At present she works as an epidemiologist with the Community Health Department of Bugando Medical Centre, Mwanza, Tanzania.

Awene Gavyole received an M.D. at the University of Dar es Salaam in 1978. He also obtained a Master's degree in PHC Management in Rome in 1992. He has worked for the Ministry of Health in Tanzania as general duty medical officer (six years), district medical officer (seven years), and regional medical officer in Mwanza Region (three years). He is now the AMREF project manager in Mwanza.

Heiner Grosskurth graduated from medical school at the University of Kiel, Germany, in 1978. After further training in surgery, general medicine and venereology he worked in clinics in Peru and Sierra Leone, and in PHC projects in Sudan and Cameroon. From 1991–1995 he worked for AMREF as the programme manager of the STD/HIV intervention and research programme in the Lake Victoria Zone of Tanzania. This included a large community-based intervention trial in collaboration with the London School of Hygiene and Tropical Medicine, and various other institutions. Since 1995 he has been a senior lecturer in the Department of Epidemiology at the London School of Hygiene and Tropical Medicine.

Balthazar Gumodoka holds an MD. and MMed (Obstetrics and Gynaecology) from the University of Dar es Salaam, Tanzania. He obtained an MPH from the Institute of Tropical Medicine in Antwerp, Belgium, in 1988. He has worked as a district medical officer, and regional obstetrician and gynaecologist in Mara Region, Tanzania, and has also been attached to the TANESA project on a part-time basis. He is currently the head of the Department of Obstetrics and Gynaecology at Bugando Medical Centre, Mwanza.

Christoph Hamelmann was trained in Germany as an MD He also has a diploma in Tropical Medicine and an M.Sc. in Molecular Biology. He has worked as clinician and researcher in various developed and developing countries. He is currently coordinator of the AIDS/STD/Sexual and Reproductive Health Programme of AMREF Tanzania.

Jumanne Hema has worked as a head teacher in various primary schools for more than ten years. Since 1993 he has been attached to the TANESA project to coordinate and implement health education at primary schools in Magu District, Tanzania.

Samuel Kalluvya qualified as a medical doctor in 1978, and completed his postgraduate studies in Internal Medicine in 1984, both at the University of Dar es Salaam. He received further training in endocrinology and metabolic medicine at the University of Newcastle Upon Tyne in the UK in 1990–1991. Since 1986 he has worked as head of the Department of Internal Medicine at Bugando Medical Centre, Mwanza, Tanzania.

Arnoud Klokke obtained an MSc in Biochemistry and Endocrinology at the University of Utrecht in 1969. Since then he has worked in hospital laboratories in the Netherlands, Zaire and Tanzania, including three years as head of the Muhimbili Medical Centre Clinical Chemistry Department in Dar es Salaam. Since 1989 he has been head of Pathology at Bugando Medical Centre in Mwanza, with responsibilities which include supervision of HIV testing, quality control of the medical laboratory and blood banking.

Mathias Lefi was trained as an assistant medical officer and joined the National Tuberculosis and Leprosy Programme in 1988. He is regional coordinator for this programme in Tabora Region and Mwanza Region.

Deo Luhamba holds an advanced diploma in Community Development. He has worked as a community development worker, and later as district training officer, for 13 years. Since 1993 he has been attached to the TANESA project as a community health educator in Magu District, Tanzania, focusing on fishing villages on the shores of Lake Victoria.

Eva Masesa obtained a diploma in nursing in 1984 and an advanced diploma in nursing education in 1992, both in Dar es Salaam. She has worked as a nursing officer in charge in district and regional hospitals in Tanzania, and since 1993 has been attached to the TANESA project as a Coordinator for training health workers.

Zaida Mgalla was trained as a teacher and obtained a Master's degree in Education from Murdoch University in Australia. She worked for the Ministry of Education for four years and has worked with the TANESA project in Mwanza since 1994, mainly in the areas of gender and youth programmes.

Martin Mkuye holds a BA in Education (1976) and an MA in Political Science and Public Administration (1983), both from the University of Dar es Salaam. He has worked for the Institute of Adult Education in Dar es Salaam and the South African Extension Unit (educational programmes for South African refugees). Since 1989 he has been working with AMREF Dar es Salaam, and is the project leader of the Kibiti-Dar-Songea High Transmission project.

Wences Msuya graduated as a Clinical Officer in 1977 and attended additional courses in health education, training and management. He has worked in rural health centres and hospitals in Tanzania and Mozambique, and as a health educator at the Centre for Educational Development in Health (CEDHA) in Arusha and later with the Red Cross in Kagera Region. In 1991 he joined AMREF Mwanza to coordinate STD/HIV projects, and is currently project leader for Reproductive Health Services for refugees in western Tanzania.

Bartimayo Mujaya obtained a BEd from the University of Dar es Salaam and an MSc in Education Management and Administration from Morray House, Edinburgh, Scotland. He has held different teaching and administrative positions in various regions of Tanzania, including head teacher, district adult education officer and regional academic officer. At present, he is regional education officer in Mwanza Region.

Ezra Mwijarubi is a clinical officer, specialized in STD control. He was seconded to AMREF by the Ministry of Health, and is now the project leader for the Regional STD Control Programme in Mwanza Region.

Blastus Mwizarubi holds an MA in Education from the University of Dar es Salaam and joined AMREF in 1990. He is project leader of the national HIV high transmission areas project in Tanzania, which involves five organizations and focuses on truck stops.

Japheth Ng'weshemi obtained an MD at the University of Dar es Salaam in 1972 and an MPH at Loma Linda University, USA, in 1976. He has made his career in the Ministry of Health of Tanzania, working in various posts including district medical officer (three years), regional medical officer (five years), senior medical officer epidemiology in charge of vector-borne diseases (five years) and head of the Department of Community Health at Bugando Zonal Consultant Hospital in Mwanza. He was seconded to AMREF for one year as a resident tutor for an international course for PHC managers in Rome, Italy. He has been TANESA project manager since 1994.

Clinton Nyamuryekunge obtained an MB and BS degree from the College of Medicine, University of Lagos, Nigeria, in 1978, an MMed (surgery) from the University of Dar es Salaam in 1984, and an MSc in community health in developing countries from the London School of Hygiene and Tropcial Medicine in 1992. Following nine years of clinical work he was head of the National AIDS Control Programme from 1988–1992. In 1992 he joined AMREF to become the AIDS Control Programme associate manager. Recently, he joined UNAIDS as the country coordinator in Ethiopia.

Venance Nyonyo was trained as a clinical officer. He has worked in clinical services, as a trainer of trainers in the Water for Health Project (HESAWA), and as district AIDS control coordinator in the municipality of Mwanza. Since 1994 he has been attached to the TANESA project as coordinator for Health Education and Campaigns.

Robert Pool obtained a PhD in medical anthropology at the University of Amsterdam in 1989. He has carried out fieldwork in India, Cameroon, Tanzania and the Netherlands. Research topics have included food taboos, traditional etiologies and interpretations of illness, witchcraft, euthanasia, and social behaviour and attitudes relating to AIDS. He is currently doing research on sexual behaviour change for the Medical Research Council in Uganda.

Dick Schapink holds a degree in social work and counselling, and obtained a MSc in survey integration for rural development in the Netherlands. He worked in the Netherlands for 11 years as a counsellor and trainer/consultant for participatory process approaches in development. He has worked for 14 years in eastern and southern Africa, including three years as a volunteer in Tanzania, seven years as team leader for district development programmes in Southern Africa and for the last four years has served as technical adviser on interventions for the Royal Tropical Institute, Amsterdam, in the TANESA project, Mwanza, Tanzania.

Veronica Schweyen holds an MA in English from Yeshiva University, New York, and an advanced degree in Counselling from Fordham University in New York. As a sister of Mary Knoll Sister's Congregation she was assigned to Tanzania as teacher and parish worker. During the last five years she has coordinated an AIDS outreach programme in Mwanza township.

James Todd received an MSc in Biometry from Reading University in 1987 after three years as a volunteer in Tanzania. He has worked as statistician at the Medical Research Laboratories in the Gambia. He is presently working with the London School of Hygiene and Tropical Medicine as a research fellow in Mwanza, Tanzania.

Eric Van Praag is a physician specialized in public health and health planning. In 1974, he started his career in Tanzania in various positions at the district level, and was senior lecturer in Community Health at the University of Dar es Salaam from 1977–1982. After leaving Tanzania, he worked in Bangladesh, in Amsterdam for the Royal Tropical Institute, and in Zambia for WHO. Since 1991 he has worked in Geneva, first as head of the Health Care & Support Unit in the Global Programme on AIDS, and now in the Office of HIV/AIDS and STD.

Mark Urassa received an MA in demography at the University of Dar es Salaam in 1994. He then joined TANESA as coordinator of research. Currently, he is at the London School of Hygiene and Tropical Medicine working on an MSc in medical demography.

Gijs Walraven is a medical doctor with a Master in Public Health from the University of Leeds and a PhD from the University of Nijmegen (on safe motherhood). He worked for seven years in Sumve hospital, Mwanza Region, as medical officer, and was coordinator of the Mwanza Archdiocese in Mwanza Region for several years. He is currently working as clinical epidemiologist and head of Farafenni Field Station, Medical Research Council Laboratories, the Gambia.

Lilian Wambura holds a BSc in Home Economics and Human Nutrition from Sokoine University of Agriculture, Tanzania. She works as a researcher on Reproductive Health Issues in the TANESA project, Mwanza, Tanzania.